Epidemiology Kept Simp

To Linda

Contents

Preface

Things should be made as simple as possible, but not any simpler.
—Albert Einstein

WHO STUDIES EPIDEMIOLOGY AND WHY THEY BOTHER

What Is Epidemiology?

Epidemiology studies the causes, transmission, incidence, and prevalence of health and disease in human populations. Medical and public health disciplines use epidemiologic study results to solve and control human health problems.

Who Studies Epidemiology?

Traditionally, epidemiology has been studied as the core science of public health. As such, it provided the objective basis for disease prevention and health promotion. Public health professionals of all types must communicate risk and read epidemiologic information. Epidemiology provides the tools to evaluate health problems and policies on a population basis. Epidemiology is also included in many undergraduate and graduate programs in medicine, the allied health professions, community health, environmental health, occupational health and industrial hygiene, health education, and health services administration. Because of its power and utility, epidemiology continues to gain a still wider audience.

Epidemiology as a Liberal Art

The study of epidemiology also belongs in the liberal arts. A liberal arts education provides general knowledge and develops overall intellectual capacities. Epidemiology fits nicely into an undergraduate liberal arts course of study because (Fraser, 1987):

- It uses the scientific method.
- It develops and improves one's ability to reason inductively (reasoning from the specific to the general).
- It develops and improves one's ability to reason deductively (logical conclusion that follows from a premise).
- It develops and improves one's ability to reason by analogy.
- It develops one's concern for aesthetic values (appreciation of elegance, beauty, simplicity, grace).
- It emphasizes investigative method rather than arcane knowledge and specialized investigative tools.

Moreover, epidemiologists benefit from studying the humanities. By studying the humanities, epidemiologists learn who they are, what is right, and how to think and act. Studying the humanities encourages epidemiologists to focus their skills on the people they serve while increasing flexibility of perspective, encouraging nondogmatisms, improving critical thinking skills, and promoting a better balance of values and ethics (Weed, 1995).

Other Reasons to Study Epidemiology

There are still other reasons to study epidemiology. One such reason is to better understand the mounting epidemiologic information we receive on a regular basis. Much of this information is confusing and some of it is apparently contradictory. To effectively use epidemiologic information, we must understand its basis, its strengths, and its limitations. Without understanding the basis of epidemiologic research, we cannot make informed health decisions for ourselves and others.

Moreover, as involved citizens and voters, we often need to evaluate potential risks and benefits of public and private interventions and policies. For example, we may be called upon to vote on regulations to allow the construction of an industrial facility in our community. To make an informed decision, we must compare the potential economic benefits of the development to the potential environmental hazards it might present. Issues like this respond to epidemiologic analysis by preparing us to weigh the risks and benefits of an intervention on a population basis.

Finally, today's job market seeks people with epidemiologic competencies, such as those associated with data collection, risk/benefit analysis, survey methodology, and outcomes evaluation. These epidemiologic job skills might be useful in your current job and are transferable to other jobs as well.

And, yes, there is another reason to study epidemiology: it is inherently interesting. The challenges of disease detectives have captured the public's interest, as I hope this book will capture yours.

B. BURT GERSTMAN
San José, California

REFERENCES

Fraser, D. W. (1987). Epidemiology as a liberal art. *New England Journal of Medicine,* 316, 309–314.

Weed, D. L. (1995). Epidemiology, the humanities, and Public Health. *American Journal of Public Health,* 85, 914–918.

Acknowledgments

I am greatly indebted to my teachers of epidemiology, for without them this book would not have been possible. I thank Lawrence Glickman for introducing me to epidemiology when I was a veterinary student at Cornell University. Without Dr. Glickman's inspiration, encouragement, and provision of a strong technical foundation, I would, perhaps, have chosen another field. I am also grateful to the fine epidemiologists I encountered while studying for my M.P.H. at the University of California, Berkeley, especially Bill Reeves, Nick Jewel, Warren Winkelstein, Mary Claire-King, Allan Smith, Len Syme, and Aaron Antonovsky. My doctoral work at the University of California, Davis, was also very important to me. For this I thank Calvin Schwabe, James Beaumont, Steve Samuels, and the many fine statisticians I encountered there, especially Jessica Utts and Hari Mukerjee.

I owe a great deal to my epidemiologic mentors at the Food and Drug Administration: Joyce Piper and Frank Lundin. Although Joyce passed away all too young, her great intelligence and spirit remain inspirational. I am very grateful to Frank for teaching me about the underlying basis of observational research—that the variability of risk *over time* is central to all study designs, even case-control studies.

I would like to acknowledge selected published works that were inspirational and helpful to me when I was learning epidemiology. Notable in this regard are *Epidemiologic Research* by Kleinbaum, Kupper, and Morgenstern (1982, Van Nostrand Reinhold), various published articles by Olli Miettinen, *Epidemiologic Analysis with a Programmable Calculator* by Rothman and Boyce (1979, NIH Publication No. 79-1649), *Foundations of Epidemiology* by Lilienfeld and Lilienfeld (1980, Oxford), and Alvan Feinstein's instructional articles on clinical epidemiology. Also very helpful were the excellent training materials prepared by Richard Dicker and his colleagues at the Centers for Disease Control and Prevention.

My assistants on this project were invaluable. I thank Karen Gracida-Ankele for her work as my research assistant and for her constant encouragement and support. Jean Shiota of the Instructional Resource Center at San José State University was a wizard with the illustrations. Also creditable were Dane Carlson for his technical writing assistance and Nancy MacAllister for her unique brand of Feldenkrais instruction. I would like to thank all the fine folks at John Wiley & Sons for the excellent job they did editing and managing the work, and I must surely acknowledge my students at San José State University for their tolerance and helpful input as I experimented with early drafts of this book.

Chapter 15 owes special thanks to Consuelo M. Beck-Sagué, Associate Director for Minority and Women's Health, National Center for Infectious Diseases, CDC, and Carol M. Knowles, Systems Operation and Information Branch, Division of Public Health Surveillance and Informatics, Epidemiology Program Office, CDC, for advice on the SAS system.

Provision of general career and administrative support is often overlooked when acknowledging support for a project like this one. Let me not be negligent in this regard by acknowledging the support of Lynn Bosco, Chuck Anello, and Jerry Faich of the Food and Drug Administration and Rose Tseng, Helen Ross, Michael Ego, and Bill Washington of San José State University.

Finally, I express my deepest appreciation to my family, who endured long hours of my absence while I worked on this book. Writing this book took away much family time and required a great deal of sacrifice on the part of my wife, Linda, and, to a lesser degree, on the part of my son, Jordan. There's good news now—Daddy's home.

B. B. G.

1

Epidemiology Past and Present

This chapter considers fundamental epidemiologic and public health definitions, discusses the scientific and social aspects of epidemiology, provides a brief historical context for the study of epidemiology, and introduces selected mortality trends in the United States.

1.1 EPIDEMIOLOGY, HEALTH, AND PUBLIC HEALTH

What Is Epidemiology?

The word **epidemiology** is based on the Greek roots *epi* (upon), *demios* (the people, as in "democracy" and "demography"), and *logia* (from *legein*, to speak). Today, epidemiology is the study of the distribution, determinants, and occurrence of disease and health-related conditions in populations.

As the name implies, the discipline of epidemiology has its roots in the study of **epidemics.** Not too long ago, the term epidemic applied only to the rapid and extensive spread of an infectious disease within a defined geographic region. Now, however, the term has evolved to apply to any disease or event that occurs in clear excess of normal expectancy. For instance, one may hear mention of a "smoking epidemic among teenagers," a "breast cancer epidemic," or an "epidemic of violence." This broader use of the term reflects modern epidemiology's expansion into areas beyond infectious disease to include the study of chronic diseases, injuries, and other health-related conditions. Nonetheless, epidemiology still focuses on the *group*. Both **pathogenic** (disease-causing) and **salutogenic** (health-causing) factors are studied for the purpose of enhancing our understanding of the biology and pathogenesis of disease and the improvement of health.

In many ways, the epidemiologist's objectives are similar to those of the clinician. However, the clinician's main unit of concern is the individual patient, whereas the epidemiologist's unit of concern is the group or "an aggregate of human beings" (Greenwood, 1935). An often cited public health metaphor compares clinical medicine to epidemiology as follows. Imagine a torrential flood contributed to by a failure in a levee system. This inundating flood is washing away citizens in record numbers. In such circumstances, it is the physician's task to offer life-jackets to citizens one at a time. The epidemiologist, on the other hand, attempts to find the flaw in the levee system to prevent further flooding. To carry this metaphor one step further, fixing the flaw in the levee is a matter of public health.

What is Public Health?

The first edition of *A Dictionary of Epidemiology* defined **public health** as "a form of political and social activism that aims to protect, promote and restore the people's health" (Last, 1983). Later editions expanded this definition to include references to the sciences, skills, and beliefs directed toward improvements of health, as well as the programs, services, and institutions involved in the process (Last, 1988, 1995). The Institute of Medicine (1988) defines public health as "organized community effort to prevent disease and promote health." By any definition, the goals of public health are to reduce the burden of disease, disability, and premature death in the population. Public health is a group of activities; epidemiology is a science—the core science of public health.

Public health is composed of many different disciplines, examples of which are epidemiology, biostatistics, community health planning, health policy development, public health administration, laboratory sciences, environmental health, occupational health and safety, injury control, family planning, reproductive health, maternal and child health, veterinary public health, nutrition, and health education.

What Is Health?

Health, itself, is difficult to define. According to mainstream medicine, health is the absence of disease. "Dis-ease," the opposite of "ease," is literally when something is wrong with a bodily function. The words "disease," "illness," and "sickness" are often used interchangeably, although they may not be entirely synonymous (Susser, 1973). **Disease** is a medically definable physiological or psychological dysfunction, **illness** is what the patient experiences, and **sickness** is the state of dysfunction of the social role of a person with a disease.

Optimal health may go beyond the mere absence of disease. The World Health Organization in the preamble to its 1948 constitution defines health as "a state of complete physical, mental, and social well-being and not merely the absence of disease or infirmity." However, other definitions of health exist. For example, the Chinese system of Tai-Chi defines health in terms of "chi." This idea, admittedly foreign, points to the facts that there are many belief systems regarding health, some of which might be culturally specific.

Walt Whitman, in his poetic way, defined health as follows (cited in Diamond, 1979, pp. 55–56):

> the condition [in which] the whole body is elevated to a state by other unknown—inwardly and outwardly illuminated, purified, made solid, strong, yet buoyant. A singular charm, more than beauty, flickers out of, and over, the face—a curious transparency beams in the eyes, both in the iris and the white—the temper partakes also. The play of the body in motion takes a previously unknown grace. Merely *to move* is then a happiness, a pleasure—to breathe, to see, is also. All the beforehand gratifications, drink, spirits, coffee, grease, stimulants, mixtures, late hours, luxuries, deeds of the night seem as vexatious dreams, and now the awakening; many fall into their natural places, wholesome, conveying diviner joys.

Morbidity and Mortality

In viewing health and disease on a population basis, epidemiologists study both **morbidity** (events and factors related to or caused by disease or disability) and **mortality** (events and factors related to death). To gain insight into factors that increase or decrease morbidity and mortality, it is often necessary to first establish the usual or **endemic** level of disease in the population. Only then are we able to recognize **epidemics** (occurrences in clear excess of normal expectancy) and **pandemics** (epidemics that affect several countries or continents). These and other selected epidemiologic terms are briefly defined in Table 1.1.

1.2 EPIDEMIOLOGIC THINKING

The Scientific Method

> *A theory is scientific if it is falsifiable.*
> —Karl Popper

Epidemiology is an eclectic science that has recently gained greater acceptance and popularity. It draws on the methods and knowledge of many different scientific disciplines, including but not limited to all the basic biomedical sciences, the clinical arts and sciences, statistics, sociology, cultural anthropology, demography, and psychology. Whatever its underlying discipline, epidemiology relies on the scientific method.

The **scientific method** has been used by the natural sciences since the Scientific Revolution of the 17th century. It is characterized by systematic observation, experimentation, measurement, and a multistep process that advances from theory to conclusion using a rigorous system of hypothesis generation, hypothesis testing, and hypothesis refinement (Fig. 1.1).

Before the Scientific Revolution, logic and philosophy, rather than observation and measurement, were used to determine what was true. In summarizing the profound impact brought about by the Scientific Revolution, Ariel and Will Durant (1961, p. 601) write (as cited in Niederhoffer, 1997, p. 71):

> Science now began to liberate itself from the placenta of its mother, philosophy. It . . . developed its own distinctive methods, and looked to improve the life of man on the earth. This movement belonged to the heart of the Age of Reason, but it did not put its faith in "pure reason"—reason independent of experience and experiment. Reason, as well as tradition and authority was now to be checked by the study and record of lowly facts; and whatever "logic" might say, science would aspire to accept only what could be quantitatively measured, mathematically expressed, and experimentally proved.

TABLE 1.1. Selected Epidemiologic Definition

Epidemiology: the study of the causes, transmission, incidence, and prevalence of disease and health-related events in populations
Public health: organized community effort to prevent disease and promote health
Endemic: occurring at or near the usual rate of occurrence.
Epidemic: the occurrence of disease in clear excess of normal expectancy
Pandemic: an epidemic that affects several countries or continents
Morbidity: related to disease or disability
Mortality: related to death

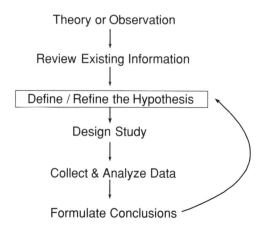

Figure 1.1. *Idealized sequence of scientific inquiry.*

Some of the features common to scientific work are measuring, sequencing, classifying, grouping, confirming, observing, formulating, questioning, identifying, generalizing, experimenting, modeling, testing, and revising.

A frequently cited parable that illustrates the scientific method goes as follows. Two professors, one science-minded, the other less so, observe a flock of white swans around a campus pond. Being thoughtful academic types, they begin to wonder about the color of swans. The nonscientific professor concludes that all swans are white, this being the basis of his observation. In contrast, the science-minded professor notes his observation but draws no further conclusions. Instead, he formulates a working hypothesis suggesting all swans are white and goes in search of swans of a different color. If he finds even one non-white swan, his initial hypothesis is rejected, or at least revised.

The science-minded professor in the swan story uses a process called **hypothetico-deductive reasoning.** The nonscientific professor bases his conclusion on observation alone. Hypothetico-deduction is a process of hypothesis generation followed by rigorous attempts at trying to disprove the hypothesis—a process based on **falsification.** By that, failure to refute the hypothesis provides the best possible support for its verity. Because the absence of disproof is a demonstration of support, the value of a hypothesis depends on the degree to which it is "disprovable." As Sherlock Holmes once noted, "when you have eliminated the impossible, whatever remains, however improbable, must be the truth."

Empiricism is a way of gaining knowledge that is primarily guided by experience and observation. Its formal consideration dates back to Francis Bacon (1561–1626), John Locke (1632–1704), and David Hume (1711–1776). In contrast to strict deduction, empiricism may pay only secondary regard to systems and theories. It also differentiates itself from deduction in that hypotheses need not be entirely preordained. Empiricists thus believe that perceptions of natural phenomena provide the source of ultimate knowledge. The crux of empiricism can be summarized by the following quote from James Madison: "Experience is the oracle of truth."

Epidemiologists have recently debated the proper roles of deduction and empiricism in gaining scientifically valid epidemiologic information. Whereas some epidemiologists believe that epidemiologic knowledge can be assured only through a fully deductive process, others believe that empirically derived results without deductive confirmation are also warranted, especially when findings are unanticipated. Some of this debate can be settled if we view deduction and empiricism as complementary processes rather than competitive methods. In fact, there may be no such thing as *the* scientific method as it applies to epidemiology or any other scientific discipline. Scientists rely on the same ways of reasoning that are common to all problem solving. According to Bridgeman, "the scientific method, as far as it is a method, is nothing more than doing one's damnedest with one's mind, no holds barred" (as cited in Wallis and Roberts, 1962, p. 13). Einstein said, "If you want to know the essence of the scientific method, don't listen to what a scientist may tell you, watch what he does." Astronomer Carl Sagan (1996) concludes: "We should not imagine that science is something erudite. . . . The keypoint of science is criticism, debate, open inquiry, the willingness to systematize knowledge, to withhold belief until the evidence is compelling, and to listen seriously to criticism."

In the end, "science" is only a Latin word meaning "knowledge."

Hard Sciences and Soft Sciences

We may hear reference to a distinction between "hard sciences" (e.g., physics) and "soft sciences" (e.g., psychology). Although this distinction is not entirely clear-cut, correlates of hard and soft science do emerge. Two of these correlates are:

- Hard sciences are characterized by the use of objective measures, often collected by means of specialized equipment; soft sciences tend to use more subjective criteria. Therefore, hard sciences are less susceptible to biases and inconsistencies on the part of the observer.
- Scholars of the hard sciences are more likely to study inanimate and nonhuman objects; scholars of soft sciences are more likely to study human phenomena directly. The tendency to focus on hard rather than soft measures can result in biomedical research that is potentially dehumanizing and potentially irrelevant (Feinstein, 1972).

Epidemiology contains elements of both hard and soft science. Like a hard science, epidemiology increasingly relies on high-technology measurement and data analysis techniques, is often misinterpreted by nonspecialists, is used to test causal hypotheses, and is often academically based. However, like a soft science, much of epidemiology still uses relatively simple data collection methods, is accessible to the nonspecialist, is a useful and relevant hypothesis generation tool, and often deals with important social and political issues directly. This divergency in epidemiology has created an underlying tension about how best to teach epidemiology and pursue its practice. Pearce (1996) suggests that the academic focus on much of modern epidemiology may cause it to become increasingly removed from public health practice.

Mechanistic and Nonmechanistic Views of Disease

Overreliance on Nonmechanistic Environmental Explanations In a 1988 article, Vandenbrouke warns that overreliance on environmental explanation for disease without due regard for pathophysiologic mechanisms is ill-advised. He notes that the contemporary Public Health Movement and many of the sciences that deal with the promotion and preservation of health are rooted in the 19th century Hygienists Movement. The 19th century Hygienists focused their efforts on sanitation and improving environmental conditions, often with only secondary regard in trying to understand the pathophysiologic basis of disease. The Hygienists main theory of disease at the time was the **miasma theory,** a nonspecific notion that emphasized environmental pollution as the cause of most diseases. (Miasma means "bad air" or "pollution.") For example, according to this theory, cholera was due to noxious vapors, which have their highest concentrations at low elevations. The miasmaists even had impressive statistical confirmation of this theory in which they demonstrated precise correlations between predicted and observed rates of cholera based on the level of elevation above the Thames River (Langmuir, 1961).

Then came the Microbiologic Revolution. As specific agents of disease became known, microbial theory flourished while miasma theory faded. Over time, this led to increased reliance on microbiologic and mechanistic views of disease at the expense of the environmental approach. (Although microbiologists eventually incorporated environmental ways of thinking into their discipline, miasmaists were generally rigid in their thinking.)

Vandenbrouke draws several analogies between 19th century Hygienists and today's environmental cancer epidemiologists (Table 1.2). Without recognizing these similarities, environmental cancer epidemiology may become trivialized. Vandenbrouke further recommends that environmental cancer epidemiologists focus their attention on the interaction between disease mechanisms and the environment, thus avoiding overreliance on environmental explanations without regard for underlying pathophysiologic mechanisms.

Overreliance on Mechanistic Explanations   A differing view suggests that too many resources are already directed toward the study of pathogenic mechanisms of disease and their correction, thus diverting funding from applied prevention research where it might be better spent. Wynder (1994) notes that discoveries of measures to prevent a disease regularly predate discovery of the disease's specific pathogenic mechanisms, often by many years. For example, it was 44 years before the microbiologic cause of cholera (*Vibrio cholerae*) was discovered following the realization that the disease was transmitted by feces-contaminated water (see that story about John Snow in the next section of this chapter). Awaiting this discovery before taking action would have needlessly put many people in harm's way. Other historical examples in which the discovery of effective preventive measures preceded the discovery of the underlying agent and mechanism of disease are presented in Table 1.3. Indeed, there is evidence now that the "war on

TABLE 1.2. Nonmechanistic and Mechanistic Views of Disease in 19th and 20th Century Groups

	Nonmechanistic	Mechanistic
19th Century groups	Hygienists	Contagionists
Main theory of infectious disease (19th century)	Miasma	Microbiologic
20th Century groups	Environmental cancer epidemiologists	Molecular epidemiologists and biologists
Main theory of neoplastic disease (20th century)	Environmental carcinogens	Oncogenetic
Causal explanations	Social or environmental	Agent or host
Emphasis on specificity of cause	No	Yes
Point of intervention	Social and behavioral	Agent and gene

Source: Based on information in Vandenbroucke (1988).

TABLE 1.3. Discovery Dates of a Measure to Prevent a Disease Compared with the Date of Identification of the Causative or Preventive Agent

Disease	Discoverer of Preventive Measure[a]	Year of Discovery of Preventive Measure	Year of Discovery of Agent	Causative or Preventive Agent[b]	Discoverer of Agent[a]
Scurvy	J. Lind	1753	1928	(Ascorbic acid)	A. Szent-Gyorgi
Pellagra	G. Casal	1755	1924	(Niacin)	J. Goldberger et al.
Scrotal cancer	P. Pott	1755	1933	Benzo[a]pyrene	J. W. Cook et al.
Smallpox	E. Jenner	1798	1958	Orthopoxvirus	F. Fenner
Puerperal fever	J. Semmelweis	1847	1879	Streptococcus	L. Pasteur
Cholera	J. Snow	1849	1893	*Vibrio cholerae*	R. Koch
Bladder cancer[c]	L. Rehn	1895	1938	2-Napththylamine	W. C. Harper et al.
Yellow fever	W. Reed et al.	1901	1928	Flavivirus	A Stokes et al.
Oral cancer[d]	R. Abbe	1915	1974	N'-nitrosonornicotine	D. Hoffmann et al.

Source: Wynder, E. L. (1994). Studies in mechanisms and prevention: striking the proper balance. *American Journal of Epidemiology, 139*, p. 548; used with permission.

[a]References for each discovery are given in Wynder (1994).
[b]Preventive agents are listed in parentheses.
[c]Associated with aniline dye.
[d]Associated with tobacco chewing.

cancer" has been misdirected toward understanding mechanisms and discovering new treatments when, in fact, applied prevention research might have met with better results (Bailar & Gornik, 1997).

"You're Right, Too." In this author's view, many of the debates about the relative merits of environmental versus mechanistic explanations of disease might be missing the point. The following traditional Jewish tale comes to mind (as told by Zeitlin, 1997).

> Two men are arguing about the theft of a horse, and a rabbi is trying to judge the case. He listens to one man, who has a very good story and says, "You know, you're right. You're absolutely right." The rabbi then says to the other man, "OK, now let me hear your side of the story." The other man tells his side of the story, after which the rabbi says, "You know something, you're right too." At this, the exasperated wife of the rabbi—the rabbitzen—gets very upset and says, "Rabbi, rabbi, what are you talking about? You just said this guy was right and then you said the other guy was right. How could they both be right?" The rabbi pauses to think about this and then says to her, "You know, you're right too."

Perhaps, as the rabbi story suggests, apparently opposing views can both be right, each capable of contributing to (or detracting from) the scientific understanding of disease. The real basis of science involves testing clearly defined hypotheses by repeated independent observations and experiments—whether the explanation is environmental or pathomechanistic.

1.3 SELECTED HISTORICAL FIGURES AND EVENTS, BRIEFLY NOTED

Why Consider the History of Epidemiology?

The development of modern epidemiology has been varied and complex, with roots in clinical and social medicine, the microbiologic revolution, demography, sociology, and statistics. Although it is beyond the scope of this book to provide a thorough discussion of epidemiology's historical development, a brief consideration of selected events will provide the necessary context. Central to the development of epidemiologic thinking is the work of John Snow.

John Snow

John Snow (1813–1858) was one of the first physicians to realize that his obligations went beyond treating the ill and extended toward all. Through a series of theories and observations, Snow was able to show that cholera was transmitted by impure water, with his most famous investigations involving the study of the London cholera epidemic of 1854. Noting that Snow's discovery of the waterborne nature of cholera preceded the discovery of the bacterium *Vibrio cholerae* by some 32 years and preceded Pasteur's demonstration that living organisms can cause epidemics by at least a decade is important. (Pasteur proved the microbial cause of an epidemic disease in silkworms in 1865.) Still, without full elaboration of the germ theory of disease, Snow concluded that cholera was caused by fecal contamination of the water supply (see Winkelstein, 1995).

Some background will help the discussion. Water distribution in 19th century London was the purview of private companies, one of which was the Southwark & Vauxhall Company. Snow noted that cholera mortality rates were 5 to 10 times higher in households served by Southwark & Vauxhall compared with households served by other water companies (Table 1.4). Further work led Snow to note that the Southwark & Vauxhall Company derived its water from downstream, polluted sources and that waters polluted with infected human waste were the ultimate source of the yet undiscovered cholera agent.

Snow supplemented the above rate analysis by constructing a graphical display in which deaths from cholera were plotted along with the locations of the water pumps in the community (Fig. 1.2). Fatal cholera cases were shown to cluster around the now infamous Broad Street pump, further validating his waterborne disease theory.

Sometimes overlooked in Snow's work is his systematic search for cases that seemed to contradict the normal pattern of infection. For example, he discovered cholera in peo-

TABLE 1.4. Rates of Cholera Death During the 1854 London Cholera Epidemic by Water Supplier

Water Source	No. of Houses	Deaths from Cholera	Deaths per 10,000 Houses
Southwark & Vauxhall	40,046	1263	315
Lambeth	26,107	98	37
Rest of London	256,423	1422	59

Source: Snow (1855).

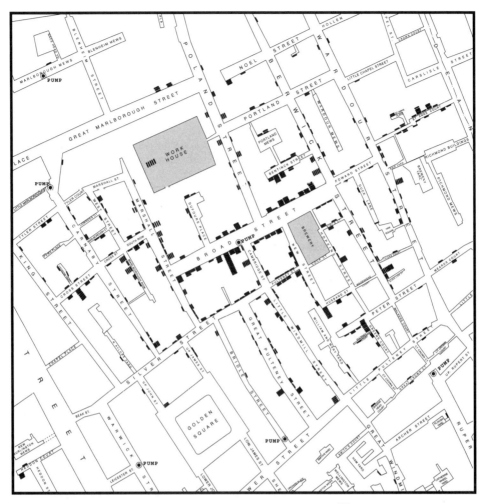

Figure 1.2. *Snow's map of the 1854 London cholera epidemic. Lines (|||||) and show deaths and bullets (●) show the location of water pumps. The map reveals a strong association between cholera mortality and the pump on Broad Street. (*Source: Snow, 1936.)

ple who resided away from the source of exposure but were exposed during their school and working hours. He also noted the low frequency of cases within Workhouse inmates and absence of cases among brewery workers who worked and lived near the pump but had alternative sources of drinking water.

To explain the presence of a case outside the epidemic area, Snow wrote:

> I was informed by this lady's son that she had not been in the neighborhood of Broad Street for many months. A cart went from Broad Street to West End every day, and it was the custom to take out a large bottle of water from the pump in Broad Street, as she preferred it. The water was taken on Thursday, 31st August, and she drank of it in the evening, and also on Friday. (Snow, 1855, pp. 44–45)

To explain the relative deficiency of cases in Workhouse inmates, Snow wrote:

> The workhouse has a pump-well on the premises, in addition to the supply from the Grand Junction Water Works, and the inmates never sent to Broad Street for water. (Snow, 1855, p. 42)

To explain the absence of cases in brewery workers, Snow wrote:

> There is a brewery in Broad Street, near to the pump, and on perceiving that no brewer's men were registered as having died of cholera, I called on Mr. Huggins, the proprietor. He informed me that there were about seventy workmen employed in the brewery, and that none of them had suffered from cholera—at least in severe form—only two have been indisposed, and that not seriously, at the time the disease prevailed. The men are allowed a certain quantity of malt liquor, and Mr. Huggins believes they do not drink water at all; and he is quite certain that the workmen never obtained water from the pump in the street. There is a deep well in the brewery, in addition to the new River Water. (Snow, 1855, p. 42)

Snow's clear and lucid combination of empirical observation and hypothetico-deductive reasoning has served as the epidemiologic *sine quo non* for the past century and a half.

Other Selected Figures and Events

A listing of selected figures and events is provided to give the reader a *brief* historical timeline of important epidemiologic events.

- **Hippocrates** (approx. 460–377 B.C.E.) is credited with laying the **foundation for scientific medicine** by freeing the study of disease from the constraints of philosophical speculation and superstition, while stressing the importance of environmental influences on health.
- The **tallying of population-based vital statistics** dates back to the reign of the black death, or bubonic plague, which killed approximately one-quarter of Europe's population between 1346 and 1352. During this period, officials began keeping records of the number of persons dying each week. The epidemiologic utility of vital statistics was further advanced by **John Graunt** (1620–1674), who, in the 17th century, collected Bills of Mortality (death certificates), which had been initiated by parish clerks in London and surrounding areas in the early 1600s. Grant used life tables to summarize the mortality experience in terms of numbers, percents, and probabilities, thus noting urban–rural differences in mortality, high mortality rates in children (one-third died before the age of 5), and discrepancies in morbidity and mortality rates in men and women (men experience higher mortality rates but lower morbidity rates that women, which, by the way, is still the case).
- In 1775, **Percival Pott** (1713–1788) wrote of the enormously elevated rates of scrotal cancer in chimney sweeps and attributed this increase to lodgment of soot in the rugae of the scrotum. Percival Pott's work provides an early example of **occupation epidemiology.**
- **Edward Jenner** (1749–1823) found, in 1798, that smallpox could be prevented by inoculation with the substance from cowpox lesions. This was the first documented case of actively preventing disease through **vaccination**.

- In 1846, **Peter Ludwig Panum** (1820–1885) took advantage of the geographic and political isolation of the Faroe Islands to study a violent outbreak of measles in native people. During his investigation, Panum used modern **infectious disease principles** to determine the extent to which the agent was infectious and found differences in host susceptibility. He also calculated the typical incubation of measles to be 13 to 14 days.

- **Jakob Henle** (1809–1885?), **Louis Pasteur** (1822–1895), and **Robert Koch** (1843–1910) are key figures credited with developing the **germ theory of disease.** The theory was first explained in the 1840 publication of Henle's treatise. This was followed by Pasteur's and Koch's experimental transmission of specific infectious disease agents in humans and animals.

- **Emile Durkheim** (1858–1917) completed a detailed study on suicide as it relates to psychopathologic states (e.g., insanity), race, heredity, climate, season, imitative behavior, egoistic factors (e.g., religion), altruism, anomie (social instability), and other social phenomena. His study, *Suicide: A Study in Sociology*, originally published in 1897, provides an early example of **social epidemiology.**

- In 1914, **Joseph Goldberger** (1874–1927) published a paper relating pellagra to diets high in cereals and canned foods and free of fresh animal products. Shortly after that, he conducted a clinical trial that proved the preventive efficacy of increasing fresh animal and leguminous protein foods in the diet. Goldberger's work is a landmark study in **nutritional epidemiology.**

- The post World War II era heralded the beginning of what some might call **modern epidemiology.** With the emergence of chronic disease as the primary causes of morbidity and mortality, the epidemiologic approach that has met with the most success is based on a biostatistical understanding of causes and contributors to the disease process. Examples of important epidemiologic events during this era are the initiation of community-based intervention trials of water fluoridation, clinical trials of the Salk polio vaccine, the Framingham Heart Study, the Report of the Advisory Committee to the Surgeon General of the Public Health Service on Smoking and Health, and recent dramatic declines in cardiovascular disease death rates.

1.4 SELECTED MORTALITY TRENDS IN THE UNITED STATES

Causes of Death

Table 1.5 lists the 10 leading causes of death in the United States in 1900 and 1990. Note that the leading causes of death have changed radically over this century. In the past, most deaths were caused by acute, infectious diseases. Today's main problems are mostly chronic and noninfectious, some of which are "life-style diseases," caused by smoking, dietary excesses, and other factors rooted in behavior.

Figure 1.3 depicts age-adjusted mortality rates for all causes combined and for six of the leading causes of death in the United States for the years 1950 through 1992. Note that rates are plotted on a logarithmic scale. This technique—equivalent to taking the logarithm of each rate and plotting it on a conventional scale—is particularly useful in assessing rates of change. A constant rate of change is indicated by a straight line with the slope of the line representing the rate of change. Thus, even relatively modest sloping lines can represent quite a large change in absolute terms. During the period of observation, the mortality rate

TABLE 1.5. Leading Causes of Death in the United States, 1900 and 1990[a]

Rank	1900[b]	1990[c]
1.	Pneumonia (all forms) and influenza [202.2]	Diseases of the heart [152.0]
2.	Tuberculosis (all forms) [194.4]	Malignant neoplasms [135.0]
3.	Diarrhea, enteritis, and ulceration of the intestines [142.7]	Unintentional injuries (includes motor vehicle crashes) [32.5]
4.	Diseases of the heart [137.4]	Cerebrovascular disease [27.7]
5.	Intracranial lesions of vascular origin [106.9]	Chronic obstructive pulmonary disease [19.7]
6.	Nephritis (all forms) [88.6]	Pneumonia and influenza [14.0]
7.	All accidents [72.3]	Diabetes mellitus [11.7]
8.	Cancer and other malignant tumors [64.0]	Suicide [11.5]
9.	Senility [50.2]	Homicide and legal intervention [10.2]
10.	Diphtheria [40.3]	Human immunodeficiency virus [9.8]

[a]Rates per 100,000 are listed in square brackets. Rates have not been age adjusted and therefore should not be directly compared.
[b]Data source: National Office of Vital Statistics (1947).
[c]Data source: National Center for Health Statistics (1995).

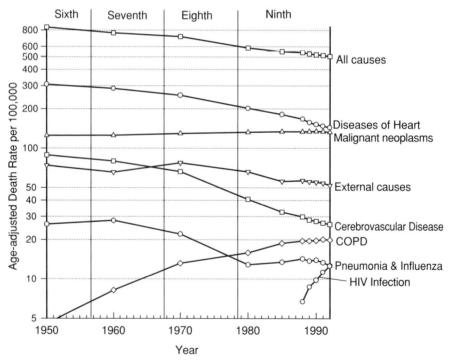

Figure 1.3. Age-adjusted mortality rates for all causes combined and the current six leading causes of death in the United States, 1950 to 1992. (Data source: National Center for Health Statistics, 1995, pp. 97–98.)

for all causes combined has decreased from 841 per 100,000 resident population to 505 per 100,000, representing an almost 40% decline. Especially important in this regard is the rapid decline in mortality due to diseases of the heart. In 1950, mortality from heart disease occurred at the rate of 307 per 100,000 residents. By 1992, this rate was cut in half to 144 per 100,000. This phenomenal decline represents one of the great successes of modern preventive medicine.

Examples of other interesting mortality trends are:

- Age-adjusted cancer mortality increased slightly between 1950 and 1990, with rates of 125 per 100,000 in 1950 and 135 per 100,000 in 1990. The rate dropped slightly thereafter, with a rate of 133 per 100,000 in 1992. Recent evidence suggests that cancer mortality has continued to decline at the modest rate of approximately 1% per year (Bailar & Gornik, 1997).

- External causes of death are important contributors to overall mortality. In 1992, the age-adjusted rate for this category was 52 per 100,000. The major contributors to this category were motor traffic crashes (16 per 100,000), other unintentional injuries (14 per 100,000), suicide (11 per 100,000), and homicide and legal interventions (11 per 100,000).

- Cerebrovascular mortality rates have decreased dramatically from 89 per 100,000 in 1950 to 26 per 100,000 in 1992.

- Chronic obstructive pulmonary disease (COPD) mortality has increased steadily, demonstrating a rate of 4 per 100,000 in 1950 and 20 per 100,000 in 1992.

- Pneumonia and influenza continue to be important causes of death. In 1992, their combined death rate was 13 per 100,000.

- HIV rates have rapidly increased, demonstrating a mortality rate of 13 per 100,000 in 1992.

Cancer trends in the United States have been of particular public concern and interest. Figure 1.4 shows age-adjusted death rates for four important types of cancer in the United States. Profound increases in respiratory cancers are apparent between 1950 and 1990. Between 1990 and 1992, however, the age-adjusted respiratory cancer mortality rates have notably declined. This decrease can further be isolated to a 4% to 5% decline in lung cancer in white and black men (National Center for Health Statistics, 1995, p. 3). Colorectal cancer death rates have decreased from 19 per 100,000 in 1950 to 13 per 100,000 in 1992, whereas age-adjusted breast cancer death rates have fluctuated only slightly, with rates of 22 per 100,000 in 1950, 23 per 100,000 in 1990, 22 per 100,000 in 1992. Age-adjusted prostate cancer death rates have increased from 13 deaths per 100,000 in 1950 to 17 per 100,000 in 1992.

Life Expectancy

Life expectancy in the United States has increased dramatically over the past century (Fig. 1.5). In 1900, the average life expectancy at birth was 47.3 years. In 1992, this value was 75.8 years. Reductions in mortality during the early part of the century were due to diminished risks in fatal infections, improved nutrition, smaller family size, better provision of uncontaminated water, control of vectors, pasteurization of milk, maternal education in the care of infants, and immunization (Doll, 1992). More recent improvements in survival can

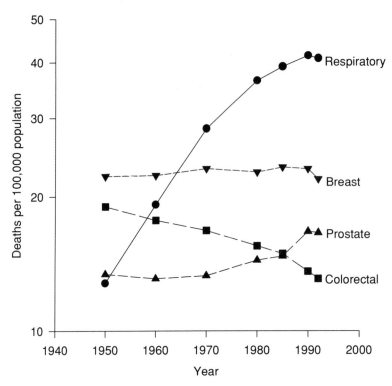

Figure 1.4. *Age-adjusted death rates for selected cancers in the United States, 1950 to 1992. (*Data source: *National Center for Health Statistics, 1995, p. 97.)*

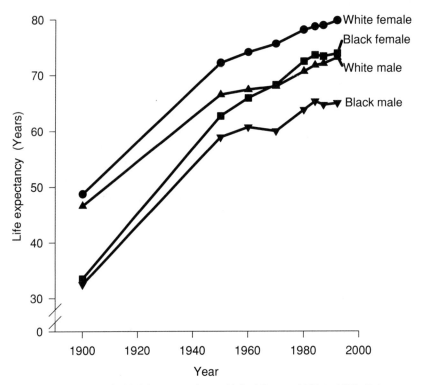

Figure 1.5. *Life expectancy at birth by sex and race, United States, 1900 to 1992. (*Data source: *Na-*

tional Center for Health Statistics, 1995, p. 96.)

be attributed to the advent of sulfa drugs and antibiotics (in 1936 and 1941, respectively), better and more effective immunization coverage, better anesthesia and postoperative care, avoiding of smoking, and reductions in heart disease through the control of high blood pressure and hyperlipidemia (Doll, 1992).

The longer average life span for females compared to males has widely been recognized since John Graunt's observation in 1665. Gender differences in mortality have been attributed to both genetic and behavioral factors. The widening gap in life expectancy between the sexes is due primarily to smoking-induced heart and respiratory disease (Doll, 1992).

The gap in life expectancy between the white and black population is still evident, but it has narrowed. In 1992, life expectancy for the white population was 6.9 years longer than for the black population (76.5 years versus 69.6 years). The life expectancy for black females now exceeds that of white males (73.9 years versus 73.2 years). However, the difference in life expectancy between white males and black males is still large (73.2 years versus 65.0 years).

SUMMARY

1. Epidemiology is the study of the distribution and determinants of disease and health-related states in populations. It draws on the knowledge and tools of many different disciplines for the purpose of discovering the causes of disease. Public health uses epidemiologic study findings to prevent and control health problems in human populations.

2. The history of epidemiology is varied and complex, with roots in clinical and social medicine, the microbiologic revolution, demography, sociology, and statistics. John Snow is a key figure in the development of modern epidemiology. Using relatively simple population-based methods. Snow was able to establish that the cholera agent was waterborne. This finding preceded isolation of the cholera bacterium by some 44 years.

3. The major causes of mortality have changed radically over the current century. In the previous century, most deaths were caused by infectious disease. Today, most fatal diseases are chronic and noncontagious. Overall age-adjusted mortality rates have decreased by 40% since the turn of the century, with life expectancy increasing by 60%. Since 1950, cardiovascular disease mortality rates have declined by more than 50%.

EXERCISES

Select the best response in each instance.

1. Which of the following statements best fits the definition of epidemiology as used in this chapter?

   (A) Epidemiology is a form of social and political activism that has as its goal the promotion of health and well-being.

   (B) Epidemiology is the study of the distribution and determinants of disease in human populations.

   (C) Epidemiology is the study of measures and interventions used to treat illness.

   (D) Epidemiology is the science that deals with the physiological and psychological effects of disease.

2. "Epidemic" means:

(A) occurring in clear excess of normal expectancy

(B) consistently present in the environment

(C) affecting a large number of countries simultaneously

(D) exhibiting regular seasonal fluctuations in occurrence

3. Currently, the leading cause of death in the United States is:

(A) malignant neoplasms (cancer)

(B) heart disease

(C) trauma

(D) chronic obstructive pulmonary disease

(E) influenza and pneumonia

4. A synonym for "relating to disease and disability" is:

(A) mortality

(B) morbidity

(C) epidemic

(D) endemic

5. Compared to soft sciences, hard sciences are relatively more likely to:

(A) use objective measures

(B) address important personal and societal issues

(C) address inanimate topics

(D) A and C

(E) A, B, and C

6. What made John Snow's work on cholera noteworthy?

(A) His work predates the demonstration that epidemics can be caused by living organisms.

(B) He was one of the first physicians to realize that his obligations went beyond treating the ill.

(C) He was one of the first persons to use methods based on population-based patterns of disease and take effective action in the prevention of future disease.

(D) A and C

(E) A, B, and C

ANSWERS TO EXERCISES

1. B   Epidemiology studies the distribution and determinants of disease in populations. Answer A is a possible definition of public health. Answers C and D describe fields of medicine, sometimes studied from an epidemiologic perspective.

2. A   An epidemic is a disease or health-related condition occurring in clear excess of normal expectancy. Definition B describes a disease that is endemic, assuming the occurrence level is more or less constant. Definition C describes a pandemic disease. Item D—normal seasonal fluctuations of a disease—is not considered epidemic.

3. B Although age-adjusted death rates from heart disease have dropped dramatically, they continue to be the number one cause of death in the United States.

4. B

5. D Although the distinction between hard science and soft science is not always clear, hard sciences tend to use more objective measures than soft sciences. They are also more likely to study inanimate subjects.

6. E

REFERENCES

Bailar, J. C. III, & Gornik, H. L. (1997). Cancer undefeated. *New England Journal of Medicine*, 336, 1569–1574.

Diamond, J. (1979). *Your Body Doesn't Lie*. New York: Warner Books.

Doll, R. (1992). Health and the environment in the 1990s. *American Journal of Public Health*, 82, 933–941.

Durant, A., & Durant, W. (1961). *The Story of Civilization, 7, The Age of Reason Begins*. New York: Simon & Shuster.

Durkheim, E. (1951). *Suicide: A Study in Sociology*. (J. A. Spaulding & G. Simpson, Trans.). New York: The Free Press. (Original work published in 1897)

Feinstein, A. R. (1972). The need for humanizing science in evaluating medication. *Lancet*, 2, 421–423.

Goldberger, J. (1914). The etiology of pellagra, the significance of certain epidemiological observations with respect to. *Public Health Reports*, 29, 1683–1686.

Graunt, J. (1939). *Natural and Political Observations Mentioned in a Following Index, and Made Upon the Bills of Mortality*. Baltimore, MD: The Johns Hopkins Press. (Original work published in 1662)

Greenwood, M. (1935). *Epidemics and Crowd-Diseases: An Introduction to the Study of Epidemiology*. London: Williams & Norgate.

Institute of Medicine. (1988). Committee for the Study of the Future of Public Health. *The Future of Public Health*. Washington, DC: National Academy Press.

Jenner, E. (1798). *An Inquiry into the Causes and Effects of the Variolae Vaccinea, a Disease Discovered in Some of the Western Counties of England, Particularly Gloucestershire, and Known by the Name of the Cow Pox*. London: Sampson Low.

Langmuir, A. D. (1961). Epidemiology of airborne infections. *Bacteriological Reviews*, 24, 173–181.

Last, J. M. (Ed.). (1983). *A Dictionary of Epidemiology*. New York: Oxford University Press.

Last, J. M. (Ed.). (1988). *A Dictionary of Epidemiology* (2nd ed.). New York: Oxford University Press.

Last, J. M. (Ed.). (1995). *A Dictionary of Epidemiology* (3rd ed.). New York: Oxford University Press.

National Center for Health Statistics. (1995). *Health, United States, 1994*. Hyattsville, MD: U.S. Public Health Service.

National Office of Vital Statistics. (1947). Deaths and Death Rates for Leading Causes of Death: Death Registration States, 1901 and 1900. Unpublished raw data.

Niederhoffer, V. (1997). *The Education of a Speculator*. New York: John Wiley & Sons.

Panum, P. L. (1940). *Observations Made During the Epidemic of Measles on the Faroe Islands in the Year 1846*. (A. S. Hatcher, Trans.). New York: Delta Omega Society. (Original work published circa 1846)

Pearce, N. (1996). Traditional epidemiology, modern epidemiology, and public health. *American Journal of Public Health*, 86, 678–683.

Pott, P. (1790). *The Chirurgical Works of Percival Pott. A New Edition, with his Last Corrections* (Vol. 3). London: J. Johnson. (Originally published as *Cancer Scroti* in 1775)

Sagan, C. (1996, Dec. 20). Carl Sagan Obituary. Bob Edwards (Host). *Morning Edition*. Washington, DC: National Public Radio.

Snow, J. (1936). *Snow on Cholera*. New York: The Commonwealth Fund. (Originally published as *On the Mode of Communication of Cholera* in 1855)

Susser, M. W. (1973). *Causal Thinking in Health Sciences*. New York: Oxford University Press.

Vandenbroucke, J. P. (1988). Are "the causes of cancer" a miasma theory for the end of the twentieth century? *International Journal of Epidemiology*, 17, 708–709.

Wallis, W. A., & Roberts, H. V. (1962). *The Nature of Statistics*. New York: The Free Press.

Winkelstein, W. (1995). A new perspective on John Snow's communicable disease theory. *American Journal of Epidemiology*, 142, S3–S9.

World Health Organization. (1984). *Health Promotion: A Discussion Document*. Copenhagen: WHO.

Wynder, E. L. (1994). Studies in mechanisms and prevention: striking a proper balance. *American Journal of Epidemiology*, 139, 547–549.

Zeitlin, S. (Guest). (1997, Apr. 20). Because God Loves Stories. *Weekend Edition*. Washington, DC: National Public Radio.

2

Selected Epidemiologic Disease Concepts

Epidemiology studies factors that change the likelihood of disease and searches for understanding the way diseases behave in individuals over time. To this end, the following topics are presented: the natural history of disease, variability in the expression of disease, causal models of disease, and the epidemiologic approach to disease investigation using time, place, and person variables.

2.1 THE NATURAL HISTORY OF DISEASE

Stages of Disease

The natural history of disease refers to the progress of a disease in an individual over time (Fig. 2.1). It includes all disease-related phenomena from before the onset of disease (i.e., the **stage of susceptibility**) until after its resolution (i.e., the **stage of recovery, disability, or death**). In the period following exposure to the etiologic agent, the prospective case enters the stage of subclinical disease. This stage corresponds to the time during which the etiologic agent is present within the body but has not yet caused discernible signs or symptoms. The subclinical stage of disease was recognized by Jacob Henle more than a century and a half ago, when he wrote: "the symptoms of disease do not appear directly after the entry of the contagious agent but rather after a certain period, which varies in the different contagions" (1840, p. 14). It is clear, therefore, that Henle understood the subclinical stage of disease much as we do today.

  Both infectious and noninfectious diseases are characterized by subclinical stages of disease. With infectious diseases, this period is called the **incubation period.** With noninfectious diseases, this period is often called the **latent period** or **induction period.** Analogous to the incubation period, the latent period of a noninfectious disease corresponds to the time between exposure to a pathogen and the emergence of its clinically discernible effects. In considering the causes of cancer, for example, the latent period corresponds to the time between exposure to the carcinogen, initiation and promotion of neoplastic

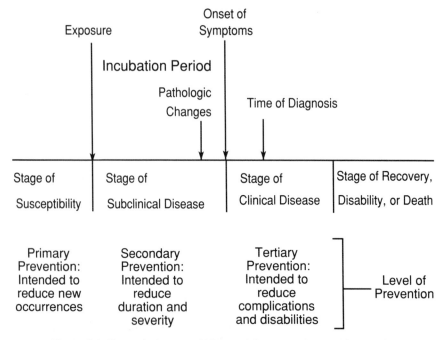

Figure 2.1. *Stages in the natural history of disease and types of prevention.*

changes, and progression of the tumor to a size or state that causes discernible signs in the patient. In considering atherosclerosis of the coronary arteries, the latent period corresponds to the cumulative time of exposure to the dietary factors associated with atherogenic changes to a point that seriously compromises cardiac function.

Incubation periods vary considerably according to agent–disease pairs. Some diseases are characterized by short incubation periods (e.g., cholera has a brief 24- to 48-hour incubation period), others by intermediate incubation periods (e.g., chickenpox has a typical incubation period of 2 to 3 weeks), and still others by extended incubation (e.g., the median incubation of acquired immunodeficiency syndrome is approximately 10 years) (Brookmeyer & Goedert, 1989; Alcabes et al., 1993). Typical incubation periods for selected infectious diseases are listed in Table 2.1.

Even for a given disease, incubation periods can vary considerably. For example, the incubation period for human immunodeficiency virus (HIV) and acquired immunodeficiency syndrome (AIDS) ranges from 3 to more than 20 years (Saag, 1994). The latent period for leukemia caused by exposure to the atomic bomb blast in Hiroshima ranged from 2 to 12 years (Cobb et al., 1959), and the incubation period for occupationally associated bladder tumors in Great Britain ranged from 5 to 40 years (Fig. 2.2). Variability in incubation and latency can be due to differences in host susceptibility, pathogenicity of the agent, and dose of exposure.

The **stage of clinical disease** begins with a patient's first symptoms and ends with either recovery, disability, or death. Depending on host factors, access to health care, and the diagnostic acumen of the clinician in charge, the lag between the onset of symptoms and diagnosis may vary considerably. Note that the onset of symptoms—not the time of diagnosis—marks the beginning of the clinical stage of disease.

TABLE 2.1. Incubation Periods for Selected Infectious Diseases

Disease	Typical Incubation Period[a]
Acquired immune deficiency syndrome	Infection to appearance of antibodies: 1–3 months; median time to diagnosis: approx. 10 years; treatment lengthens the incubation period
Amebiasis	2–4 weeks
Chickenpox	13–17 days
Common cold	2 days
Hepatitis B	60–90 days
Influenza	1–5 days
Legionellosis	5–6 days
Malaria (*Plasmodium vivax* and *P. ovale*)	14 days
Malaria (*P. malariae*)	30 days
Malaria (*P. Falciparum*)	12 days
Measles	7–18 days
Mumps	12–25 days
Poliomyelitis, acute paralytic	7–14 days
Plague	2–6 days
Rabies	2–8 weeks (depends on severity of wound)
Salmonellosis	12–36 hours
Schistosomiasis	2–6 weeks
Staphylococcal food poisoning	2–4 hours
Tetanus	3–21 days

Source: Benensen (1990).

[a]The incubation periods of some diseases vary considerably. See the latest edition of *Control of Communicable Diseases* for details.

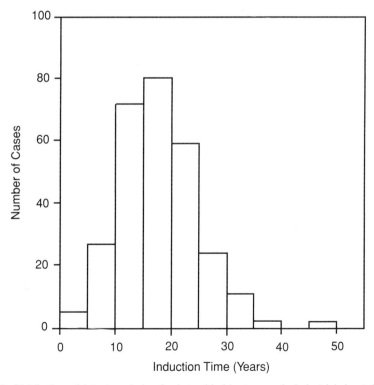

Figure 2.2. Distribution of latent periods of urinary bladder tumors in industrial dyestuff workers. (Source: Case et al., 1954, p. 85; reproduced with permission of BMJ Publishing Group.)

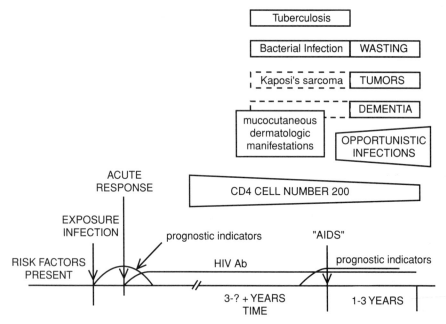

Figure 2.3. *The natural history and progression of HIV infection and AIDS. (Source: Cotton, D. J. (1995). The natural history of HIV infection: implications for clinical trials. In D. M. Finkelstein & D. A. Schoenfeld (Eds.). AIDS Clinical Trials, p. 8; Copyright © 1995 by Wiley-Liss, Inc. Reprinted by permission of Wiley-Liss, Inc., a subsidiary of John Wiley & Sons, Inc.)*

Studying the natural history of a disease is a prerequisite to understanding its epidemiology. For example, AIDS can only be understood after grasping the multifarious stages of HIV infection (Fig. 2.3). Exposure to HIV is followed by an acute response that is often accompanied by unrecognized flu-like symptoms. Although prospective cases do not exhibit detectable antibody until approximately 6 weeks following the initial infection, they can still be infectious during this acute phase. A long incubation period ensues, during which CD4+ lymphocyte counts decline, but the patient is largely free from symptoms. The risk of developing AIDS is low during the initial few years of infection but increases over time. AIDS, of course, expresses itself in many different ways (e.g., opportunistic infections, cancers, dementia).

Primary, Secondary, and Tertiary Prevention

Disease prevention efforts can be classified according to the stage of disease in which they are applied (Fig. 2.1). **Primary prevention** is directed toward the stage of susceptibility, that is, before the pathogen establishes itself in the body. Its goal is to prevent the disease from occurring, thus reducing its incidence and prevalence in the community. Examples of primary prevention are needle-exchange programs to prevent the spread of HIV, vaccination programs, and smoking cessation and prevention programs.

Secondary prevention is directed toward the subclinical stage of disease, that is, in people who carry the agent in their bodies but are not yet symptomatic. The goal of secondary prevention is to reduce the expression or severity of the disease once it emerges.

Treating asymptomatic HIV-infected patients with combinations of antiviral agents to delay the onset of AIDS is a form of secondary prevention. Screening for cervical cancer and breast cancer to detect these diseases in their early stages so that the disease is more amenable to treatment is also a form of secondary prevention.

Tertiary prevention is directed toward the clinical stage of disease. The aim of tertiary prevention is to prevent or minimize the progression of the disease or its sequelae. Screening people with diabetes for diabetic retinopathy in order to promptly treat the progression of blindness is a form of tertiary prevention. As the prevalence of chronic diseases continues to rise, tertiary prevention is taking on increasing importance as a means of preventing disabilities and minimizing the cost of care associated with prevalent, degenerative conditions.

2.2 VARIABILITY IN THE EXPRESSION OF DISEASE

Spectrum of Disease

A particular disease can display a broad scope of manifestations and severities, ranging from silent in some people to progressive and fulminating in others. When considering infectious diseases, this range of manifestation is known as the **gradient of infection.** When considering noninfectious diseases, this range of manifestation is known as the **spectrum of disease.** For example, HIV infection ranges from inapparent, to mild disease (e.g., AIDS-related complex), to severe disease (e.g., wasting syndrome), to death. Coronary artery disease might exist in the following stages: asymptomatic atherosclerosis of the coronary arteries, compromised cardiac circulation resulting in transient ischemia and angina, myocardial infarction due to lodgement of a clot in the narrowed artery, and death.

The Iceberg Metaphor

The broad range of some illnesses has been likened to an **iceberg,** in that, like an iceberg, the bulk of the problem may be hidden from view (Fig. 2.4). For example, at any given time, the number of AIDS cases represents only the tip of all HIV infections. This metaphor also applies to chronic diseases and injuries. For example, many people with atherosclerotic coronary artery disease experience no symptoms until their first heart attack. In a different way, most dog bite injuries go undetected by normal surveillance methods: for *each* U.S. dog bite fatality there are about 670 hospitalizations, 16,000 emergency department visits, 21,000 other medical visits, and 187,000 nonmedically treated bites (Weiss et al. 1998; Fig. 2.5).

Gradients of infection vary from disease to disease. For example, over 90% of poliomyelitis infections are associated with no clinically apparent signs, whereas nearly all measles cases exhibit symptoms.

Nonspecificity of Effect

A given agent can be nonspecific in its effect. For cxample, *Herpes zoster* causes both chickenpox and shingles; HIV causes AIDS-related complex, tuberculosis, dementia, Kaposi's sarcoma, and pneumocystis pneumonia; smoking causes cardiovascular disease, cancer, chronic lung diseases, and musculoskeletal disease. Thus, agents and diseases do necessarily share simple one-to-one relationships.

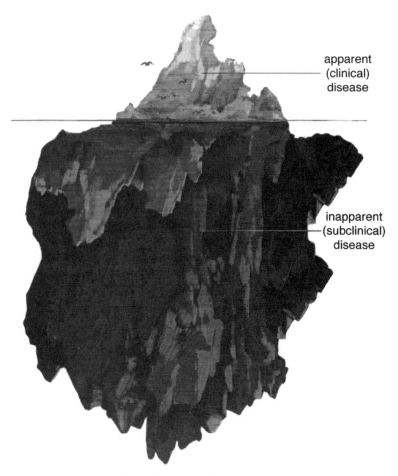

apparent
(clinical)
disease

inapparent
(subclinical)
disease

Figure 2.4. *The iceberg metaphor.*

2.3 DISEASE ETIOLOGY

Definition of "Cause"

Epidemiologists take a broad view of cause. From an epidemiologic perspective, an etiologic (causal) factor is any event, condition, or characteristic that increases the likelihood of disease, *caeteris paribus* (all other things being equal). In general, a factor is considered causal if an increase in its level is accompanied by an increase in the incidence of disease. If the factor can be eliminated or altered in such a way that the frequency of the disease declines or the severity of the problem decreases, then theories supporting the causal nature of the factor are bolstered.

Causal factors may represent single events or a complex interaction of factors. The prevention and control of a disease should thus be directed toward all relevant factors, with attention focused on those factors that are most easily influenced and that have the greatest potential impact.

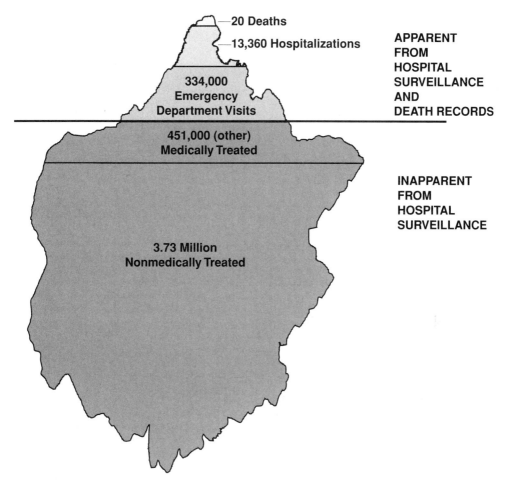

20 Deaths

13,360 Hospitalizations

334,000 Emergency Department Visits

451,000 (other) Medically Treated

3.73 Million Nonmedically Treated

APPARENT
FROM
HOSPITAL
SURVEILLANCE
AND
DEATH RECORDS

INAPPARENT
FROM
HOSPITAL
SURVEILLANCE

Figure 2.5. *Approximate yearly number of dog bite injuries in the United States. (Data source: Weiss, et al., 1998.)*

Causal Web

Cause, from an epidemiologic perspective, includes both direct cause (a factor that leads directly to pathogenic change) and indirect cause (a factor that increases the likelihood of pathology but does not lead directly to the pathologic change). Indirect and direct causes may act to form a hierarchical **causal web** of events. A complex interaction of events may ultimately determine the level of disease in a community. An excellent and well-known example of a causal-web model is shown in Figure 2.6.

Necessary, Sufficient, and Contributory Factors

Causal factors may further be classified as either necessary, sufficient, or contributory (Rothman, 1976). **Necessary factors** must be present for the disease to occur. For example, the tubercle bacillus is necessary (but not alone sufficient) to cause tuberculosis. **Sufficient**

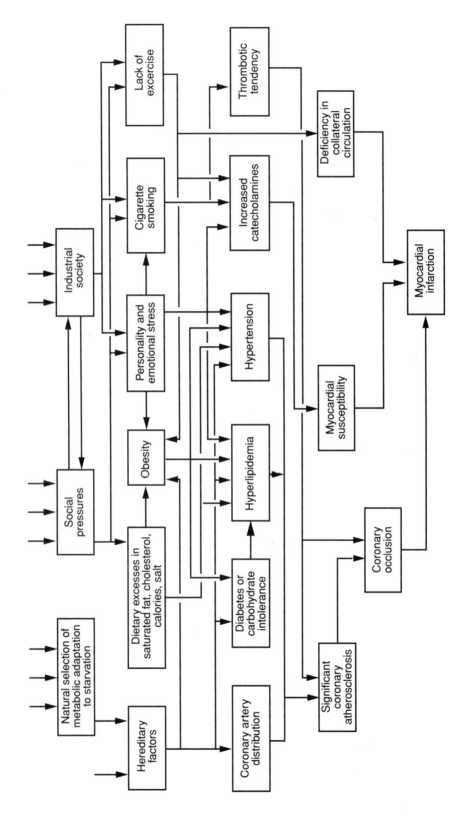

Figure 2.6. A causal-web model for myocardial infarction. (Source: Friedman, G. D. (1974). Primer of Epidemiology. New York McGraw-Hill; reproduced with permission of the McGraw-Hill Companies.)

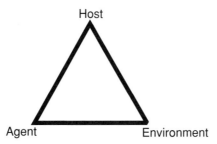

Figure 2.7. Classic epidemiologic triad.

factors always lead to disease. For example, exposure to the tubercle bacillus combined with susceptibility to the infection is usually sufficient to cause tuberculosis. Several factors may act in consort to form a sufficient cause, and a particular disease might have several different sufficient causes. **Contributing factors** are neither necessary nor sufficient but, when combined with other factors, increase the likelihood of disease occurrence.

Agent, Host, and Environment

Causal factors can be related to the agent, host, or environment (Fig. 2.7). **Agents** are biological, physical, or chemical factors whose presence, absence, or relative amount (too much or too little) are necessary for the disease to occur (Table 2.2). **Host factors** include personal characteristics and behaviors, genetic predispositions, and immunologic and other susceptibility-related factors that increase or decrease the likelihood of disease. **Environmental factors** are external conditions, other than the agent, that contribute to the disease process. Environmental factors can be physical, biological, or social in nature.

Ecology of Disease

Over time, a succession of agent, host, and environmental factors can evolve to form a steady state of **epidemiologic homeostasis.** Thus, an ecologic balance of conditions results in an endemic level of disease. Alterations in this equilibrium might result from any of the following.

- Increases in the ability of the agent to infect or enter the host (**infectivity** of the agent)

TABLE 2.2. Types of Disease-Causing Agents

Biologic	Chemical	Physical
Helminths	Nutritive (deficiencies and	Heat
Protozoan	excesses)	Light
Fungi	Poisons	Radiation
Bacteria	Drugs	Noise
Rickettsia	Allergens	Vibration
Viral		Objects
Prion		

- Increases in the ability of the agent to cause disease within the host (**pathogenicity** of the agent)
- Increases in the severity of disease caused by the agent once it has invaded the host (**virulence** of the agent)
- Increases in the proportion of susceptibles in the population
- Environmental changes that favor growth and spread of the agent
- Environmental changes that compromise host resistance

An example of the interactive balance between agent, host, and environmental factors considers the relationship between air pollution and morbidity and mortality (Munn, 1970). This work suggests that high environmental levels of sulfur dioxide and particulate air pollution can cause elevations in the overall morbidity and mortality rate in humans and animals. High pollution can be traced to industrial polluters and meteorologic conditions that favor retention of pollutants in the ecosphere (e.g., meteorologic inversions). When scrutinized further, the adverse effects of the pollution are concentrated in people and animals with preexisting cardiorespiratory disease. Thus, morbidity and mortality levels are linked to a complex interaction of agent (sulfur dioxide pollution), host (preexisting cardiorespiratory disease), and environmental (meteorologic) conditions.

The extent of HIV sexual transmission in a population can also be viewed as a function of agent, host, and environmental factors (Fig. 2.8). Agent factors include phenotypic

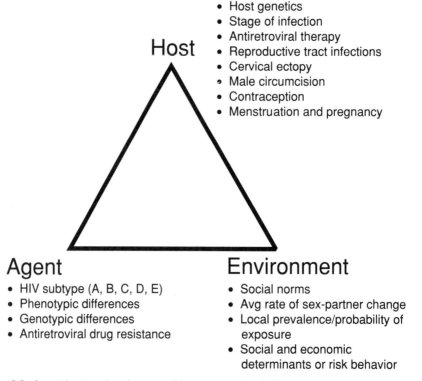

Figure 2.8. Agent, host, and environmental factors associated with the sexual transmission of HIV in a community. (Source of information: Royce et al., 1997).

and genotypic differences in the virus that influence the ability of the virus to replicate and spread. Examples of host factors are the coexistence of reproductive tract infections that produce genital ulcers (thus increasing the risk of transmission), availability of anti-retroviral therapy that decreases concentrations of HIV in bodily fluids, and contraceptive method choices (e.g., condoms and spermicides containing nonoxynol 9). Environmental factors influencing the sexual transmission of HIV include the rate of sex partner exchange, presence of unregulated commercial sex facilities, presence of crack cocaine houses, and social norms that influence these and other factors (Royce et al. 1997).

2.4 EPIDEMIOLOGIC VARIABLES

I keep six honest serving men
(They taught me all I know);
Their names are what and why and when
And how and where and who.
    —Rudyard Kipling

Descriptive and Analytic Epidemiology

One of the main functions of epidemiology is to discover groups of individuals with unusually high or low rates of disease. This allows for the rational generation of causal postulates. When searching for causal clues, it often helps to present results according to time, place, and person variables. This branch of epidemiology, often called **descriptive epidemiology,** deals with detecting high-risk groups so that educated hunches about cause and effect can be generated. This contrasts with **analytic epidemiology,** in which causal theories are tested.

Time

Analysis of disease patterns over **time** is useful in formulating hypotheses about environmental change, presence of the agent, and source of transmission. Variability of disease occurrence by time can be analyzed from different points of view, some of which are presented in Table 2.3. Observations are often organized in the form of an **epidemic curve** in which the number of cases is plotted against a time axis. Examples of temporal patterns of disease, shown in Figure 2.9, are (a) sporadic (occurring rarely and without regularity), (b) endemic (occurring predictably and with only minor or predictable fluctuations), (c)

TABLE 2.3. Examples of Epidemiologic Time References

Calendar time
Time since an event
Physiologic and hormonal cycles
Time under observation
Age (time since birth)
Circadian rhythm
Season

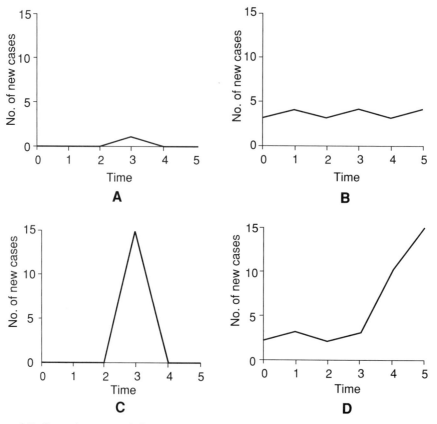

Figure 2.9. *General patterns of disease occurrence: (A) sporadic, (B) endemic, (C) point epidemic, and (D) propagating epidemic. (Source: Schwabe, C. W., Rieman, H. P., & Franti, C. E. (1977).* Epidemiology in Veterinary Practice. *Philadelphia & Febiger; reproduced with permission of Williams & Wilkins.)*

point epidemic (occurring in clear excess and rapidly returning to normal), and (d) propagating epidemic (occurring in clear excess with continuing increases over time).

Place

Place-related differences in disease patterns imply etiological differences related to host or environmental factors (see Table 2.4). We can analyze place-related difference based on geographic localities or characteristics common to localities (e.g., urbanicity, economic development, climate type). Early clues about many diseases have come from comparing geographic-specific mortality rates. This type of investigation is called an **ecological study,** because the analytic unit is the region rather than the person. A classic ecological study from cancer research considers international breast cancer mortality rates for the period 1958 to 1959 (Segi & Kurihara, 1962, pp. 30–31; Lilienfeld et al., 1967, p. 57). Data are displayed in Figure 2.10. Immediately apparent is Japan's distinctly low breast cancer mortality rate compared to other countries. This begs the question whether genetic or environmental factors are largely responsible for breast cancer. Studies of Japanese

TABLE 2.4. Host and Environmental Factors Associated with Place

Presence and level of agents
Presence of vectors
Genetic differences in residents
Physiologic and anatomic differences in residents
Geology
Climate
Population density
Nutritional practices
Occupational practices
Recreational practices
Urbanization
Economic development
Socially disruptive events (e.g., war, natural disasters)
Social norms and practices
Medical practices
Access to health care

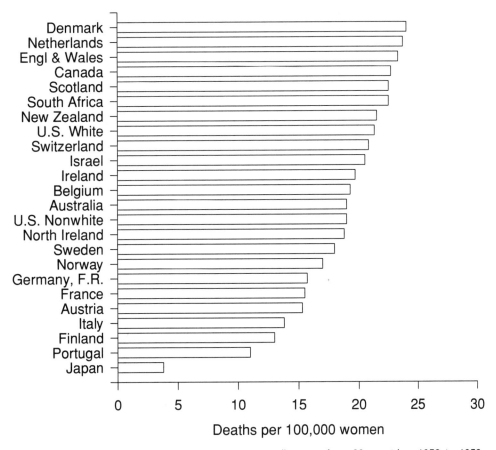

Figure 2.10. *Age-adjusted female breast cancer mortality rates from 23 countries, 1958 to 1959.* (Data source: *Segi & Kurihara, 1962, p. 31.*)

immigrants to the United States show that breast cancer rates in Japanese–American women become "Americanized" over successive generations (Buell, 1973). Additionally, steep increases in breast cancer rates in Japan over the past few decades (Wynder et al., 1991) suggest that environmental factors are important contributors to breast cancer risk. Investigators have offered a broad range of theories to help explain these observations. For example, Lilienfeld (1963) hypothesized that lengthy breast-feeding and long lactation periods among Japanese women are protective for breast cancer (a reasonable explanation given the influence of sex hormones on breast tissue). Subsequent explanations have considered variations in body weight (De Waard et al., 1977), aspects of diet (Armstrong & Doll, 1975), age at menarche (Henderson & Bernstein, 1991), and menstrual cycle length (Wang et al., 1992). Although none of these theories have been fully confirmed, this demonstrates an important feature of epidemiologic advancement: initial studies are seldom conclusive and must, therefore, be followed by further study. It is only through the combining of information from multiple sources that knowledge is advanced. Perhaps this is the reason it is said that "art is I, science is we."

Person

Examples of **person** variables studied by epidemiologists are listed in Table 2.5. Variation in disease rates by person variables suggests differences in the opportunity for exposure to the agent or differences in susceptibility once exposed. In comparing groups or people, it is important that the populations being compared should, insofar as possible, differ only with respect to the variable being examined. When differences in risk are found, characteristics that differentiate groups are said to be risk factors or risk indicators. A **risk factor** is a factor that is thought to cause the disease in question. A **risk indicator,** on the other hand, denotes a factor that is statistically associated with a disease but has not yet been

---

TABLE 2.5. Examples of Person Variables

Age
Sex
Ethnicity
Genetic predispositions
Physiologic states (e.g., pregnancy)
Concurrent disease
Immune status
Physical activity
Marital status
Dietary practices
Tobacco use
Alcohol use
Risk-taking behavior
Body mass
Response to social and physical stressors
Education level
Socioeconomic status
Occupation
Customs
Religion
Knowledge, attitude, and behaviors

---

proved to be causal. Note that not all risk indicators are risk factors, because association is not the same as causation. (This distinction will be discussed further in Chapter 12.)

SUMMARY

1. The natural history of disease refers to the progress of disease in an individual over time. It consists of stages of susceptibility, subclinical disease, clinical disease, and resolution. Prevention measures directed toward the stage of susceptibility are referred to as primary prevention; prevention measures directed toward the stage of subclinical disease are referred to as secondary prevention; prevention measures directed toward the stage of clinical disease are referred to as tertiary prevention.

2. The subclinical stage of disease corresponds to the period between the exposure to a pathogen and the emergence of the first symptoms of disease. With infectious disease, this period is called the incubation period. With noninfectious disease, this period is called the latent period. Incubation and latent periods vary considerably, depending on the pathogenic agent, dose of exposure, and resistance of the host.

3. A given disease can demonstrate a broad range of clinical manifestations and severities. When most of the disease is subclinical or undetected by normal epidemiologic means, the spectrum of disease is likened to an iceberg. Clinical signs are rarely specific for a given disease.

4. From an epidemiologic perspective, a causal factor is any agent, host, or environmental event that increases the likelihood of disease, all other things being equal. Causal factors may act directly to influence the pathogenesis of disease or may act indirectly in a causal web. Causal factors may be further classified as sufficient, necessary, or contributory.

5. The interaction of agent, host, and environmental factors contributes to the equilibrium of disease in a population. This equilibrium can be upset by changes in the infectivity, pathogenicity, or virulence of the agent, or changes in the environment that favor the agent or weaken the host.

6. Epidemiology describes disease patterns and occurrences as to time, place, and person variables. Descriptive epidemiology is used to generate causal hypotheses and is seldom conclusive in its findings. Analytic epidemiologic studies are used to test causal theories.

EXERCISES

Select the best response in each instance.

1. After infection with HIV, a period ensues during which the virus multiplies and progressively destroys immunocompetent cells. Early in this phase, there are few signs or symptoms in the host. This period of disease is called the:
    (A) susceptibility period
    (B) incubation period
    (C) clinical stage of disease
    (D) stage of recovery, disability, or death

2. Recommendations to reduce consumption of dietary fat are what form or prevention?
   (A) primary prevention
   (B) secondary prevention
   (C) tertiary prevention

3. The term "risk indicator" suggests the factor in question:
   (A) causes the disease
   (B) is statistically associated with the disease
   (C) increases the likelihood of disease, all other things being equal
   (D) is a sufficient cause

4. The "natural history of disease refers" to:
   (A) the time from which a disease is discovered until a cure is found
   (B) the time from diagnosis to recovery, disability, or death
   (C) the progress of disease in an individual over time
   (D) the time between exposure to an agent and first symptoms

5. What type of causal factor always leads to disease?
   (A) sufficient cause
   (B) necessary cause
   (C) contributing cause
   (D) all of the above

6. The x axis of an epidemic curve contains information about:
   (A) the number of cases in the population
   (B) a host characteristic
   (C) an environmental characteristic
   (D) an element of time

7. Nutritional elements in excess or deficiency can cause disease. What category of agent does this represent?
   (A) biological
   (B) chemical
   (C) physical

8. An epidemic might occur as the result of:
   (A) an increase in the pathogenicity of an agent
   (B) an increase in the susceptibility of a population
   (C) changes in the environment that favor the agent
   (D) A or C
   (E) A, B, or C

9. Women who have first-degree relatives with breast cancer are at twice the risk of developing breast cancer compared to other women. Is having a first-degree relative with breast cancer a host, agent, or environmental cause of this disease?
   (A) host
   (B) agent
   (C) environmental

10. Match each of the following terms with its definition:

infectivity

necessary factor

pathogenicity

risk factor

causal-web model

sufficient factor

virulence

(A) related to the severity of disease caused by the agent once it has entered and established itself in the host

(B) a factor or combination of factors that when introduced into the host always leads to the disease in question

(C) a factor that truly increases the occurrence of the disease in question, all other things being equal

(D) the ability of the agent to enter and establish itself in the host

(E) a theory of causality that suggests direct and indirect factors contribute to the disease process in an interrelated hierarchy of events

(F) the ability of the agent to cause disease within the host

(G) a factor that must be present for the disease to occur

ANSWERS TO EXERCISES

1. B The incubation period is the period during which the agent is in the body but has not yet caused discernible signs or symptoms.

2. A Interventions directed toward susceptible people before they develop disease are considered to be primary prevention.

3. B The term risk indicator suggests only a statistical association and not necessarily a causal one. The term risk factor is reserved for factors that are thought to be causal. Associations with risk indicators may be spurious.

4. C The natural history of disease includes all disease-related processes from before the onset of disease through the resolution of the disease.

5. A By definition, factors that always lead to disease are considered sufficient.

6. D The x axis contains an element of time.

7. B Nonliving constituents of foods are chemical in nature.

8. E The homeostatic balance of agent, host, and environmental factors that determine disease levels in a population can be upset by any one of the elements described in answers A through C.

9. A Genetic factors are inherent host characteristics.

10. (definition)   term
    (A)   virulence
    (B)   sufficient factor

(C)   risk factor
(D)   infectivity
(E)   causal-web model
(F)   pathogenicity
(G)   necessary factor

REFERENCES

Alcabes, P., Muñoz, A., Vlahov, D., & Friedland, G. H. (1993). Incubation period for human immunodeficiency virus. *Epidemiologic Reviews*, 15, 303–318.

Armstrong, B., & Doll, R. (1975). Environmental factors and cancer incidence and mortality in different countries with special reference to dietary practices. *International Journal of Epidemiology*, 15, 617–631.

Benenson, A. S. (Ed.) (1990). *Control of Communicable Diseases in Man* (15th ed.). Washington, DC: American Public Health Association.

Brookmeyer, R., & Goedert, J. J. (1989). Censoring in an epidemic with an application to hemophilia-associated AIDS. *Biometrics*, 45, 325–335.

Buell, P. (1973). Changing incidence of Breast Cancer in Japanese–American Women. *Journal of the National Cancer Institute*, 51, 1479–1483.

Case, R. A. M., Hosker, M. E., McDonald, D. B., & Pearson, J. T. (1954). Tumours of the urinary bladder in workmen engaged in the manufacture and use of certain dyestuff intermediates in the British chemical industry. Part I. The role of aniline, benzidine, alpha-naphthylamine and beta-naphthylamine. *British Journal of Industrial Medicine*, 11, 75–104.

Centers for Disease Control and Prevention [CDC]. (1992). *Principles of Epidemiology, Second Edition. Self-Study Course 3030-G*. Atlanta: Department of Health and Human Services.

Cobb, S., Miller, M., & Wald, N. (1959). On the estimation of the incubation period in malignant disease. *Journal of Chronic Diseases*, 9, 385–393.

Cotton, D. J. (1995). The natural History of HIV infection: implications for clinical trials. In D. M. Finkelstein & D. A. Schoenfeld (Eds.). *AIDS Clinical Trials* (pp. 5–19). New York: Wiley-Liss.

De Waard, F., Cornelis, J. P., Aoki, K., et al. (1977). Breast cancer incidence according to weight and height in two cities of the Netherlands and in Aichi Prefecture, Japan. *Cancer*, 40, 1269–1275.

Friedman, G. D. (1974). *Primer of Epidemiology*. New York: McGraw-Hill.

Henderson, B. E., & Bernstein, L. (1991). The international variation in breast cancer rates: an epidemiological assessment. *Breast Cancer Research and Treatment*, 18(Suppl 1), S11–S17.

Henle, J. (1840). Pathologishe Untersuchingen. In G. Rosen (Ed. and Trans.) (1938), *Henle: On Miasmata and Contagia*. Baltimore: The Johns Hopkins Press.

Kipling, R. (1987). *Just So Stories*. London: Penguin.

Lilienfeld, A. M. (1963). The epidemiology of breast cancer. *Cancer Research*, 23, 1503–1513.

Lilienfeld, A. M., Pedersen, E., & Dowd, J. E. (1967). *Cancer Epidemiology: Methods of Study*. Baltimore, MD: The Johns Hopkins Press.

Munn, R. E. (1970). Air quality for sulfur oxides. *Biometeorologic Methods*. Washington, DC: Academic Press.

Rothman, K. J. (1976). Causes. *American Journal of Epidemiology*, 104, 587–592.

Royce, R. A., Sena, A., Cates, W., & Cohen, M. S. (1997). Sexual transmission of HIV. *New England Journal of Medicine*, 336, 1072–1078.

Saag, M. (1994). Natural history of HIV-1 disease. In S. Broder, T. C. Merigan, & D. Bolognesi (Eds.), *Textbook of AIDS Medicine* (pp. 45–53). Baltimore, MD: Williams & Wilkins.

Segi, M., & Kurihara, M. (1962). *Cancer Mortality for Selected Sites in 24 Countries, No. 2 (1958–1959).* Sendai, Japan: Department of Public Health, Tohoku University School of Medicine.

Schwabe, C. W., Rieman, H. P., & Franti, C. E. (1977). *Epidemiology in Veterinary Practice.* Philadelphia: Lea & Febiger.

Wang, S. Q., Ross, R. K., Yu, M. C., et al. (1992). A case–control study of breast cancer in Tianjin, China. *Cancer Epidemiology, Biomarkers, and Prevention*, 1, 435–439.

Weiss, H. B., Friedman, D. I. & Coben, J. H. (1998). Incidence of dog bite injuries treated in emergency departments. *JAMA*, 279, 51–53.

Wynder, E. L., Fujita, Y., Harris, R. E., et al. (1991). Comparative epidemiology of cancer between the United States and Japan. *Cancer*, 67, 746–763.

3

Elements of Infectious and Chronic Disease Epidemiology

This chapter considers two distinct types of epidemiology: infectious disease epidemiology and chronic disease epidemiology. The discipline of epidemiology initially focused on infectious diseases. However, as chronic diseases became more prevalent, epidemiologists turned their attention to these entities as well. The first section of this chapter addresses the infectious disease process. The second section introduces epidemiologic elements more often associated with chronic disease epidemiology.

3.1 THE INFECTIOUS DISEASE PROCESS

Reasons to Study Infectious Disease Epidemiology

Studying infectious disease epidemiology is important for two different reasons. First, infectious disease epidemiology provided the original model for the study of epidemiology. Many of its general principles, therefore, have been adopted by other fields of epidemiology. Second, many infectious diseases—such as HIV, tuberculosis, hantavirus, Lassa fever, Rift Valley fever, Yellow fever, and dengue—have emerged or resurged to imperil the public's health (Centers for Disease Control, 1994). Infectious and parasitic diseases remain the leading cause of morbidity and mortality worldwide (World Health Organization, 1992; National Institute of Allergy and Infectious Disease, 1992). Therefore, studying infectious disease epidemiology in its own right has once again taken on increased relevance.

Components of the Infectious Disease Process

As an introduction to infectious disease epidemiology, we consider the following components of the infectious disease process:

- Agents
- Reservoirs
- Portals of entry and exit

- Transmission
- Host immunity

Agents

Infections are caused by entry and multiplication of microorganisms and parasites in the body of humans and animals. However, "infection" is not synonymous with **infectious disease,** since many infections remain inapparent throughout their course. In addition, the presence of living infectious agents on the exterior of the body or on an article of clothing is not infection, but contamination of a surface.

Infectious agents may be classified according to their size, structure, and physiology. The major categories of infectious disease agents (from structurally largest to smallest) are:

- Helminths (parasitic worms)
- Fungi and yeast (parasitic lower plants that lack chlorophyll)
- Protozoans (minute unicellular organisms often having complex life cycles)
- Bacteria (microscopic unicellular organisms capable of independent reproduction)
- Rickettsia (microscopic intracellular organisms transmitted by *Ixodes* ticks)
- Viruses (submicroscopic infectious agents containing their own genetic material but incapable of multiplication external to a host)
- Prions (poorly understood infectious proteins, without discernible nucleic acids, that cause central nervous system infections)

Examples of important infectious diseases from each of these categories are listed in Table 3.1

TABLE 3.1. Examples of Important Diseases from Each Category of Infectious Agent

Disease	Agent Type	Microbiologic Discipline	Comment
Schistosomiasis	Helminth	Parasitology	Causes hundreds of thousands of deaths in circumscribed areas of Asia, Africa, and South America
Cryptococcosis	Fungus	Mycology	Causes problems in immunocompromised patients
Malaria	Protozoan	Protozoology	Continues to affect millions of people in specific areas of Asia, Africa, and South America
Acute diarrheal and respiratory diseases	Bacteria	Bacteriology	A leading cause of mortality worldwide, especially troublesome among infants and children in countries with undeveloped economies
Typhus fever	Rickettsia	Bacteriology or virology	Louse-borne disease, historically a concomitant of war and famine. Endemic in mountainous regions of Mexico, Central and South America, central Africa, and numerous countries in Asia
Acquired immunodeficiency syndrome (AIDS)	Virus	Virology	AIDS, caused by the human immunodeficiency virus, is becoming an increasingly important cause of mortality in developing nations
Creutzfeldt–Jakob disease	Prion	Virology	Progressive subacute spongiform infection of the central nervous system; related to "mad cow disease"

Reservoirs

The **reservoir** of an agent is the normal habitate in which it lives, multiplies, and grows. Without a reservoir, the agent cannot perpetuate itself in nature.

There are many types of reservoirs. These are:

- Symptomatic cases
- Carriers
    Inapparent carriers
    Incubatory carriers
    Convalescent carriers
- Animals (zoonoses)
    Direct zoonoses
    Cyclozoonoses
    Metazoonoses
    Saprozoonoses
- Inanimate objects
    Water
    Food
    Soil
    Air
    Fomites

Symptomatic Cases **Symptomatic cases** are people with apparent signs of infection. Examples of human diseases in which the primary reservoirs are acute cases include influenza, measles, and smallpox. However, we should not automatically assume that the acutely ill individual always fulfills the role of a reservoir in nature; in many diseases, acute cases might represent biological dead ends in which an essential phase of the agent does not develop or, for some other reason, transmission is disabled. Even when acutely ill individuals are capable of transmitting the agent, they are not necessarily efficient in doing so; acutely ill individuals might be less likely to circulate in the general population of susceptibles and engage in activities necessary for transmission. In fact, it is often the silent carrier that provides the most efficient means of transmission.

Carriers **Carriers** are people who harbor the infectious agent, manifest no discernible signs of infection, yet are potential sources of infection. There are three types of carriers:

- Inapparent carriers
- Incubatory carriers
- Convalescent carriers

Inapparent carriers remain free of the disease throughout the course of infection, yet are still capable of shedding the agent. An example of a disease in which transmission occurs primarily through inapparent carriers is poliomyelitis. For every 100 poliomyelitis infections, only 1 becomes paralyzed, 4 develop nonparalytic disease, and 95 remain disease-free. Nevertheless, all infected individuals may transmit the agent. An additional example of a disease in which inapparent carriers play a crucial role in perpetuating infection is hepatitis A; only 10% of hepatitis A infected children demonstrate jaundice, yet fully half are contagious.

Incubatory carriers transmit the agent prior to the onset of disease. Examples of infectious diseases with large incubatory carrier pools include acquired immunodeficiency syndrome (AIDS) and hepatitis B. During the long incubatory phase of AIDS, HIV carriers are contagious. Hepatitis B carriers are infectious for an average of 3 months before signs appear.

In the case of **convalescent carriers,** infected persons have recovered from the disease in question but still harbor the agent. A well known case of a convalescent carrier was Mary Mallon—the infamous "Typhoid Mary." Typhoid Mary was free of typhoid symptoms yet continued to harbor and shed the typhoid bacilli throughout her life. She is, perhaps, the world's best known chronic convalescent carrier, having infected at least 53 persons, resulting in three known deaths (Gordon, 1986). However, Typhoid Mary was hardly unique. In general, 1 typhoid patient in 20 continues to shed the infectious agent for at least a year after recovery. Some, like Mary, excrete the typhoid bacilli for life. Convalescent carriers who continue to harbor infection for more than a year are called **chronic carriers.** For some bacterial diseases, incomplete treatment with antibiotics increases the likelihood of the convalescent carrier state. This is why it is important to complete the full course of antibiotic therapy, even after symptoms have abated.

Animal Carriers **Zoonoses** are infections naturally transmitted between lower vertebrate animals and humans. A less anthropocentric view of zoonoses suggests that they are infections in which the agent is *shared* between species. Zoonoses constitute a large and diverse group of diseases (over 150 such diseases exist under natural conditions), many of which still cause substantial morbidity and mortality worldwide.

Many zoonotic disease agents have complex life cycles with mandatory intermediate hosts and insect vectors. Accordingly, the following classification scheme for zoonoses has been established:

Direct zoonoses require only a single animal reservoir species to maintain the agent's infectious life cycle. Examples of direct zoonoses are rabies, brucellosis, and trichinosis.

Cyclozoonoses require at least two vertebrate species to complete their infection cycle. Examples of cyclozoonoses are infections with tapeworms and hydatid cysts (larval stages of the *Echinococcus* tapeworm).

Metazoonoses are transmitted to vertebrate hosts by invertebrates, requiring invertebrate vectors or intermediate hosts. Examples of important metazoonoses are schistosomiasis, Lyme disease, arthropod-borne viral diseases (e.g., Yellow fever), and plague. Schistosomiasis has a snail intermediate host, Lyme disease is transmitted by an *Ixodes* tick, arthropod-borne viral diseases are transmitted by mosquitoes, and plague is transmitted by a flea.

Saprozoonses are zoonoses that require inanimate reservoirs in addition to their animal reservoirs. An example of a saprozoonosis is coccidioidomycosis (Valley fever), which is caused by a fungus that grows in the soil as a saprophytic mold. It infects humans, cattle, cats, dogs, horses, sheep, wild desert rodents, and other animal species.

Inanimate Objects Some infectious agents are free-living in the environment, growing in inanimate objects such as water, food, soil, air, and other inert substances. Examples of infectious agents with inanimate reservoirs are legionellosis (in which the gram-negative bacillus grows and multiplies in pools of water such as those produced by cooling towers and evaporative condensers), histoplasmosis (a fungal disease with a soil reservoir), and staphylococcal food poisoning (in which the agent multiplies in food, producing toxins capable of causing gastroenteritis).

Portals of Entry and Exit

For an infectious agent to propagate itself in nature, it must leave one host and enter another. Exit and entry sites for pathogens are called **portals.** There are six portals in the body:

- Respiratory tract (upper and lower)
- Conjunctiva (mucous membranes surrounding the eye)
- Urogenital tract (urinary tract, sexual genitalia and organs)
- Gastrointestinal tract (upper and lower)
- Skin (both intact and broken skin)
- Placenta (vertical transmission to offspring)

Blocking an agent's portal can effectively prevent its transmission. Thus, condoms are recommended for the prevention of sexually transmitted diseases and rubber gloves are recommended for the prevention of **nosocomial** (hospital-borne) infections. Inadvertent transdermal transmission of HIV and hepatitis B can be prevented by exercising sufficient care in the disposal of needles and other sharp clinical and surgical instruments.

In general, agents exhibit preferred portals of entry and exit. For example, tuberculosis bacilli and influenza viruses enter and exit through the respiratory tract, schistosomiasis enters through the skin of humans and exits through the urine or feces (depending on species), and gonorrhea is generally transmitted though the urogenital tract. However, there are some agents that use multiple routes of entry and exit. For example, HIV may enter and exit through the urogenital tract (vagina or penis), gastrointestinal tract (rectal mucosa), skin, and placenta (mother to child).

Transmission

Mode of Transmission **Transmission** refers to any mechanism by which an infectious agent is spread to another host. In order for an agent to pass from one host to another, the gap between portals must be bridged. Transmission of infection can be accomplished by means of direct and indirect **contact,** by **vectors** (animate objects), and by **vehicles** (inanimate objects). A classification scheme for the modes of transmission is as follows:

- Contact
    Direct (requiring physical contact between hosts)
    Indirect (contact with relatively fresh bodily fluids or tissue)

Droplets (large infectious particles sprayed from a respiratory portal of an infected host to a susceptible host propelled over a short distance by sneezing or coughing)

Droplet nuclei (small aerosolized particles suspended in air and capable of traveling considerable distances)

· Vectors (animate intermediaries)

Mechanical transmission (no multiplication of the agent in the vector)

Developmental transmission (the infectious organism undergoes a necessary period of development or maturation in the vector)

Propagative transmission (the organism undergoes multiplication in the vector)

Cyclopropagative transmission (the organism multiplies and undergoes development in the vector)

· Vehicles (inanimate intermediates)

Mechanical transmission

Developmental transmission

Propagative transmission

Cyclopropagative transmission

Examples of diseases transmitted by contact are sexually transmitted diseases, mononucleosis, surgical wound infections, and most respiratory diseases. Examples of vector-borne transmission are malaria (mosquito-borne), Lyme disease (tick-borne), and plague (flea-borne). Examples of diseases transmitted by vehicles are foodborne diseases (e.g., salmonellosis) are waterborne diseases (e.g., cryptosporidiosis).

Dynamics of Transmission   Diseases can be transmitted by means of a common vehicle or by serial transfer. **Common vehicle spread** refers to transmission of an agent through a common source. Examples of common vehicles that may serve this purpose are air, water, food, and drugs. Examples of common vehicle transmission are foodborne disease outbreaks spread by the ingestion of a single contaminated food source or beverage, respiratory disease outbreaks spread by common vehicle transmission through inhalation of air from a contaminated environment (e.g., legionellosis disease), and needle sharing serving as a common vehicle for bloodborne pathogens.

Serial transfer refers to transmission from human to human, human to animal to human, and human to environment to human in sequence. Examples of serially transmitted diseases are measles (spread by the respiratory route from infected to susceptible individuals), sexually transmitted diseases, and any of the diseases requiring person-to-contact (e.g., AIDS).

Infectious Cycle in Nature   Many infectious agents have complex **biological cycles,** requiring specific transfers between hosts of different species and within the body of a given host. For example, schistosomiasis (the human blood worm) is acquired from water contaminated with larval forms. The eggs of the worm leave the mammalian host either with the urine or feces (depending on species). Eggs hatch in water, liberating a larval form (miracidium) that enters a suitable freshwater snail host. A different larval phase (cercariae) emerges from the snail and penetrates the human skin while the human host is immersed in a contaminated water source. The cercariae enter the bloodstream, are carried to the lungs, and migrate to the liver, where they develop to maturity. The mature worm migrates to the mesenteric and pelvic veins where eggs are deposited and eventually escape to the lumen of the bladder *(Schistosoma haematobium)* or bowel (other *Schistosoma* species). The complex life cycle of *Schistosoma* species is illustrated in Figure 3.1.

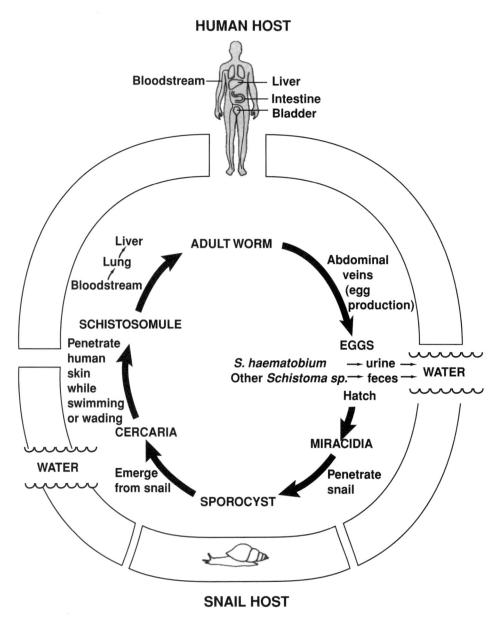

Figure 3.1 *Life cycle of* Schistosoma *species (inner circle) and location of the parasite in the host and environment (outer circle).*

Understanding the **natural history of the infectious agent within the host** may also be useful in minimizing the risk of transmission. For example, the infectivity of HIV is determined by its stage of development within the infected host. The natural history of HIV infection is summarized in Figure 3.2. During the acute phase of infection, hosts demonstrate high virus titers and associated high levels of infectiousness, even though an antibody response is lacking (Jacquez et al., 1994; Koopman, 1996; Piatak et al., 1993; Royce et al., 1997). This is followed by a period of low viral titers and, hence, low infectivity. During the latter stages of HIV infection—indicated by symptoms of disease—the host is highly infectious as a result of high viral titers (de Vincenzi, 1994; Lazzarin et al., 1991; Lee et al., 1996; Royce et al., 1997).

Host Immunity

Types of Immunity **Immunity** refers to all factors that alter the likelihood of infection and disease in the host once the agent is encountered. There are two categories of immunity: innate immunity and acquired immunity. **Innate immunity** refers to physical, chemical, cellular, and other physiologic barriers to disease and infection. **Acquired immunity** refers to resistance developed by a host as a result of previous exposure to a natural or artificial pathogen or foreign substance.

Innate Immunity Innate immunity includes those barriers that prevent invading pathogens from entering the body and thus establishing themselves within the host. It also includes nonspecific chemical, cellular, and inflammatory bodily reactions that are present from birth.

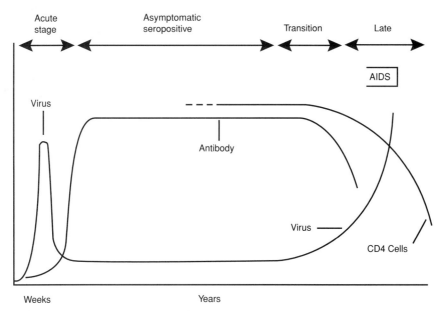

Figure 3.2. *The course of HIV infection. (Source: Institute of Medicine, 1988, reprinted with permission from* Confronting AIDS: Update 1988. *Copyright 1988 by the National Academy of Sciences. Courtesy of the National Academy Press, Washington, D.C.)*

Examples of innate **physical barriers** to infection are:

· Intact skin
· Mucosa linings of organs and body cavities
· Mucus sheaths on mucosal surfaces
· Cilia in the respiratory tract
· Cough and gag reflex

Examples of innate **chemical barriers** to infection are:

· Acidity of the stomach and vagina
· Hydrolytic and proteolytic enzymes in saliva and of the intestines
· Miscellaneous biologically active substances, such as enzymes, lipids, and other molecules (e.g., interferons), that create a hostile environment for invading pathogens

Examples of innate **cellular and physiologic barriers** to infection are:

· Macrophages (large, motile, phagocytic cells found in tissue)
· Polymorphonuclear cells (neutrophils and other white blood cells with deeply lobed nuclei capable of chemotaxis, adherence to immune complexes, and phagocytosis)
· Reticular endothelial cells (circulating monocytes and stationary phagocytic cells distributed widely throughout the body)
· Natural killer cells (cells that release extracellular lytic enzymes)
· Inflammation (the body's nonspecific response to injury, including the biologic injury due to infecting pathogens)
· Fever

Innate immunity forms the first line of defense before acquired immunity gets a chance to respond to specific pathogens. These factors are genetically determined but can be modified by host attributes such as age, hormonal status, nutritional status, and physiologic states such as pregnancy and emotional distress.

Acquired Immunity   **Acquired immunity** is the result of a highly specific and evolved response on the part of the host that begins when the host is exposed to a foreign pathogen or substance. Acquired immunity comprises cellular (**immunocytes**) and fluid (**humoral**) components. There are two types of immunocytes:

· Lymphocytes (mononuclear white blood cells found in the lymph, blood, and lymphoid tissue)
· Bone marrow stem cells (progenitors of other immunocytes)

There are two kinds of lymphocytes: B-lymphocytes and T-lymphocytes. **B-lymphocytes** (so named because they originate in the bone marrow) synthesize **antibodies** (biochemical proteins that attach themselves to the surface of invading agents), which are secreted into the bloodstream. **T-lymphocytes** (so named because they mature in the thymus) help

B-cells in producing antibodies, neutralize invaders, and regulate other aspects of the immune response through substances called lymphokines. The two forms of immunity—innate and acquired—work closely together to mount the total immunologic response of the host (Fig. 3.3).

Immunization **Immunization** is the act of acquiring immunity through contact with a foreign substance or agent. There are three types of immunization: active immunization, passive immunization, and adoptive immunization.

Active immunization is a product of the host derived as a result of natural or artificial exposure to **antigens** (foreign proteins associated with the agent or by-products of the agent). **Vaccines** represent artificial exposures that elicit an immune response. Vaccines come in several general forms: **killed vaccines** represent agent proteins incapable of replicating themselves; **modified live vaccines** comprise nonvirulent strains of the agent modified to be nonpathogenic but still capable of stimulating the immune response; **toxoids** are harmless derivatives of microbiologic toxins that stimulate production of antibodies and immunocytes to counter the negative effects of a toxin released by a pathogen or other poisonous source.

Passive immunization is derived from maternal and therapeutic sources. **Maternally derived passive immunity** is acquired through the placenta and colostrum (first milk). **Therapeutic derived immunity** is acquired through the use of immune serums, cytokines, and antitoxins.

Adoptive immunization involves the transfer of immunocytes from one individual to another. It represents a new technology that holds promise for the future but has few current applications.

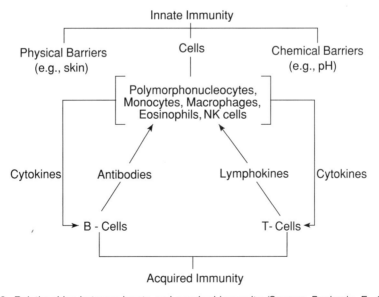

Figure 3.3. *Relationships between innate and acquired immunity. (Source: Benjamin, E., Sunshine, G., & Leskowitz, S. (1996). Immunology. A Short Course (3rd ed.). New York: Wiley-Liss, p. 38; reprinted by permission of Wiley-Liss, Inc., a subsidiary of John Wiley & Sons, Inc.)*

3.2 INTRODUCTION TO CHRONIC DISEASE EPIDEMIOLOGY

Chronic diseases are diseases of long duration that seldom entirely resolve sponta-neously. Because they often result in a loss of function, impairment, and long-term dis-ability, chronic diseases are also called **degenerative diseases.** In public health practice, the term **chronic disease epidemiology** generally excludes diseases that are thought to be contagious (e.g., AIDS) or within the domain of agencies outside the health department (e.g., mental disorders). Examples of important chronic diseases studied by epidemiolo-gists include:

- Cardiovascular disease
- Cancer
- Chronic lung disease
- Diabetes and other metabolic diseases
- Liver disease
- Musculoskeletal disease
- Neurological disorders

In fact, many of the above disease categories represent large and diverse groups of dis-eases with different etiologies and manifestations. In addition to the problem of uncertain etiology, many chronic diseases are characterized by insidious onset, occurring only after prolonged exposure to the etiologic factor. This makes it all the more important to under-stand the natural history and range of clinical expression of these diseases. Despite these difficulties, epidemiologists have identified modifiable risk factors that may be manipu-lated to control the occurrence or severity of many of the chronic diseases (Table 3.2). Note, however, that many of the known risk factors for chronic diseases are not amenable to modification or manipulation (e.g., genetic factors). Nonetheless, the goals of chronic disease epidemiology remain the same: to uncover modifiable risk factors and develop in-terventions that reduce the incidence and severity of these diseases.

The epidemiologic approach that seems to have met with the most success in these en-deavors is the biostatistical approach. **Statistics** is the discipline concerned with the treat-ment of numerical data derived from groups of individuals. **Biostatistics** is the applica-tion of statistical methods to biological data. Many of the advanced biostatistical methods of studying chronic disease were motivated by the lack of success met by other ap-proaches in identifying the causes and predictors of increasingly prevalent chronic dis-eases. Biostatistical epidemiologic research includes methods for:

- Describing the frequency of conditions in the population
- Designing and conducting studies to identify and quantify the relative importance of various risk factors
- Evaluating the accuracy of descriptive and analytic studies
- Determining whether the apparent associations between various factors and diseases are causal or artifactual
- Communicating findings of risk to scientific and lay communities
- Assessing whether attempts at prevention and control are effective and, if so, how much morbidity and mortality can be prevented

TABLE 3.2. Chronic Diseases and Their Relationship to Selected, Modifiable Risk Factors, United States

	Cardiovascular Disease	Cancer	Chronic Lung Disease	Diabetes	Cirrhosis	Musculoskeletal Diseases	Neurologic Disorders
Tobacco use	+	+	+			+	?
Alcohol use	?	+			+	+	+
High cholesterol	+						
High blood pressure	+						
Diet	+	+	?	?		+	?
Physical inactivity	+	+		+		+	
Obesity	+	+		+		+	+
Stress	?	?					
Environmental tobacco smoke	?	+	+				
Occupation		+	+		?	+	
Pollution		+	+				+
Low socioeconomic status	+	+	+	+	+	+	

Source: Brownson et al. (1993), p. 4; reproduced with permission of the American Public Health Association.

+ = Established risk factor.

? = Possible risk factor.

In its practice and application, biostatistical epidemiology is fundamentally an investigative or research-based discipline. An awareness of the different study designs at the epidemiologist's disposal, plus the strengths and limitations of each investigation, is a prerequisite for understanding the nature of this discipline. It is to this end that many biostatistical methods are presented and illustrated throughout the remainder of this book.

SUMMARY

1. This chapter considers two distinct forms of epidemiology: infectious disease epidemiology and chronic disease epidemiology. Many epidemiological principles evolved from the study of infectious diseases. However, as chronic disease became more important in modern society, biostatistical approaches were needed to deal with increasingly complex patterns of disease occurrence.

2. Infectious disease epidemiology searches to understand the infectious process in terms of agents, reservoirs of infection, portals of entry and exit of the agent, modes and dynamics of transmission, and host immunity. The classes of infectious disease agents are helminths, fungi and yeasts, protozoans, bacteria, rickettsia, viruses, and prions. The four types of reservoirs in nature are infectious cases, carriers, animals, and inanimate objects. Portals are the entry and exit sites for the pathogen. Transmission of infectious agents may occur through contact, vectors, and vehicles. Immunity refers to all factors that influence the likelihood of disease once a pathogen is encountered. Immunity comes in two basic forms: innate immunity and acquired immunity. Innate immunity is present from birth and is composed of physical, chemical, and cellular barriers to infection. Acquired immunity requires a response on the part of the host and is achieved as a result of natural or artificial exposure to antigens.

3. Chronic diseases are diseases of long duration in which complete cures are rare. The epidemiologic approach that seems to have met with the most success in addressing these diseases relies on biostatistical methods to describe disease occurrence patterns and identify modifiable risk factors.

EXERCISES

1. Which of the following items *cannot* serve as a portal of entry or exit?

(**A**) cardiovascular system

(**B**) skin

(**C**) respiratory tract

(**D**) genitourinary tract

2. Which of the following is *not* an innate factor of immunity?

(**A**) gastric acid

(**B**) cilia in the respiratory tract

(**C**) antibodies

(**D**) mucous membranes

3. Toxoids confer:

    (A) innate immunity

    (B) natural immunity

    (C) active immunity

    (D) passive immunity

4. Passage of maternal antibodies from mother to child through the placenta confers which kind of immunity?

    (A) innate immunity

    (B) natural immunity

    (C) active immunization

    (D) passive immunization

5. Which of the following can act as a reservoir?

    (A) inanimate objects

    (B) animals

    (C) carriers

    (D) acute cases

    (E) only A and C

    (F) only A and B

    (G) A, B, and C

    (H) A, B, C, and D

6. Which type of carrier may result from incomplete treatment with antibiotics?

    (A) incubatory carrier

    (B) inapparent carrier

    (C) convalescent carrier

7. Name the type of carrier that remains free of disease throughout the course of infection.

    (A) chronic carrier

    (B) inapparent carrier

    (C) incubatory carrier

    (D) convalescent carrier

8. The transmission of the malaria protozoan through the bite of a mosquito is an example of which mode of transmission?

    (A) vehicle borne

    (B) direct contact

    (C) airborne

    (D) vector borne

9. A zoonotic disease requiring only a single animal reservoir and no inanimate reservoir to maintain its life cycle is best classified as a:

    (A) direct zoonosis

    (B) cyclozoonosis

(C) metazoonosis

(D) saprozoonosis

ANSWERS TO EXERCISES

1. A   A portal is an entry or exit site for the agent. Agents cannot enter directly through the cardiovascular system.

2. C   Antibodies are not innate. They are acquired as a result of exposure to a specific antigen.

3. C   Toxoids invoke active responses to specific toxic antigens.

4. D   Maternal transfers are a form of passive immunization.

5. H   All of the items listed may serve as reservoirs.

6. C   Incomplete treatment with antibiotics causes the increased likelihood of the convalescent carrier state.

7. B   Inapparent carriers remain disease-free throughout infection. Incubatory carriers are yet to demonstrate signs of disease. Chronic and convalescent carriers have recovered from the disease in question.

8. D   Animate transmitters of infectious agents are called vectors.

9. A   By definition, direct zoonoses have a single animal reservoir. Cyclozoonoses require two vertebrates species to complete their life cycle; metazoonoses require an invertebrate host or vector in addition to the vertebrate reservoir; and saprozoonoses require an inanimate reservoir in addition to their animal reservoirs.

REFERENCES

Benjamini, E., Sunshine, G., & Leskowitz, S. (1996). *Immunology. A Short Course* (3rd ed.). New York: Wiley-Liss.

Brownson, R. C., Remington, P. L., & Davis, J. R. (Eds.). (1993). *Chronic Disease Epidemiology and Control*. Washington, DC: American Public Health Association

Centers for Disease Control and Prevention. (1994). *Addressing Emerging Infectious Disease Threats: A Prevention Strategy for the United States*. Atlanta: U.S. Department of Health and Human Services, Public Health Service.

de Vincenzi, I. (1994). A longitudinal study of human immunodeficiency virus transmission by heterosexual partners. *New England Journal of Medicine*, 331, 341–346.

Gordon, R. (1986). *Great Medical Disasters*. New York: Dorset Press, Chap. 16.

Institute of Medicine, National Academy of Sciences. (1988). *Confronting AIDS: Update 1988*. Washington, DC: National Academy Press.

Jacquez, J. A., Koopman, S. J., Simon, C. P., & Longini, I. M. Jr. (1994). Role of primary infection in epidemics of HIV infection in gay cohorts. *Journal of Acquired Immune Deficiency Syndrome and Human Retrovirology*, 7, 1169–1184.

Koopman, J. (1996). Emerging objectives and methods in epidemiology. *American Journal of Public Health*, 86, 630–632.

Lazzarin, A., Saracco, A., Musicco, M., & Nicolosi, A. (1991). Man-to-woman sexual transmission of the human immunodeficiency virus: risk factors related to sexual behavior, man's infectiousness, and woman's susceptibility. *Archives of Internal Medicine*, 151, 2411–2416.

Lee, T. H., Sakahara, N., Fiebig, E., Busch, M. P., O'Brien, T. R., & Herman, S. E. (1996). Correlation of HIV-1 RNA levels in plasma and heterosexual transmission of HIV-1 from infected transfusion recipients. *Journal of Acquired Immune Deficiency Syndrome and Human Retrovirology*, 12, 427–428.

National Institute of Allergy and Infectious Disease. (1992). *Report of the Task Force on Microbiology and Infectious Disease*. Bethesda: U.S. Department of Health and Human Services, Public Health Service, National Institutes of Health, NIH Publication 92-3320.

Piatak, M. Jr., Saag, M. S., Yang, L. C., et al. (1993). High levels of HIV-1 in plasma during all stages of infection determined by competitive PCR. *Science*, 259, 1749–1754.

Royce, R. A., Sena, A., Cates, W., & Cohen, M. S. (1997). Sexual transmission of HIV. *New England Journal of Medicine*, 336, 1072–1078.

World Health Organization. (1992). *Global Health Situations and Projections, Estimates 1992*. Geneva: WHO.

4

Identification of Disease, Part I (Reproducibility and Validity)

Accurate discrimination of people with and without disease is essential in all aspects of epidemiologic work. This chapter considers the accuracy of a diagnostic instrument and its implications for population-based screening.

4.1 INTRODUCTION

Data Collection

The accuracy of a reported condition is a function of the method used to collect information. Data can be collected by personal interview, questioning of a surrogate, through a written questionnaire, scrutinizing preexisting records, or direct examination. Generally, direct examination is more likely to give accurate results than direct or indirect questioning (Table 4.1).

Symptoms, Signs, and Tests

Identification of disease by examination is based on symptoms, signs, and diagnostic test results. **Symptoms** are subjective sensations, perceptions, and observations made by the patient. Examples of symptoms are pain, nausea, fatigue, and dizziness. **Signs** are perceptions and observations made by an examiner. Observations may be based on the clinician's senses (sight, hearing, smell, taste, feel), imaging techniques (e.g., X-ray), and microbiologic techniques. Although signs tend to be more objective than symptoms, they are still influenced by the skill and judgment of the examiner. **Diagnostic tests** are quantifiable measures of physiologic, immunologic, and biochemical processes. Tests can range from the mundane (e.g., body temperature) to arcane (e.g., clinical chemistry values). Although medical tests tend to be objective, they too have their sources of error.

TABLE 4.1. Comparison of Prevalence Estimates of Selected Chronic Conditions as Determined by Household Interviews and Clinical Evaluations, All Ages Combined

	Prevalence per 1000	
Condition	Household Interview	Clinical Evaluation
All heart disease[a]	25	96
Hypertension and hypertensive heart disease	36	117
All arthritis[b]	47	75
All neoplasms	8	55

Source: Adapted from Lilienfeld & Lilienfeld (1980), p. 150; original data from Commission on Chronic Illness (1957).

[a]For interview data, includes rheumatic fever.

[b]For interview data includes rheumatism.

Reproducibility and Validity

The accuracy of an examination is affected by two factors:

- The **reproducibility** of an observation made by the same examiner or separate examiners
- The **validity** of an observation, or its ability to discriminate between people with and without disease

We consider these factors separately.

4.2 REPRODUCIBILITY

Reproducibility Defined

Reproducibility refers to the repeatability, consistency, or stability of a measure or test from one use to the next. A perfectly reproducible method of disease ascertainment would produce the same results every time it was used in the same patient. A test that fails to reproduce consistent results is inherently unreliable.

For example, if you had your blood pressure taken and it read in the hypertensive range, you had it taken again and it read in the nonhypertensive range, you repeated the process and it read in the hypertensive range, then the blood pressure measurement would not be very reproducible. If, however, in a series of blood pressure measurements you consistently got the same diagnosis (say, "hypertension"), your diagnosis would be reproducible—even if it were not accurate and you were really normotensive.

Agreement Statistics

A classic 1966 study of epidemiologic nonreproducibility by Lilienfeld and Kordan found a significant number of discrepancies in the interpretation of chest X-rays read by two radiologists. Using six diagnostic categories, diagnostic agreement was a modest 65.1% (Table 4.2). When the diagnostic classification scheme was simplified to form only two

TABLE 4.2. Comparison of Two Different Radiologists' Interpretations of Chest X-Ray Films: Highlighted Numbers Represent Areas of Diagnostic Agreement

Radiologist A	Radiologist B						
	SN	OSPA	CV	NSA	NEG	TU	Total
SN	61	16	1	9	8	0	95
OSPA	70	1,320	63	861	367	33	2,714
CV	19	151	1,322	369	1,880	62	3,803
NSA	25	407	43	1,716	1,656	40	3,887
NEG	28	157	91	680	8,475	50	9,481
TU	0	2	0	4	47	0	53
Total	203	2,053	1,520	3,639	12,433	185	20,033

Source: Lilienfeld & Kordan (1966), p. 2147; reproduced with permission of the American Association for Cancer Research.

Abbreviations: SN = suspect neoplasm; OSPA = other significant pulmonary abnormality; CV = cardiovascular abnormality; NSA = nonsignificant abnormality; NEG = negative; TU = technically unsatisfactory X-ray film.

$$\text{Overall agreement} = \frac{\text{total no. of agreements}}{\text{total no. of satisfactory films}} = \frac{61 + 1320 + 1322 + 1716 + 8475}{20,333 - (185 + 53)} = .651$$

diagnostic categories—significant pulmonary lesion, yes or no—diagnostic agreement improved to 89.4% (Table 4.3). This value is all the less impressive when one considers that among the 3558 X-rays labeled as positive by at least one of the radiologists, agreement was present in only 1467 (41.2%)—and this does not account for agreement due to chance.

TABLE 4.3. Comparison of Two Different Radiologists' Interpretations of Chest X-Ray Films. Diagnostic Categories Have Been Combined to Indicate Either Presence or Absence of a Significant Pulmonary Abnormality

Radiologist A	Radiologist B		Total satisfactory films
	+	−	
+	1,467	1,309	2,776
−	782	16,232	17,014
Total satisfactory films	2,249	17,541	19,790

Source: Lilienfeld & Kordan (1966), p. 2147.

+ = Suspected neoplasm or other significant pulmonary abnormality.

− = Cardiovascular abnormality, nonsignificant abnormality, negative.

X-ray films that were related technically unsatisfactory by either reviewer are eliminated from this analysis.

$$\text{Overall agreement} = \frac{1467 + 16232}{19790} = .894$$

Agreement in subjects labeled positive by at least one radiologist

$$= \frac{\text{total no. of agreements}}{\text{total no. X-rays with at least positive diagnosis}}$$

$$= \frac{1467}{1467 + 1309 + 782} = .412$$

TABLE 4.4. Types of Disease-Causing Agents

Range of Values for Kappa	Interpretation
.>75	Excellent agreement
.40 to .75	Fair to good agreement
<.40	Poor agreement

Kappa Statistic

The **kappa statistic** (κ) was developed as a measure of the percent agreement between two raters that occurs beyond chance. If there is complete agreement between raters, $\kappa = +1$. If the observed agreement is greater than or equal to that expected due to chance, $\kappa \geq 0$. If agreement is less than or equal to chance agreement, $\kappa \leq 0$. Rules of thumb for characterizing different values of kappa are shown in Table 4.4.

To calculate kappa for data in which there are only two diagnostic categories (condition present or absent), data are converted to proportions and laid out in a two-by-two table, with notation shown in Table 4.5. *Note that entries in this table represent proportions of subjects, not counts.* Using this notation, the kappa statistic is

$$\kappa = \frac{2(ad - bc)}{p_1 q_2 + p_2 q_1} \tag{4.1}$$

where a represents the proportion of subjects in which both raters offer a positive diagnosis, b represents the proportion of subjects in which rater A offers a positive diagnosis and rater B offers a negative diagnosis, c represents the proportion of subjects in which rater B offers a positive diagnosis and rater A offers a negative diagnosis, d represents the proportion of subjects in which both raters offer negative diagnosis, p_1 represents the proportion of rater A's diagnoses that are positive, q_1 represents the proportion of rater A's diagnoses that are negative, p_2 represents the proportion of rater B's diagnoses that are positive, and q_2 represents the proportion of rater B's diagnoses that are negative (Fleiss, 1981, p. 217).

The X-ray interpretation data presented in Table 4.3 are displayed in Table 4.6. The kappa statistic for these data is

$$\kappa = \frac{2[(.0741)(.8202) - (.0661)(.0395)]}{(.1403)(.8864) + (.1136)(.8597)} = .5240$$

This indicates fair to good agreement between the radiologists' diagnoses.

TABLE 4.5. Notation for Measuring Agreement for a Single Diagnostic Category: Entries in the Table Represent Proportions, not Counts

Rater A	Rater B +	−	
+	a	b	p_1
−	c	d	q_1
	p_2	q_2	1

TABLE 4.6. Agreement of X-Ray Diagnoses: Data from Table 4.3 Displayed in the Format Required to Calculate the Kappa Statistic. Data Represent Proportions

		Rater B		
Rater A	+	−		
+	.0741	.0661	.1403	
−	.0395	.8202	.8597	
	.1136	.8864	1	

Even Objective Measures Can Vary

Even objective, quantifiable tests may exhibit nonreproducibility of results. To evaluate the accuracy of blood glucose determinations in Swedish clinical laboratories, Björkhem et al. (1981) sent a pooled blood specimen to 64 different hospital and clinical laboratories. Routine clinical chemistry values derived by each lab were compared to the true value determined by a definitive technique with no known sources of error (isotope dilution–mass spectrometry). The glucose determinations at the 64 labs exhibited a mean result of 5.72 mmol/L with a range of 4.46–6.78 mmol/L. The definitive value (the true biologic value) determined by the state-of-the-art isotope dilution–mass spectrometry method was 5.79 mmol/L. Ahlbom and Norell (1990) selected data from 10 of these labs in which each lab performed 16 analyses on the same sample. Data are displayed in Figure 4.1. This figure shows results to vary considerably, both within labs and between labs. Moreover, individual values frequently differ from the actual biological value (indicated by the dashed line).

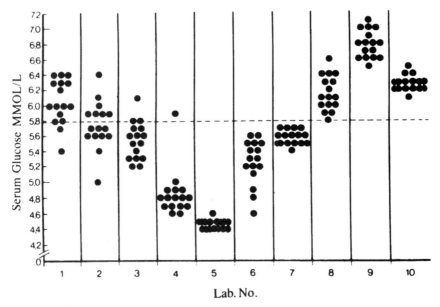

Figure 4.1. Blood glucose determinations of a pooled sample of blood according to 10 clinical laboratories in Sweden. The horizontal dashed line represents the actual glucose level of the samples as determined by isotope dilution–mass spectrometry. (Data source: Björkhem et al., 1981; Graphic source: Ahlbom & Norell, 1990, p. 17; reproduced with permission of Epidemiology by Resources, Inc., Newton, Massachusetts.)

If the accuracy of routine data collection methods are suspect, we might ask why the definitive method is not used in every instance. Herein lies the problem: limitations on time and money inevitably lead to suboptimal data collection practices, especially in investigations that study large groups of people. Nonetheless, the investigator must (a) take all practical steps to increase the reproducibility and validity of results by standardizing the conditions under which data are collected and (b) take all necessary steps to understand deviations from the true biological state of affairs, whenever possible.

4.3 VALIDITY

Diagnostic Discrimination

Validity is a term used to describe a measurement instrument or test that measures what it is supposed to measure. A perfect method of disease ascertainment would correctly discriminate between people with and without disease without fail. In other words, a perfect test would be perfectly valid. A test that fails to produce the correct results is inherently inaccurate or biased.

We will discuss four measures of diagnostic test validity: sensitivity, specificity, predictive value positive, and predictive value negative. To calculate these measures, we must first classify test results into one of the following four possible categories:

- **True positives** (*TP*) have the disease in question and show positive test results.
- **True negatives** (*TN*) do not have the disease in question and show negative test results.
- **False positives** (*FP*) do not have the disease in question but show positive test results.
- **False negatives** (*FN*) have the disease but show negative test results.

This, of course, assumes that a "gold standard" means of identifying individuals who definitely have and do not have these disease is available by which to make these comparisons. After test results are classified into one of the above four categories, the frequency of test results is cross-tabulated to form a table similar to the one shown in Table 4.7.

Sensitivity and Specificity

Sensitivity (*SEN*) is the probability that a test result will be positive when the test is administered to people who actually have the disease or condition in question. Using conditional probability notation, we define sensitivity as

$$SEN = Pr(T+|D+)$$

TABLE 4.7. Notation for Calculating Sensitivity, Specificity, Predictive Value Positive, and Predictive Value Negative

	Disease +	Disease −	Total
Test +	TP	FP	TP + FP
Test −	FN	TN	FN + TN
	TP + FN	FP + TN	n

where *Pr* denotes "probability," *T+* denotes "test positive," *D+* denotes "disease positive," and the vertical line (|) denotes "conditional upon" or "given." Thereby, $Pr(T+|D+)$ is read as "the probability of being test positive conditional upon being disease positive."

Sensitivity is calculated by administering the test to a random sample of subjects who have the disease in question. The number of diseased people who test positive is divided by the total number of diseased people tested:

$$SEN = \frac{TP}{\text{all those with the disease}} = \frac{TP}{TP + FN} \tag{4.2}$$

Specificity (*SPEC*) is the probability that a test will be negative when administered to people who are free of the disease or condition in question. In other words, specificity is the probability of being test negative conditional upon being disease negative:

$$SPEC = Pr(T-|D-)$$

Specificity is calculated by administering the test to a random sample of disease-free subjects. The number of people testing negative is divided by the total number of disease-free people tested:

$$SPEC = \frac{TN}{\text{all those without the disease}} = \frac{TN}{TN + FP} \tag{4.3}$$

Illustration   To illustrate sensitivity and specificity, let us consider a hypothetical survey of teen smoking. Initially, we plan on using a questionnaire as a screening instrument to help determine whether subjects smoke. We are concerned, however, that many teen smokers may feel compelled to falsely answer in the negative. To quantify the accuracy of the questionnaire, we compare its results to a more reliable method of ascertainment based on testing for cotinine in the saliva of study subjects. (Cotinine, a major detoxication product of nicotine, is a reliable indicator of recent smoking.) Thus, the questionnaire serves as a rapid and inexpensive screening instrument and the salivary cotinine test serves as the definitive ("gold standard") method with which to compare the questionnaire's results. Let us assume that the questionnaire is positive in 65 of the 100 confirmed smokers who test positive on the salivary cotinine test (Table 4.8, left column). The sensitivity of the questionnaire is therefore .650. The questionnaire is negative in 99 of the 100 nonsmokers who test negative on the cotinine test (Table 4.8, right column). By that, the specificity of the questionnaire is .990.

Predictive Value Positive and Predictive Value Negative

Although sensitivity and specificity quantify a test's accuracy in the presence of known disease status, they are unable to predict the performance of the test in the population. To accomplish this objective, the alternative indices of predictive value positive and predictive value negative are needed.

The **predictive value positive (*PVP*)** of a test is the probability that a person with a positive test will actually have the disease in question. In other words, the predictive value positive is the probability of being disease positive conditional upon being test positive:

$$PVP = Pr(D+|T+)$$

TABLE 4.8. Results of a Smoking Survey Questionnaire and Definitive Salivary Cotinine Test: Hypothetical Illustration Data

		Salivary Cotinine Test ("Gold Standard")		
		+	−	Total
Response to Questionnaire	+	65	1	66
(Screening Instrument)	−	35	99	134
		100	100	200

$$SEN = \frac{TP}{TP + FN} = \frac{65}{65 + 35} = .650$$

$$SPEC = \frac{TN}{TN + FP} = \frac{99}{99 + 1} = .990$$

$$PVP = \frac{TP}{TP + FP} = \frac{65}{65 + 1} = .985$$

$$PVN = \frac{TN}{TN + FN} = \frac{99}{99 + 35} = .739$$

$$P = \frac{TP + FN}{n} = \frac{65 + 35}{200} = .500$$

$$P^* = \frac{TP + FP}{n} = \frac{65 + 1}{200} = .330$$

This statistic is calculated by dividing the number of true positives by all those people who test positive:

$$PVP = \frac{TP}{\text{all those who test positive}} = \frac{TP}{TP + FP} \tag{4.4}$$

The **predictive value negative (PVN)** is the probability that a person who shows a negative test will be disease negative—the probability of disease negative "given" test negativity:

$$PVN = Pr(D-|T-)$$

The predictive value negative is calculated by dividing the number of true negatives by all those people who test negative:

$$PVN = \frac{TN}{\text{all those who test negative}} = \frac{TN}{TN + FN} \tag{4.5}$$

The distinction between sensitivity/specificity and predictive value positive/predictive value negative may at first appear confusing. This becomes less confusing if one remembers that sensitivity and specificity quantify a test's accuracy given the known disease status of study subjects, whereas predictive values quantify a test's accuracy given only the test results.

Illustration   Let us return to our smoking questionnaire illustration. In this analysis, we have 65 true positives and 1 false positive (Table 4.8, top row). The predictive value positive is therefore .985. This means that the probability that a positive responder is actually a smoker is almost 99%. The questionnaire identified 35 false negatives and 99 true negatives (Table 4.8, bottom row). Since 99 of the 134 people who responded to the questionnaire in the negative are actual nonsmokers, the predictive value negative of the questionnaire is .739. This means that the probability that a negative responder is a nonsmoker is a little less than 74%.

4.4   RELATIONSHIP BETWEEN PREVALENCE OF DISEASE AND PREDICTIVE VALUE OF A TEST

True Prevalence and Apparent Prevalence

The prevalence of disease can be calculated on the basis of the true number of people with the disease in the population or the apparent number of people with the disease based on screening test results. The **true prevalence** of the disease (P) represents the proportion of people who actually have the disease or condition:

$$P = \frac{\text{all those with the disease}}{\text{all those tested}} = \frac{TP + FN}{n} \tag{4.6}$$

where TP represents the number of true positives, FN represents the number of false negatives, and n represents all those tested.

The **apparent prevalence** of a disease ($P*$) represents the proportion of people who test positive on a screening test:

$$P* = \frac{\text{all those who test positive}}{\text{all those tested}} = \frac{TP + FP}{n} \tag{4.7}$$

where TP represents the number of true positives, FP represents the number of false positives, and n represents all those tested.

The apparent prevalence and true prevalence differ when the screening test is imperfect. In our smoking survey illustration, the true prevalence of smoking is .500 and apparent prevalence is .330 (see Table 4.8). The discrepancy between the true prevalence and apparent prevalence is due to underreporting of smoking based on the questionnaire results.

Future references to prevalence in this chapter assume we are dealing with true prevalence values.

Relationship Between Prevalence and Predictive Value Positive

Determinants   The predictive value positive of a test depends on the sensitivity of the test, the specificity of the test, and the prevalence of the disease in the population in which the test is being used. Although the first two determinants of predictive value (sensitivity and specificity) are expected, many students are surprised by the important role prevalence plays in determining predictive value. In general, if the prevalence of disease is low, the predictive value positive will be low. If the prevalence of disease is high, the predictive value positive will be high. This relationship holds for all diagnostic tests that fall short of perfection.

Illustration of How an Identical Test Used in Two Different Populations Can Have Quite Different Predictive Values Consider a hypothetical screening test with a sensitivity of .99 and specificity of .99 that is used in two different populations: population A has a .10 prevalence of disease and population B has a .001 prevalence of disease. Each population consists of 1,000,000 people.

Since the number of people with disease ("cases") is equal to the prevalence times the population size, population A has (.1 × 1,000,000 =) 100,000 cases and population B has (.001 × 1,000,000 =) 1000 cases. In population A, the test correctly identifies 99,000 (99%) of the 100,000 cases, leaving 1000 false negatives. The test also correctly identifies 891,000 (99%) of the 900,000 noncases as true negatives in population A, leaving 9000 false positives. The resultant distribution of test results is displayed in Table 4.9, population A. Using these data, the predictive value positive of the test in population A is .917.

In population B, the test correctly identifies 990 (99%) of the 1000 cases, leaving 10 false negatives. The test also correctly identifies 989,010 (99%) of the noncases as true negatives in population B, leaving 9900 false positives. The predictive value positive of the test in population B is therefore .090 (Table 4.9, population B). Thus, the predictive value positive of the same test is substantially less in population B than in population A. This is because even a specific test will identify many false positives when the disease is rare.

TABLE 4.9. Test Results of a Screening Test in Two Different Populations: Sensitivity = .99, Specificity = .99

Population A (Prevalence = 100,000/1,000,000 = .10)

	Disease +	Disease −	Total
Test +	99,000	9,000	108,000
Test −	1,000	891,000	892,000
	100,000	900,000	1,000,000

Standard calculation of predictive value positive:

$$PVP = TP/(TP + FP) = 99{,}000/(99{,}000 + 9{,}000) = .917$$

Bayesian calculation of predictive value positive:

$$PVP = \frac{(P)(SEN)}{(P)(SEN) + (1 - SPEC)(1 - P)} = \frac{(.1)(.99)}{(.1)(.99) + (1 - .99)(1 - .1)} = .917$$

Population B (Prevalence = 1000/1,000,000 = .001)

	Disease +	Disease −	Total
Test +	990	9,990	10,980
Test −	10	989,010	989,020
	1,000	999,000	1,000,000

Standard calculation of predictive value positive:

$$PVP = TP/(TP + FP) = 990/(990 + 9{,}900) = .090$$

Bayesian calculation of predictive value positive:

$$PVP = \frac{(P)(SEN)}{(P)(SEN) + (1 - SPEC)(1 - P)} = \frac{(.001)(.99)}{(.001)(.99) + (1 - .99)(1 - .001)} = .090$$

Bayesian Formula

The predictive value positive of a test can be calculated directly from its sensitivity, specificity, and the prevalence of disease in the population it is being used in, if these quantities are known, according to the formula:

$$PVP = \frac{(P)(SEN)}{(P)(SEN) + (1 - SPEC)(1 - P)} \qquad (4.8)$$

where *PVP* represents predictive value positive, *P* represents (true) prevalence, *SEN* represents sensitivity, and *SPEC* represents specificity. Because formula 4.8 is derived using Bayes's Law of Probability, it is called the "Bayesian formula for predictive value positive."

This formula can be used to calculate the predictive value positive of the illustrative smoking questionnaire. Given a sensitivity of .650, specificity of .990, and prevalence of .500, the predictive value positive is

$$PVP = \frac{(P)(SEN)}{(P)(SEN) + (1 - SPEC)(1 - P)}$$
$$= \frac{(.500)(.650)}{(.500)(.650) + (1 - .990)(1 - .500)} = .985$$

This value matches the previously calculated value as determined by formula 4.4.

The Bayesian formula for predictive value positive allows us to plot predictive value positive as a function of prevalence, sensitivity, and specificity. Figure 4.2 plots this relationship for three different diagnostic tests. The sensitivity of all three tests is held constant at .99. Specificity varies between .80 and .99, as labeled on the figure. This figure suggests the following:

- All three tests have low predictive value positive when used in populations with low disease prevalence.
- Predictive value positive increases as a function of prevalence.
- Increases in predictive value positive are most pronounced in the prevalence range of 0 to .20 (or thereabouts).
- Tests of low specificity add little new information about the population if the prevalence of disease is low.

Relationship Between Prevalence and Predictive Value Negative

As was the case with predictive value positive, the predictive value negative of a test also depends on the sensitivity and specificity of the test and prevalence of disease in the population in which the test is being used. The Bayesian formula relating these factors is

$$PVN = \frac{(1 - P)(SPEC)}{(1 - P)(SPEC) + (1 - SEN)(P)} \qquad (4.9)$$

where *PVN* represents predictive value negative, *P* represents (true) prevalence, *SEN* represents sensitivity, and *SPEC* represents specificity.

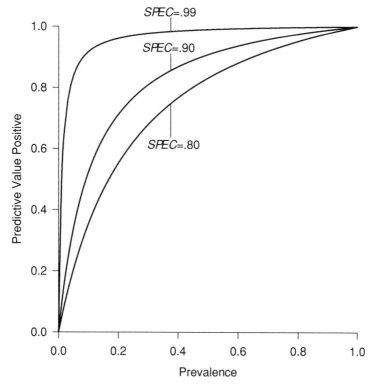

Figure 4.2. *Predictive value positive as a function of prevalence. All three tests have a sensitivity of .99. Tests of three specificities are considered (indicated by* SPEC*).*

Application of this formula to the illustrative teen smoking data results in

$$PVN = \frac{(1 - P)(SPEC)}{(1 - P)(SPEC) + (1 - SEN)(P)}$$

$$= \frac{(1 - .500)(.990)}{(1 - .500)(.990) + (1 - .650)(.500)} = .739$$

Figure 4.3 plots the relationship between prevalence and predictive value negative for three different diagnostic tests. Each test has a specificity of .99. The sensitivity varies between .80 and .99, as labeled on the figure. This figure suggests the following:

- Predictive value negative decreases as a function of prevalence.
- Decreases are most pronounced when the disease is common (i.e., prevalence is high).
- There is a direct correlation between sensitivity and predictive value negative; low sensitivity is associated with low predictive value negative.
- Tests of low sensitivity add little new information on populations in which the prevalence of the condition is already high (as is the case in our illustrative teen smoking data).

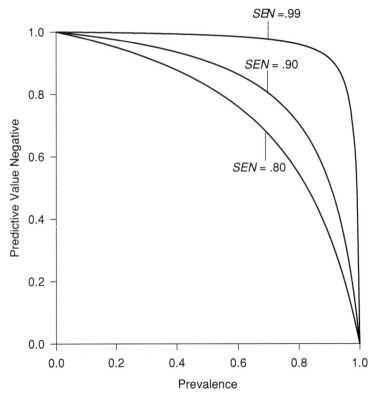

Figure 4.3. *Predictive value negative as a function of prevalence. All three tests have a specificity of .99. Tests of three sensitivities are shown (indicated by* SEN*).*

4.5 SELECTING A CUTOFF POINT FOR POSITIVE AND NEGATIVE TEST RESULTS

Many diagnostic test results are based on a continuum of values that must be converted to either "positive" or "negative" results in order to be interpreted. For example, enzyme-linked immunosorbent assay methods used to detect the presence of human immunodeficiency virus (HIV) indicate the presence of the HIV antibody by fluorescing. Higher concentrations of HIV antibody are associated with greater levels of immunofluorescence. The degree of immunofluorescence is read on a numerical optical density ratio (ODR) scale that demonstrates a range of ODRs associated with positive tests. Due to nonspecific immunologic reactions, sera from people free from HIV infection also demonstrate a range of immunofluorescence upon testing. It would be convenient if the distributions of ODR values for HIV-positive and HIV-negative populations did not overlap. Unfortunately, this is not the case. As a result, sera from some HIV-negative people demonstrate higher ODR readings than their HIV-positive counterparts (Fig. 4.4). Selecting a low cutoff point by which to determine positive tests would identify all people carrying HIV as positive. However, in so doing, many false positives will be identified. The resulting test will have high sensitivity but low specificity (Fig. 4.4A). Selecting an intermediate cutoff results in a test that identifies fewer false positives, but some false negatives will now be identified. The resulting test will have intermediate sensitivity and intermediate specificity

A.

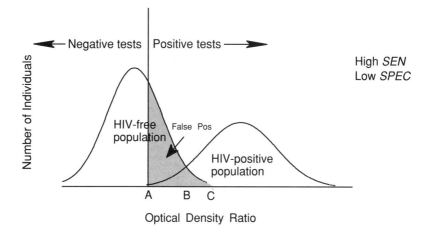

B.

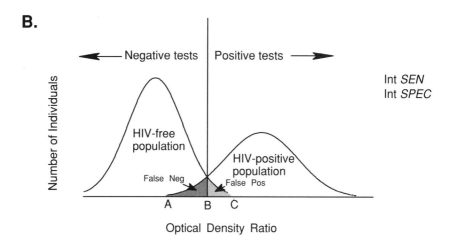

C.

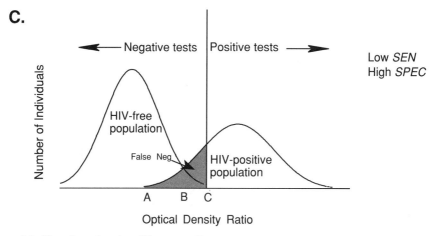

Figure 4.4. *The effect of setting different cutoffs on the sensitivity and specificity of an enzyme-linked immunosorbent HIV assay—hypothetical data.*

(Fig. 4.4B). Selecting a high cutoff point eliminates false positives; however, now many more false negatives will be identified. The resulting test will have high specificity but low sensitivity (Fig. 4.4C). Thus, the selection of a cutoff point must be determined by the purpose of the test. When attempting to avoid false negatives, a low cutoff point is used (Fig. 4.4A). When attempting to minimize overall error, an intermediate cutoff point is used (Fig. 4.4B). When attempting to avoid false positives, a high cutoff point is used (Fig. 4.4C). Each strategy has its place, as well as its consequences.

Given the inherent trade-offs in sensitivity and specificity, a multistage screening program must be used to accurately identify cases. In its simplest form, a two-stage process is used. If we hope to avoid false negatives, the first stage of screening uses a highly sensitive test. In using a highly sensitive test, false negatives are avoided, but false positives may be commonplace. Thus, a second stage of screening is needed. This second stage sorts out true positives and false positives using a test of high specificity. This process is analogous to casting a wide net and sorting out what you want to keep and what you don't want to keep later (Fig. 4.5). Because the purpose of screening is to identify cases for early diagnosis and treatment, noncases are periodically reexamined to determine whether disease has developed since the last screening procedure.

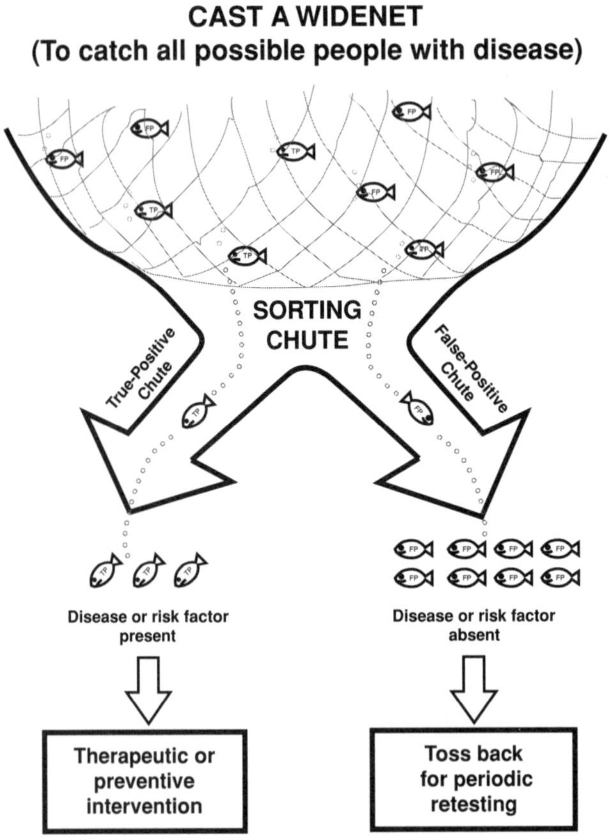

Figure 4.5. Fishing metaphor for two-stage screening. The first stage of screening casts a wide net to identify all possible cases (i.e., uses a test of high sensitivity). The second stage uses a test of high specificity to sort out true positives from false positives.

SUMMARY

1. The accuracy of an instrument used to identify disease is affected by two factors: (a) the reproducibility of an observation and (b) the ability of a test to discriminate between people with and without disease (validity). The investigator must take all practical steps to increase the reproducibility and validity of results by standardizing the conditions under which data are collected. Furthermore, she must take all necessary steps to quantify and understand deviations from the true biological state of affairs, whenever possible.

2. The kappa statistic is a chance-corrected measure of reproducibility. For most purposes, kappa values greater than .75 may be taken to represent excellent reproducibility beyond chance, values between .40 and .75 may be taken to represent fair to good reproducibility beyond chance, and values of less than .40 may be taken to represent poor agreement beyond chance.

3. Sensitivity, specificity, predictive value positive, and predictive value negative are measures of diagnostic test validity. Using conditional probability notation, these terms are defined as follows:

Sensitivity $= Pr(T+|D+)$

Specificity $= Pr(T-|D-)$

Predictive value positive $= Pr(D+|T+)$

Predictive value negative $= Pr(D-|T-)$

4. The predictive value of a test is a function of its sensitivity and specificity, and the prevalence of the disease in the population on which it is used. Predictive value positive results can be low when the disease is uncommon.

5. In selecting a cutoff point for determining a positive test result, there are trade-offs in opting for either a sensitive or specific test. To circumvent this problem, screening programs use multiphasic procedures, using an initially sensitive test to identify all possible cases followed by a specific test to sort out true positives and false positives.

NOTATION AND FORMULA REFERENCE

Diagnostic Test Reproducibility Statistics

a Proportion of subjects in which both raters offer a positive diagnosis

b Proportion of subjects in which rater A offers a positive diagnosis and rater B offers a negative diagnosis

c Proportion of subjects in which rater B offers a positive diagnosis and rater A offers a negative diagnosis

d Proportion of subjects in which both raters offer negative diagnoses

p_1 Proportion of rater A's diagnoses that are positive

q_1 Proportion of rater A's diagnoses that are negative

p_2 Proportion of rater B's diagnoses that are positive

q_2 Proportion of rater B's diagnoses that are negative

κ Kappa statistic (formula 4.1)

Diagnostic Test Validity Statistics

TP   True positive
TN   True negative
FP   False positive
FN   False negative
n   Sample size
SEN   Sensitivity (formula 4.2)
SPEC   Specificity (formula 4.3)
PVP   Predictive value positive (formulas 4.4 and 4.8)
PVN   Predictive value negative (formulas 4.5 and 4.9)
P   True prevalence (formula 4.6)
P*   Apparent prevalence (formula 4.7)

EXERCISES

1. Determine whether each of the following is primarily a symptom, sign, or test.

 (A) chills

 (B) fever of 104.6°F

 (C) sore throat

 (D) visibly swollen and reddened pharyngeal mucosa

2. An epidemiologic study based on a self-administered questionnaire finds a higher rate of disabilities related to activities of daily living (e.g., difficulty sitting down or getting up from a chair) in Dutch Trappist and Benedictine monks than in other comparably aged Dutch men (Mackenbach et al., 1993). Can we explain these results in terms of differences unrelated to the risk of disability? If so, how?

3. We wish to compare the results of a new screening test (test B) to the current gold standard method (test A). Data appear in Table 4.10.

 (A) How many false positives did test B ascertain?

 (B) How many false negatives were evident?

TABLE 4.10. Results from the Current Gold Standard Procedure (Test A) and a New Screening Test (Test B): Exercise 3 Data

Specimen Number	Test A ("Gold Standard")	Test B (Screening Test)
1	−	+
2	+	+
3	−	−
4	+	+
5	−	−
6	+	+
7	−	−
8	−	−
9	−	+
10	+	−

TABLE 4.11. Tabulated results; Data for Exercise 4

		Definitive Clinical Exam		
		+	−	
Screening Test	+	40	25	65
	−	10	125	135
		50	150	200

(C) Parse the data into a two-by-two sensitivity/specificity table.

(D) What is the sensitivity of test B?

(E) What is the specificity of test B?

4. To characterize the sensitivity and specificity of a simple and inexpensive screening test, 200 people simultaneously participate in a study in which they receive the screening test while simultaneously undergoing a definitive clinical examination. Results are tabulated in Table 4.11.

(A) What is the sensitivity of the screening test?

(B) What is the specificity of the screening test?

(C) What is the *PVP* of the screening test?

(D) What is the *PVN* of the screening test?

5. A screening program aimed at the early detection of a cancer uses a screening test that demonstrates a sensitivity of .95 and specificity of .90. Of those attending the screening program, 1 per 1000 (.001) actually has the cancer in question. What proportion of those who screen positively have the cancer in question?

6. Suppose 5% of the people in a study population use illicit drugs. We employ a test that is 95% "accurate" in that the test will be positive in 95% of drug users and negative in 95% of nonusers. If a person selected at random from the population demonstrates a positive test result, what is the likelihood that the person is actually a drug user?

ANSWERS TO EXERCISES

1. A   Chills, as subjective sensations of the patient, are *symptoms*.
   B   Body temperature in degrees Fahrenheit is a *test*.
   C   Soreness, as reported by the patient, is a *symptom*.
   D   Swelling and redness as observed by a clinician is a *sign*.

2. Yes. Monks might be less hesitant to report disabilities than other comparably aged men. (On the other hand, there is no evidence to suggest this is indeed the case.)

3. A   There are two false positive specimens: #1 and #9.
   B   There is one false negative specimen: #10.
   C   Table 4.12.
   D $SEN = TP/(TP + FN) = 3/4 = .750$.
   E $SPEC = TN/(TN + FP) = 4/6 = .667$.

4. A $SEN = 40/50 = .800$.
   B $SPEC = 125/150 = .833$.

TABLE 4.12. Answer to Exercise 3C

		Test A (Gold Standard) +	Test A (Gold Standard) −	Total
Test B	+	3	2	5
(Screening Test)	−	1	4	5
		4	6	10

C $PVP = 40/65 = .615.$
D $PVN = 125/135 \doteq .926.$

5. $PVP = \dfrac{(P)(SEN)}{(P)(SEN) + (1 - SPEC)(1 - P)}$

$= \dfrac{(.001)(.95)}{(.001)(.95) + (1 - .90)(1 - .001)} = .0094$

Less than 1% of people testing positive on the screening test will actually have the cancer in question.

6. The problem implies a prevalence of .05, sensitivity of .95, and specificity of .95. The question requests the predictive value positive of a test. According to formula 4.8.

$PVP = \dfrac{(P)(SEN)}{(P)(SEN) + (1 - SPEC)(1 - P)}$

$= \dfrac{(.05)(.95)}{(.05)(.95) + (1 - .95)(1 - .05)} = .50$

Therefore, only half of the people testing positive will actually be drug users.

REFERENCES

Ahlbom, A., & Norell, S. (1990). *Introduction to Modern Epidemiology* (2nd ed.). Chestnut Hill, MA: Epidemiology Resources.

Björkhem, I., Bergman, A., Falk, O., Kallner, A., Lantto, O., Svensson, L., Äkerlöf, E., & Blomstrand, R. (1981). Accuracy of some routine methods used in clinical chemistry as judged by isotope dilution–mass spectrometry. *Clinical Chemistry*, 27, 733–735.

Commission on Chronic Illness. (1957). *Chronic Illness in the United States Vol. IV, Chronic Illness in a Large City:The Baltimore Study.* Cambridge, MA: Harvard University Press.

Fleiss, J. L. (1981). *Statistical Methods for Rates and Proportions* (2nd ed.). New York: John Wiley & Sons.

Landis, J. R., & Koch, G. G. (1977). The measurement of observer agreement for categorical data. *Biometrics*, 33, 159–174.

Lilienfeld, A. M., & Kordan, B. (1966). A study in the variability in the interpretation of chest X-rays in the detection of lung cancer. *Cancer Research*, 26, 2145–2147.

Mackenback, J. P., Kunst, A. E., de Vrij, J. H., & van Meel, D. (1993). Self-reported morbidity and disability among Trappist and Benedictine monks. *American Journal of Epidemiology*, 138, 569–573.

CHAPTER ADDENDUM (CASE STUDY): SCREENING FOR ANTIBODIES TO THE HUMAN IMMUNODEFICIENCY VIRUS

Source   Centers for Disease Control. *1992 EIS Course.*

Authors   L. Peterson, G. Birkhead, and R. Dicker

Objectives

After completing this case study, the student should be able to:

1. Define and perform calculations of sensitivity, specificity, predictive value positive, and predictive value negative.
2. Describe the relationship between prevalence and predictive value.
3. Discuss the trade-offs between sensitivity and specificity.
4. List the principles of a good screening program.

Part I

In December 1982, a report in the *Morbidity and Mortality Weekly Report* (MMWR) described three persons who had developed acquired immunodeficiency syndrome (AIDS) but who had neither of the previously known risk factors for the disease: homosexual/bisexual activity with numerous partners and intravenous drug use. These three persons had previously received whole-blood transfusions. By 1983, widespread recognition of the problem of transfusion-related AIDS led to controversial recommendations that persons in known high-risk groups voluntarily defer from donating blood. In June 1984, after the discovery of the human immunodeficiency virus (HIV), five companies were licensed to produce enzyme-linked immunosorbent assay (EIA, then called ELISA) test kits for detecting HIV antibody. A Food and Drug Administration spokesperson stated that "getting this test out to the blood banks is our No. 1 priority." Blood bank directors were anxiously waiting to start screening blood with the new test until March 2, 1985, the date the first test kit was approved by the FDA.

In the prelicensure evaluation, sensitivity and specificity of the test kits were estimated using blood samples from four groups: those with AIDS by CDC criteria, those with other symptoms and signs of HIV infection, those with various autoimmune disorders and neoplastic diseases that could give a false-positive test results, and presumably healthy blood and plasma donors.

Numerous complex issues were discussed even before licensure. Among them were agreeing on the significance of a negative blood test, determining the percentage of antibody-positive persons who were capable of transmitting the virus, understanding the magnitude of the problem of false-positive test results, and determining whether test-positive blood donors should be notified.

It is now March 2, 1985, and you are the State Epidemiologist of State Y. The first HIV antibody test kits will arrive in blood banks in your state in a few hours. Meeting with you to discuss the appropriate use of this test are the Commissioner of Health, the medical director of the regional blood bank, and the chief of the State Y Drug Abuse Commission.

To help in your discussions, you turn to prelicensure information regarding the sensitivity and specificity of test kit A. The information indicates that the sensitivity of test kit A is 95.0% (.95) and the specificity is 98.0% (.98).

Question 1   With this information, by constructing a two-by-two table, calculate the predictive value positive and predictive value negative of the EIA in a hypothetical population of 1,000 blood donors. Using a separate two-by-two table, calculate *PVP* and *PVN* for a population of 1000 drug users. Assume that the actual prevalence of HIV antibody among blood donors is 0.04% (.0004) and that of intravenous drug users is 10.0% (.10).

The blood bank director wants your assistance in evaluating the EIA as a test for screening donor blood in State Y. In particular, she is concerned about the possibility that some antibody-positive units will be missed by the test, and she wonders about false-positive test results since she is under pressure to develop a notification procedure for EIA-positive donors.

Question 2   Do you think that the EIA is a good screening test for the blood bank? What would you recommend to the blood bank director about notification of EIA-positive blood donors?

The chief of the State Y Drug Abuse Commission has noticed a dramatic increase in AIDS among clients of his intravenous-drug-abuse treatment programs. He wants to do a voluntary HIV antibody seroprevalence survey of intravenous-drug-abuse clients for planning purposes and would like to assess the feasibility of using the test as part of behavior modification counseling.

Question 3   Do you think that the EIA performs well enough to justify informing test-positive clients in the drug-abuse clinics that they are positive for HIV?

Question 4   If sensitivity and specificity remain constant, what is the relationship of prevalence to predictive value positive and predictive value negative?

Part II

EIA results are recorded as optical density ratios (ODRs). The ODR is a ratio of absorbance of the tested sample to the absorbance of a control sample. The greater the ODR, the more "positive" is the test result. The EIA, as with most other screening tests, is not perfect; there is some overlap of optical density ratios of samples that are actually antibody positive and those that are actually antibody negative. This is illustrated in Figure 4.4 (p. 67).

Establishing the cutoff value to define a positive test result from a negative one is somewhat arbitrary. You initially decide that optimal density ratios greater than "B" on Figure 4.4 are positive.

Question 5a   In terms of sensitivity and specificity, what happens if you raise the cutoff from "B" to "C"?

Question 5b   In terms of sensitivity and specificity, what happens if you lower the cut-off from "B" to "A"?

Question 6   From what you know now, what is the relationship between sensitivity and specificity of a screening test?

Question 7   What would the blood bank director and the head of drug treatment consider in deciding where the cutoff point should be for each program? Who would probably want a lower cutoff value?

Part III

You are concerned that because of the low predictive value of the EIA in the blood donor population, the blood bank personnel cannot properly inform those who are EIA positive of their actual antibody status. For this reason, you wish to evaluate the Western blot test as a confirmatory test for HIV antibody.

The Western blot test identifies antibodies to specific proteins associated with the human immunodeficiency virus. The Western blot is the most widely used secondary test to detect HIV antibody because its specificity exceeds 99.99%; however, it is not used as a primary screening test because it is expensive and technically difficult to perform. Its sensitivity is thought to be lower than that of the EIA.

Because the Western blot test is not generally available, the blood bank director is wondering whether the initial EIA-positive results can be confirmed by repeating the EIA and by considering persons to have the antibody only if results of both tests are positive.

You decide that you want to compare the performance of the repeat EIA and the Western blot as confirmatory tests. To do this, use your earlier hypothetical sample of 1,000,000 blood donors. Assume that serum specimens that are initially positive by EIA are then split into two aliquots; a repeat EIA is performed on one portion and a Western blot on the other portion.

Question 8   What is the actual antibody prevalence in the population of persons whose blood samples will receive confirmatory testing?

Question 9   Calculate the predictive value positive of the two sequences of tests: EIA–EIA and EIA–Western blot. Assume that the sensitivity and specificity of the EIA are 95.0% and 98.0%, respectively. Assume that the sensitivity and specificity of the Western blot are 80.0% and 99.99%, respectively.

Question 10   Why does the predictive value positive increase so dramatically with the addition of a second test? Why is the predictive value positive higher for the EIA–WB sequences than for the EIA–EIA sequence?

Part IV

It is now July 1987 and the Governor has asked you to evaluate a proposed premarital HIV-antibody-screening program. A bill to establish the program is to be presented to the

TABLE 4.13. Results of Initial EIA Test in People Getting Married

		Actual Antibody Status		Total
		+	−	
Initial EIA	+	23	120	143
	−	1	59,856	59,857
		24	59,976	60,000

state legislature tomorrow. You estimate that 60,000 people will get married in your state in the next year. The proposed legislation requires that each prospective bride and groom submit a blood sample for EIA testing. Those positive EIA test results will then receive a Western blot test.

You decide that a goal of the screening program is to decrease inadvertent perinatal or sexual HIV transmission by determining who among those to be married are probably infected with the virus.

Question 11 What criteria would you consider in evaluating this proposed screening program?

Tables 4.13 and 4.14 show the results of the testing, assuming that persons getting married have the same actual HIV-antibody prevalence as blood donors (0.04%). In 1987 the sensitivity and specificity of the currently available version of EIA Test Kit A were 97.0% and 99.8%, respectively. The Western blot sensitivity and specificity were 95.0% and 99.99%, respectively.

With sequential testing, the sensitivity is 92%, the specificity is 100%, and predictive value positive is 100%.

Question 12 Compute the cost of the screening program. Assume a cost of $50.00 for every initial EIA test ($10.00 lab fee and $40.00 health-care-provider visit) and an additional $100.00 for EIA-positive persons who will need additional testing. What is the cost of the screening program in the next year? What is the cost per identified antibody-positive person?

Question 13 What is your final recommendation to the Governor?

TABLE 4.14. Results of Follow-up Western Blot Test in People Getting Married

		Actual Antibody Status		Total
		+	−	
Initial EIA	+	22	0	22
	−	1	120	121
		23	120	143

Additional Information

The following 10 principles of good mass screening programs were proposed by Wilson and Jungner of the World Health Organization in 1968:

1. The condition being sought is an important health problem for the individual and the community.
2. There is an acceptable form of treatment for patients with recognizable disease.
3. The natural history of the condition, including its development from latent to declared disease, is adequately understood.
4. There is a recognizable latent or early symptomatic stage.
5. There is a suitable screening test or examination for detecting the disease at the latent or early symptomatic state, and this test is acceptable to the population.
6. The facilities required for diagnosis and treatment of patients revealed by the screening program are available.
7. There is an agreed policy on which to base treatment of patients.
8. Treatment at the presymptomatic, borderline stage of a disease favorably influences its course and prognosis.
9. The cost of the screening program (which would include the cost of diagnosis and treatment) is economically balanced in relation to possible expenditure on medical care as a whole.
10. Case-finding is a continuing process, not a "once and for all" project.

Bibliography—Screening for HIV

Check, W. A. (1983). Preventing AIDS transmission: would blood donors be screened? *JAMA*, 249, 567–570.

Cleary, P. D., Barry, M. J., Mayer, K. H., et al. (1987). Compulsory premarital screening for the human immunodeficiency virus: technical and public health considerations. *JAMA*, 258, 1757–1762.

Goldsmith, M. F. (1985). HTLV-III testing of donor blood imminent; complex issues remain. JAMA, 253, 173–181.

Marwick, C. (1985). Use of AIDS antibody test may provide more answers. *JAMA*, 253, 1694–1699.

Schwartz, J. S., Dans, P. E., & Kinosian, B. P. (1988). Human immunodeficiency virus test evaluation, performance, and use: proposals to make good tests better. *JAMA*, 259, 2574–2579.

Sivak, S. L., & Wormser, G. P. (1986). Predictive value of a screening test for antibodies to HTLV-II. *American Journal of Clinical pathology*, 85, 700–703.

Sloand, E. M., Pitt, E., Chiarello, R. J., & Nemo, G. J. (1991). HIV testing: state of the art. *JAMA*, 266, 2861–2866.

Turnock, B. J., & Kelly, C. J. (1989). Mandatory premarital testing for human immunodeficiency virus: the Illinois experience. *JAMA*, 261, 3415–3418.

Ward, J. W., Grindon, A. J., Feorino, P. M., Schable, C., Parvin, M., & Allen, J. R. (1986). *JAMA*, 256, 357–361.

Bibliography—General Concepts of Screening

Seilker, H. P. (1986). Clinical prediction rules. *New England Journal of Medicine*, 314, 714.

Tyler, J. W., & Cullor, J. S. (1989). Titers, tests, and truisms: rational interpretation of diagnostic serologic testing. *Journal of the American Veterinary Medical Association*, 194, 1550–1558.

ANSWERS TO CASE STUDY: SCREENING FOR ANTIBODIES TO THE HUMAN IMMUNODEFICIENCY VIRUS

Part I

Answer 1
Blood Bank Calculations

Given: $N = 1,000,000$

EIA sensitivity 95.0%

EIA specificity 98.0%

Blood donor prevalence of 0.04% (.0004)

See Table 4.15 for numerical results.

$$PVP = 380/20,372 = .019$$

$$PVN = 979,608/979,628 = .99998$$

Notes

- The left column is the total number who are antibody-positive, which is $1,000,000 \times .0004 = 400$.
- Right column total is $1,000,000 - 400 = 999,6000$, total antibody-negative.
- The "A" cell is the number who are truly positive and who test positive, and is calculated as the left column total times sensitivity, or $400 \times .95 = 380$.
- The "C" cell can be calculated as $400 - 380 = 20$.
- The "D" cell is the number who are truly negative and who test negative, and is calculated as the right column total times specificity, or $999,6000 \times .98 = 979,608$.
- The "B" cell can be calculated as $999,600 - 979,608 = 19,992$.
- Row totals are next: 20,372 and 979,628.
- Now review formulas for *PVP* and *PVN* and calculate them.

Drug Clinic Calculations

Given: EIA sensitivity 95.0%

EIA specificity 98.0%

Drug user prevalence of 10% (.10)

TABLE 4.15. Screening in Blood Bank Population

	Disease +	Disease −	Total
Test +	380	19,992	20,372
Test −	20	979,608	979,628
	400	999,600	1,000,000

TABLE 4.16. EIA Screening in Drug Clinic Population

	Disease +	Disease −	Total
Test +	95	18	113
Test −	5	882	887
	100	900	1,000

See Table 4.16 for numerical results.

$$PVP = 95/113 = .841$$

$$PVN = 882/887 = .994$$

Answer 2   At the blood bank, the primary concern is the safety of the blood supply. The EIA is a good but not perfect screening for the blood bank. Ninety-five percent (380/400) of the antibody-positive units will be screened out, and 2% (20,372/1000,000) of the donated units will need to be discarded.

Because only 1.9% of the test-positive persons will actually have the antibody (predictive value positive = .019), test-positive blood donors should *not* be notified on the basis of this test alone.

Answer 3   For the drug-clinic clients, persons with a positive test will have a 84.1% chance of actually having the antibody (predictive value positive), while those with a negative test will only have a 0.6% chance of having the antibody ($1 - PVN$). Although the EIA is much more useful in separating those with and without antibody in the drug clinic than in the blood bank, 16% ($1 - PVP$) of drug-clinic clients with a positive test result will not actually have the antibody (false-positive).

Note, however, that regardless of the tests results, counseling of this population is important because they are engaging in high-risk behavior.

Answer 4   If the prevalence is high, the predictive value positive will be high, and the predictive value negative will be low. If the prevalence is low, the predictive value positive will be low, and the predictive value negative will be high (see Figures 4.2 and 4.3, pp. 65–66).

Part II

Answer 5a   Moving the cutoff from "B" to "C" will decrease the sensitivity and will increase the specificity of the test.

Answer 5b   Moving the cutoff from "B" to "A" will increase the sensitivity and will decrease the specificity of the test.

Answer 6   By changing the cutoff, if the sensitivity is increased, the specificity is decreased. Conversely, if the sensitivity is decreased, the specificity is increased.

Answer 7   The blood bank director's primary goal is to screen out antibody-positive (probably capable of transmitting the infection) blood at almost any cost. Therefore, she would choose to have a very sensitive test. The cost will be a lower specificity; hence there will be more false-positive test results, and more blood will be discarded because of false-positive results.

Because of the severe ramifications of notifying a person that he/she has the antibody, when, in fact, he/she does not (false-positive), the director of drug treatment will want a test with high specificity in order to maximize the predictive value positive.

For these reasons, the blood bank director will probably want a lower cutoff.

Part III

Answer 8 In this problem, all persons with a positive EIA result will receive Western blot confirmatory testing. From the hypothetical 1,000,000-person blood-donor population in Question 1, 20,372 persons will have a positive test result. Of these 20,372 persons, 380 (1.9%) will actually have the antibody.

Answer 9 In this problem, we are assuming that both tests are independent—the results of the first test do not affect the results of the second test. This is generally not true with series of screening tests; the second test will not perform as well in a population that has already been screened with an initial test. Therefore, our calculations in this problem will overestimate the predictive value positive.

An example of nonindependence is the repeat EIA. On the initial EIA, some of the false-positive test results will be due to laboratory errors that will be unlikely to be repeated, such as incorrect recording of results. Other initial false-positive test results will be likely to be repeated; for example, if there was a biological reason for the initial false-positive test results (such as antibody cross-relativity), the repeat test will probably yield a false-positive result as well. In other words, a person who has had one false-positive test result will have a greater chance of having another false-positive test result.

The population of those who actually do not have the antibody in the unscreened population and the population of those who actually do not have the antibody and are being retested are different: those to be retested all had initial false-positive test results. From this, we can see that on repeat testing a larger percentage of those who actually do not have the antibody will have positive test results because these persons all had one initial false-positive test result. Therefore, the specificity of the repeat EIA will be lower than the specificity of the initial EIA in the unscreened population.

For each confirmatory test, the population to be tested consists of those who were initially EIA-positive from the hypothetical 1,000,000-person blood donor population. From Question 8, the population to have confirmatory testing comprises 20,372 persons, of whom 380 actually have the antibody.

EIA–EIA

Given: EIA sensitivity 95.0%
        EIA specificity 98.0%

See Table 4.17 for numerical results.

Persons are considered to be test-positive only if results of both the initial EIA and the repeat EIA are positive. Because only those with an initial positive EIA were included in the above table, the 761 persons with a repeat positive EIA were positive in both the ini-

TABLE 4.17. EIA–EIA Testing

	Disease +	Disease −	Total
Test +	361	400	761
Test −	19	19,592	19,611
	380	19,992	20,372

tial and repeat tests. However, of these 761 persons, only 361 actually have the antibody. Therefore, the predictive value positive is 47.4% (361/761).

EIA–WB

Given: WB sensitivity 80.0%
   WB specificity 99.9%

See Table 4.18 for numerical results.

Persons are considered to be test-positive only if results of both the initial EIA and the confirmatory Western blot are positive. Because only those with an initial positive EIA were included in the above table, the 306 persons with a positive Western blot were positive on both tests. Of these 306 persons, 304 actually had the antibody. Therefore, the predictive value positive is 99.3% (304/306).

Note: Currently, the sequence many blood banks use for notification purposes is EIA–EIA–Western blot (i.e., the original EIA, a repeat EIA, then a Western blot only for those positive on both EIAs). Table 4-19 shows the results of subjecting those blood specimens that are positive on both EIAs to a Western blot test.

EIA–EIA–WB

Given: WB sensitivity 80.0%
   WB specificity 99.9%

See Table 4.19 for numerical results.

Predictive value positive = 289/289 = 100%
Number missed = 400 − 289 = 111
Sensitivity of the entire EIA–EIA–WB sequence = 72%
Specificity of the entire EIA–EIA–WB sequence = 100%, because "b" cell = 0

TABLE 4.18. EIA–WB Testing

	Disease +	Disease −	Total
Test +	304	2	306
Test −	76	19,990	20,066
	380	19,992	20,372

TABLE 4.19. EIA–EIA–WB Testing

	Disease +	Disease −	Total
Test +	289	0	289
Test −	72	400	472
	361	400	761

Answer 10 From these two examples, we can see that the two most important factors in determining predictive value positive are the prevalence of the disease and the specificity of the test. In the EIA–EIA example, the predictive value positive increased from 1.9% after the initial EIA to 47.4% after the repeat EIA, even though the sensitivity and specificity were the same for both initial and repeat tests. This improvement resulted from the higher prevalence of the antibody in the retested population. For the unscreened population, the prevalence was 0.04%, while for the population being retested, the prevalence was 1.9%.

In the EIA–WB example, the predictive value positive after the Western blot test was 99.3%—a marked improvement over repeating the EIA ($PVP = 47.4\%$). This improvement was a result of Western blot's very high specificity (99.9%), even though the sensitivity of the Western blot was much lower than that of the EIA (80% and 98%, respectively).

Answer 11 The criteria to be used in evaluating this screening program include:

1. **Validity.** How well does the test measure what it is supposed to measure? In our premarital program, we are concerned about differentiating those who are infected and those who are not infected. The best scientific evidence to date indicates that those who are exposed to HIV, and hence are antibody-positive, probably remain infected for life. Therefore, an actual antibody-positive person is probably currently infected. It is unknown, however, which infected persons are capable of transmitting the infection.

2. **Reproducibility.** If you repeat the test on the same person, will you get the same result?

3. **Test performance.** What is the yield of the test in terms of sensitivity, specificity, and predictive value?

4. **Cost.** What is the cost of the program?

5. **Follow-up.** Will there be a mechanism to follow up on those with a positive test result?

6. **Acceptance.** Will those who are to be screened accept the program, and will the program be accepted by those performing the follow-up services?

7. **Confidentiality.**

8. **Public health impact.** Does notification affect behavior?

9. **Prevalence of HIV infection.**

10. **Feasibility.** What resources and technology are available? What other activities would the screening program displace?

11. **Other benefits.** Source of surveillance data.

12. **Alternatives.** Are there are other programs that would meet the same objectives?

13. **Coverage.** Does the program address those at risk?
14. **Consequences of misclassification.**

Answer 12   The costs are:

$3,000,000   Initial screening for all (60,000 × $50.00)
$14,300   Confirmatory testing of those who are initially EIA positive (143 × $100,00)

Answer 13   This question is intended to provoke discussion. (There is no consensus answer.) However, most would probably not recommend the screening program to the Governor. In considering the criteria in question 11, the screening program probably meets the criteria of validity, reliability, and yield (high sensitivity, specificity, and predictive value). The program is definitely not cost-effective; the $3 million anticipated cost for this program that would identify 22 antibody-positive persons exceeds the total AIDS budget for most states. The program is likely to be only marginally acceptable to the general population, and there is no proposed mechanism for follow-up of antibody-positive persons. It is also unknown whether notification of antibody-positive persons will cause them to change their sexual practices to reduce the risk of sexual transmission or whether notification will deter them from having children. The program only tests persons at one point in time, shortly before marriage. Therefore, the program would miss persons who have children out of wedlock and those who became antibody-positive after marriage.

5

Identification of Disease, Part II (Case Definitions and Disease Classification)

This chapter continues our consideration of the identification of disease started in the previous chapter. In this chapter, we consider criteria for defining cases, the standardized system of disease nomenclature known as the ICD, and artifactual fluctuation in reported rates of disease due to changes in coding practices and surveillance case definitions.

5.1 CASE DEFINITIONS

Establishing a Case Definition

A **case definition** is a set of objective, uniform, and consistent criteria by which to decide whether an individual should be classified as having the disease under investigation. Use of carefully researched and constructed standardized case definitions enhances diagnostic reproducibility and validity and allows for comparisons of epidemiologic study results among different studies.

Case definitions are composed of clinical criteria, other indicators of underlying pathophysiology, and epidemiologic restrictions based on person, place, and time criteria. Whenever possible, case definition criteria should be based on simple and objective measures. Examples of simple objective clinical criteria are:

- Fever greater than or equal to 38.6°C
- Bowel movements that conform to the shape of their container (a case definition for diarrhea)
- Force expiratory volumes less than X liters/second
- Elevated antibody titers
- Fatigue severe enough to limit daily activities

Case definitions may include epidemiologic restrictions based on person, place, and time factors. For example, cases can be restricted to people of a specified age range, to resi-

dents living within the epidemic area, or to cases with the onset of illness within a specified time. Criteria must be applied consistently throughout the study, without exception. A
new case definition can be adapted, however, if it is equally applied to both previous and
future cases.

Multiple Choice Criteria

Carefully constructed case definition alternatives can be built on multiple criteria. Diagnosis of myocardial infarction in the Framingham study, for example, was generally made
in the presence of clinical documentation and established electrocardiographic changes.
In cases lacking a clinical history of myocardial infarction, evidence of a "silent" heart attack was accepted only if an unequivocal pattern of myocardial infarction had developed
since the previous electrocardiographic tracing was obtained. For some analyses, the
presence of prolonged acute coronary insufficiency with electrocardiographic abnormali-
ties was included as cases (Kannel et al., 1961).

A common case definition approach is to combine diagnostic criteria in an "either/or"
fashion. This has been likened to a Chinese menu, for, like a Chinese menu, criteria can
be satisfied using different combinations of choices. (Historically, Chinese restaurants offered dinners in which one could choose one from column A or one from column B, and
so on). An example of a Chinese menu case definition for myocardial infarction, used by
Henning and Lundman (1975), was to meet two of the criteria listed in A, B, or C (below), *or* criterion D alone.

- Criterion A: chest pain, pulmonary edema, syncope, or shock
- Criterion B: pathologic changes detected in the electrocardiogram
- Criterion C: changes observed in ASAT and ALAT blood chemistry values
- Criterion D: autopsy findings of myocardial necrosis of an age consistent with the
  onset of symptoms

The either/or aspect of the "Chinese menu" allows for adjustment to the case definition
by either broadening or restricting criteria. A broad case definition is useful during the
early phases of an investigation when one needs to gather information on all possible
cases. The case definition can later be tightened to allow a sharper focus for testing causal
hypotheses.

Chronic Fatigue Syndrome, as an Example

Chronic fatigue syndrome has no known cause and is characterized by chronic fatigue
and an array of nonspecific signs and physical symptoms. No laboratory test to confirm
the existence of the disease is available, and diagnostic criteria for the syndrome have not
been uniformly applied. Researchers, therefore, have lacked adequate tools for assessing
the severity and functional limitations of the illness and its response to therapy (Klonoff,
1992). Moreover, without a consistent method for identifying cases, progress in understanding the epidemiology and clinical correlates of this syndrome have been hampered.

Recognizing these limitations, a group of epidemiologists and academic researchers
developed a working case definition based on major and minor clinical and physical criteria (Table 5.1). According to these criteria, a case of chronic fatigue syndrome must fulfill
two major diagnostic criteria and eight minor criteria (six or more symptom criteria and

TABLE 5.1. Working Case Definition of Chronic Fatigue Syndrome

A case of Chronic Fatigue Syndrome must first fulfill both of the major criteria. In addition, six or more of the symptom criteria plus two or more of the physical criteria must be fulfilled.

Major Criteria

1. New onset of persistent or relapsing, debilitating fatigue or easy fatigability in a person with no previous history of similar symptoms. The fatigue must be severe enough to reduce or impair daily activity below 50% of the patient's premorbid activity level for a period of at least 6 months.

2. Other clinical conditions that produce similar symptoms must be excluded by thorough evaluation, based on history, physical examination and appropriate laboratory findings. (Examples of conditions that must be excluded are malignancy, autoimmune disease, localized infection, chronic or subacute bacterial disease, fungal disease, parasitic disease, diseases related to HIV, chronic psychiatric disease, chronic inflammatory disease, neuromuscular disease, endocrine disease, drug dependency or abuse, side effects of chronic medication or other toxic agents, or other known or defined chronic pulmonary, cardiac, gastrointestinal, hepatic, renal, or hematolic diseases.)

Minor Criteria

Symptom Criteria

1. Chills or mild fever (oral temperature between 37.5°C and 38.6°C, if measured by the patient; oral temperatures greater than 38.6°C are less compatible with chronic fatigue syndrome and should prompt studies for other causes of illness).
2. Sore throat.
3. Painful lymph nodes in the anterior neck or armpit regions.
4. Unexplained generalized muscle weakness.
5. Muscle pain or myalgia.
6. Prolonged (greater than 24 hours in duration) generalized fatigue after modest levels of exercise that would have easily been tolerated in the patient's premorbid state.
7. Generalized headaches (of a type, severity, or pattern different from headaches the patient experienced in the premorbid state).
8. Migratory joint pain without swelling or redness.
9. Neuropsychologic complaints (one or more of the following: photophobia, transient visual scotomata, forgetfulness, excessive irritability, confusion, difficulty thinking, inability to concentrate, or depression).
10. Sleep disturbance (hypersomnia or insomnia).
11. Description of the main symptom complex as initially developed over a few hours to a few days. (This is not a true symptom but may be considered equivalent to the above symptoms in meeting the requirements of the case definition.)

Physical Examination Criteria

1. Low-grade fever (oral temperature between 37.5°C and 38.6°C or rectal temperature between 37.8°C and 38.8°C)
2. Nonexudative pharyngitis.
3. Palpable or tender anterior or posterior cervical or axillary lymph node (*Note:* Lymph nodes greater than 2 cm in diameter suggest other causes warranting further evaluation.)

Source: Holmes et al. (1988).

two or more of the physical criteria). In 1991, a national workshop updated this case definition by excluding specific psychiatric diagnoses and postinfectious disease fatigue that could explain the patient's symptoms (Schluederberg et al., 1992). Because chronic fatigue syndrome is not a homogeneous abnormality and no single pathogenic mechanism is known, this update further emphasized the need to delineate patient subgroups for separate data analyses. These standards now serve as the basis for conducting clinical and epidemiologic studies of chronic fatigue syndrome, thus providing a rational basis for evaluating patients and discovering the syndrome's cause.

Evolution of the AIDS Case Definition, as an Example

Case definitions often evolve over time as our understanding of the pathophysiology of disease increases and diagnostic technologies advance. For example, the surveillance case definition of acquired immunodeficiency syndrome (AIDS) has evolved to adapt to our increased understanding of its pathogenesis. Initially, in 1986, the Centers for Disease Control and Prevention (CDC) defined AIDS through the occurrence of a dozen opportunistic infections (e.g., *Pneumocystis carinii* pneumonia) and several cancers (e.g., Kaposi's sarcoma). These diseases—diagnosed by standard clinical, microbiologic, and histopathologic techniques—were considered sufficiently specific to suggest the underlying immunodeficiency, assuming other known causes for the immunodeficiency had been ruled out. In 1987, the CDC revised the surveillance case definition for AIDS to include additional indicator diseases (e.g., wasting syndrome) and to accept as a presumptive diagnosis other indicator conditions if laboratory tests showed concurrent evidence of HIV infection.

The CDC last revised the surveillance case definition of AIDS in 1992 to include HIV-infected people who have less than 200 CD4+ T-lymphocytes per microliter of blood or a CD4+ T-lymphocyte percentage of total lymphocytes of less than 14 (Table 5.2). In addition, three new clinical conditions (pulmonary tuberculosis, recurrent pneumonia, and invasive cervical cancer) were added to the surveillance case definition, while retaining the

TABLE 5.2. 1993 Revised Classification System for HIV Infection and the Expanded AIDS Surveillance Case Definition for Adolescents and Adults. The Shaded Cells Represent the Expanded AIDS Surveillance Case Definition. People with AIDS Indicator Conditions (Clinical Category C) and Those with CD4+ T-Lymphocyte Counts Less than 200/µL Are Reportable as AIDS Cases in the United States

	Clinical Categories		
CD4+ T-Cell Count	(A) Asymptomatic, Acute (Primary) HIV Infection or PGL[a]	(B) Symptomatic, Not (A) or (C) Conditions[b]	(C) AIDS Indicator Condition[c]
(1) ≥ 500/µL	A1	B1	
(2) 200–499/µL	A2	B2	
(3) <200/µL			

Source: CDC (1992a), table 1.
[a]PGL = persistent generalized lymphadenopathy.
[b]Category B clinical conditions (partial list) include bacillary angiomatosis, mild forms of candidiasis, cervical dysplasia/cervical carcinoma (*in situ*), persistent fever or diarrhea (longer than 1 month in duration), oral hairy leukoplakia, at least two episodes of shingles, idiopathic thrombocytopenia, listeriosis, pelvic inflammatory disease, and peripheral neuropathy.
[c]Category C (AIDS indicator) conditions include severe forms of candidiasis (e.g., of lungs), severe forms of coccidioidomycosis, HIV-related encephalopathy, chronic and severe *Herpes simplex* infections, disseminated histoplasmosis, Kaposi's sarcoma, several specific forms of lymphoma, several specific forms of *Mycobacterium* infection, pneumocystis pneumonia, recurrent pneumonia, progressive multifocal leukoencephalopathy, recurrent *Salmonella* septicemia, toxoplasmosis of the brain, and HIV-related wasting syndrome.

23 AIDS-defining conditions published by the CDC in 1987. These changes were made to fit the clinical importance of CD4+ lymphocyte level as part of the pathogenesis and medical management of HIV infection. It also simplified identification and reporting of cases and more accurately reflected HIV-related morbidity.

Classification of Case Status Based on Certainty

Investigators might choose to classify cases as confirmed, probable, or possible, whenever uncertainty exists. **Confirmed cases** usually require laboratory or special clinical pathologic study verification. **Probable cases** usually have typical clinical features but do not have laboratory or other supporting pathologic confirmation. **Possible cases** have fewer typical clinical features but have a clinical history consistent with the disease in question. CDC *Self-Study Course 3030-G* (1992b, p. 358) presents the following examples of confirmed, probable, and possible case definitions for an outbreak of hemolytic-uremic syndrome caused by infection with *Escherichia coli* O157:H7:

- Confirmed case: *E. coli* O157:H7 isolated from a stool culture or development of hemolytic-uremic syndrome in a school-age child resident of the county, with gastrointestinal symptoms beginning between November 3 and November 8, 1990.
- Probable cause: Bloody diarrhea, with the same person, place, and time restrictions as above.
- Possible case: Abdominal cramps and diarrhea (at least three stools in a 24-hour period) in a school-age child with onset during the same period as above.

Classifying cases as probable or possible allows the investigator to keep track of potential cases pending confirmation by means of laboratory results. It may also offer economic and practical advantages, especially when dealing with diseases with characteristic clinical pictures (e.g., measles) or when the diagnostic test in question is expensive or difficult to obtain. At times, confirming each case as definite may be unnecessary. For example, in investigating a foodborne outbreak, it is only necessary to isolate the agent from a few afflicted cases. Other descriptive epidemiologic and compatible clinical features will confirm the source and transmission of the agent, making isolation of the agent from each case superfluous.

5.2 THE INTERNATIONAL CLASSIFICATION OF DISEASE

Since 1948, the World Health Organization (WHO) has published the International Classification of Disease (ICD). This scheme provides standardized nomenclature necessary for coding and classifying the causes of morbidity and mortality for regional, national, and international use while helping to enhance diagnostic concordance and reliability. The ICD is currently in its 10th revision (WHO, 1990), although the 9th revision is still widely used in some environments (e.g., Health Care Financing Administration, 1989). The ICD meets the epidemiologist's need for consistency in coding required for rational comparisons of disease trends worldwide.

The 9th revision of the ICD is organized around 17 categories of diseases grouped according to similarities of cause, pathogenesis, and anatomical location. The 17 major categories are:

1. Infectious and Parasitic Diseases (codes 0–139)
2. Neoplasms (140–239)
3. Endocrine, Nutritional, and Metabolic and Immunity Disorders (240–279)
4. Diseases of the Blood and Blood-Forming Organs (280–289)
5. Mental Disorders (290–319)
6. Diseases of the Nervous System and Sense Organs (320–389)
7. Diseases of the Circulatory System (390–459)
8. Diseases of the Respiratory System (460–519)
9. Diseases of the Digestive System (520–579)
10. Diseases of the Genitourinary System (580–629)
11. Complications of Pregnancy, Childbirth, and the Puerperium (630–679)
12. Diseases of the Skin and Subcutaneous Tissue (680–709)
13. Diseases of the Musculoskeletal System and Connective Tissue (710–739)
14. Congenital Anomalies (740–759)
15. Certain Conditions Originating in the Perinatal Period (760–779)
16. Symptoms, Signs, and Ill-Defined Conditions (780–799)
17. Injury and Poisoning (800–999)

Beyond the 17 main categories, supplementary classifications are based on factors influencing health status and contact with health services (V codes) and external causes of injury and poisoning (E codes)

The coding hierarchy of the ICD is achieved by sequencing categories, headings, and subheadings according to clinical detail. For example, the category Diseases of the Circulatory System (390–459) has the following organization:

390–392	Acute rheumatic fever
393–398	Chronic rheumatic heart disease
401–405	Hypertensive disease
410–414	Ischemic heart disease
415–417	Diseases of pulmonary circulation
420–429	Other forms of heart disease
430–438	Cerebrovascular disease
440–448	Diseases of arteries, arterioles, and capillaries
451–459	Diseases of veins and lymphatics, and other diseases of circulatory system

Diseases within subcategories are further organized to provide a basis for indexing and analysis. For example, the individual subcategory Ischemic heart disease (410–414) includes the following three-digit headings:

410	Acute myocardial infarction
411	Other acute and subacute forms of ischemic heart disease
412	Old myocardial infarction
413	Angina pectoris
414	Other forms of chronic ischemic heart disease

Additional specificity is achieved by fourth and fifth digits following a decimal point. For example, the codes under Acute myocardial infarction (410) are:

410.0	Of the anterolateral wall
410.1	Of other anterior wall
410.2	Of inferolateral wall
410.3	Of inferoposterior wall
410.4	Of other inferior wall
410.5	Of other lateral wall
410.6	True posterior wall infarction
410.7	Subendocardial infarction
410.8	Of other specified sites
410.9	Unspecified site

Thus, in this case, ultimate subcategories provide the specific anatomic location of the injury.

5.3 ARTIFACTUAL FLUCTUATIONS IN REPORTED RATES

Artifactual changes in reported morbidity and mortality rates can result from changes in coding and reporting practices. Moreover, the completeness of reported rates varies from study to study and according to region, cause, and other factors. We must be careful when comparing reported rates of disease over time and among studies, especially whenever the ICD is revised and coding practices change.

For example, before 1949, all death certificates that mentioned diabetes as either the immediate cause of death, underlying cause of death, or other significant condition contributing to death were coded as a death due to diabetes. After 1949, this practice changed so that only death certificates listing diabetes as the underlying cause of death were coded as death due to diabetes (Gordis, 1996). This caused an artifactual decline in diabetes death rates (Fig. 5.1).

Additional examples of artifactual fluctuations are seen when AIDS surveillance case definitions were changed in 1987 and, again, in 1993. The surveillance case definition was revised in October 1987 to include additional illnesses and diagnostic criteria. In 1993, the surveillance case definition was again changed, this time to include HIV-infected people with CD4+ lymphocyte counts of less than 200 cells/μL but who do not necessarily have an AIDS indicator disease. This resulted in artifactual large influxes in cases with apparent spikes in reporting rates (Fig. 5.2).

SUMMARY

1. The case definition is the standard set of criteria that epidemiologists use for deciding whether an individual should be classified as having the disease or condition under investigation. It is based on simple and objective clinical and epidemiologic criteria. Combinations of criteria can be used to either broaden or restrict the case definition, as dictated by the needs of the investigation. Case definitions evolve over time as our understanding of the pathophysiology of disease increases and diagnostic technologies advance.

2. The International Classification of Disease (ICD) provides a widely accepted, standardized nomenclature for coding and classifying the causes of morbidity and mortality worldwide. It is currently in its 10th revision, although the 9th revision is still used in some en-

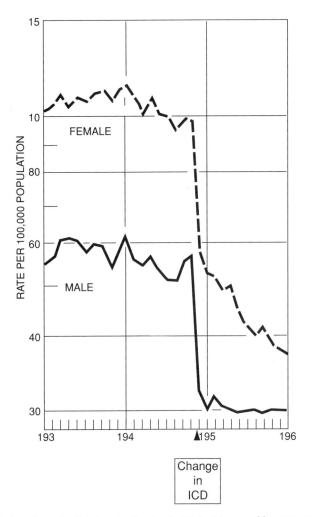

Figure 5.1. *Artifactual drops in diabetes death rates in 55- to 64-year white men and women, United States, 1930–1960.* (Source: *National Center for Health Statistics, 1964, p. 36.*)

vironments. The ICD is organized around 17 categories of diseases, grouped according to similarities of cause, pathogenesis, and anatomical location. Consistency in coding is required for rational comparisons of disease trends across various times and regions.

3. Sudden increases or decreases in the reported rates of disease might be due to changes in coding practices or case definitions. Artifactual fluctuations in the rate of a disease are especially likely when the ICD is revised and when surveillance case definitions are altered.

REFERENCES

Centers for Disease Control and Prevention [CDC]. (1986). Classification system for human T-lymphotropic virus type III/lymphadenopathy-associated virus infection. *MMWR*, 35, 334–339.

Centers for Disease Control and Prevention [CDC]. (1987). Revision of the CDC surveillance case definition for acquired immunodeficiency syndrome. *MMWR*, 36, 1S–15S.

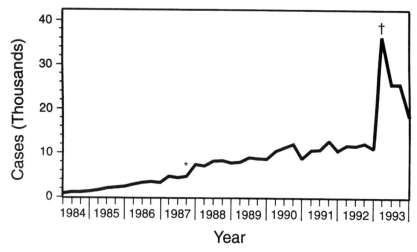

Figure 5.2. AIDS cases by quarter year of report, United States, 1984–1993. (Source: CDC, 1994, p. 827.) *Case definition revised in October 1987 to include additional illnesses and to revise diagnostic criteria. †Case definition revised in 1993 to include CD4+ criteria and three additional illnesses.

Centers for Disease Control and Prevention [CDC]. (1992a). 1993 Revised classification system for HIV infection and expanded surveillance case definition for AIDS among adolescents and adults. *MMWR*, 41, No. RR-17.

Centers for Disease Control and Prevention [CDC]. (1992b). *Principles of Epidemiology. Self-Study Course 303-G* (2nd ed.). Atlanta: U.S. Department of Health and Human Services.

Centers for Disease Control and Prevention [CDC]. (1994) Update: trends in AIDS diagnosis and reporting under the expanded surveillance definition for adolescents and adults—United States, 1993. *MMWR*, 43, 826–827.

Gordis, L. (1996). *Epidemiology*. Philadelphia: W. B. Saunders.

Health Care Financing Administration. (1989). *The International Classification of Diseases—9th Revision–Clinical Modification (ICD-9-CM)* (3rd ed.) (DHHS Publication No. PHS 89-1260). Washington, DC: U.S. Government Printing Office.

Henning, R., & Lundman, T. (1975). Swedish co-operative CCU study. A study of 2008 patients with acute myocardial infarction from twelve Swedish hospitals with coronary care units. *Acta Medica Scandinavica*, Supplement 586.

Holmes, G. P., Kaplan, J. E., Gantz, N. M., Komaroff, A. L., Schonberger, L. B., Straus, S. E., et al. (1988). Chronic fatigue syndrome: a working case definition. *Annals of Internal Medicine*, 108, 387–389.

Kannel, W. B., Dawber, T. R., Kagan, A., Revotskie, N., & Stokes, J. III. (1961). Factors of risk in the development of coronary heart disease—six-year follow-up experience. The Framingham Study. *Annals of Internal Medicine*, 55, 33–50.

Klonoff, D. C. (1992). Chronic fatigue syndrome. *Clinical Infectious Diseases*, 15, 812–823.

National Center for Health Statistics. (1964). *Vital and Health Statistics. Analytic Studies. The Change in Mortality Trend in the United States*. (U.S. Public Health Service Publication No. 1000, Series 3, Number 1). Washington, DC: U.S. Government Printing Office.

Schluederberg, A., Straus, S. E., Peterson, P., Blumenthal, S., Komaroff, A. L., Spring, S. B., et al. (1992). Chronic fatigue syndrome research: definition and medical outcome assessment. *Annals of Internal Medicine*, 117, 325–331.

World Health Organization [WHO]. (1990). *Tenth Revision of the International Classification of Diseases*. Geneva: World Health Organization.

6

Measures of Disease Frequency

Quantifying disease frequency is central to modern epidemiologic practice. Epidemiologists use two main measures of disease frequency: prevalence and incidence. Prevalence is the proportion of people having a disease or condition at a particular time. Incidence may be measured as a proportion (cumulative incidence) or rate (incidence density) and represents the likelihood of developing a disease or condition over a given period of time.

6.1 BACKGROUND

The Inadequacy of Simple Counts

As a background to our discussion of prevalence and incidence, we must first address the inadequacy of a simple count of cases. A simple count of cases without some meaningful reference is seldom useful in epidemiology. For example, suppose we find that there are more fatal motor vehicle accidents in green cars than in cars of any other color. Does this imply that green cars present a greater driving hazard? Probably not. It may simply reflect the greater number of green cars on the road. To derive a meaningful result, we must convert the count to a proportion or rate. Only then can rational comparisons be made.

Wallis and Roberts (1962) provide additional illustrations of the essential nature of proportions and rates:

> During World War II, about 375,000 people were killed within the United States by accidents, and about 480,000 were killed in the armed forces. From these figures, it has been argued that it was not much more dangerous to be overseas in the armed forced than to be at home. A more meaningful comparison, however, would consider risk, not mere numbers of deaths, and would further consider the age distributions within each group. This comparison would reflect adversely on the safety of the armed forces during the war—in fact, the armed forces death rate (about 12 per thousand men per year) was 15 to 20 times as high as the overall civilian death rates from accidents (about 0.7 per thousand per year). Peacetime versions of the same fallacy are also common: "Homes are more dangerous than places of work,

since more accidents occur at home." "Beds are the most dangerous things in the world, because more people die in bed than anywhere else." "Sick people are more likely to die when cared for in hospitals than when cared for at home." (p. 103)*

This does not imply that case counts are always useless; there are valid ways to use counts, but every case count must have a valid reference, and a valid reference must be placed in proper context.

Probability of Selected Events

The probability of an event describes its relative frequency in the population. Without the quantification of probabilities, perceptions of day-to-day hazards are often misinformed. Consider the data reported in Table 6.1. This table provides several guideposts by which to judge hazards and risks. For instance, most people would agree that being struck by lightning is a rarity of little day to day concern. This is because it occurs in only 1 in 2 million people per year. In contrast, death due to any cause occurs in 1 in 110 per year.

TABLE 6.1. Risks of Selected Events

Event	Annual Risk		
	per 100,000	Unicohort[a]	Logarithmic[b]
Kidnaping by strangers[c]	0.02	1 in 5,000,000	−6.7
Aircraft fatality on scheduled U.S. carriers[d]	0.04	1 in 2,500,000	−6.4
Death by lightning[e]	0.05	1 in 2,000,000	−6.3
Death by bicycle crash[e]	1	1 in 100,000	−5.0
Death by homicide, United Kingdom, 1964[f]	1	1 in 100,000	−5.0
Death by homicide and legal intervention, United States, 1992[g]	10	1 in 10,000	−4.0
Death by motor vehicle crash, United States, 1988[h]	20	1 in 5,000	−3.7
Premature death due to smoking, United States[c]	120	1 in 830	−2.9
Death by heart disease, United States, 1992[g]	287	1 in 350	−2.5
Death, any cause, United States, 1992[g]	870	1 in 110	−2.1

[a]Average number of people needed to find one case = 1/risk. Unicohort risks are reported using two-significant-figure accuracy.
[b]The logarithm of a number is the power to which 10 must be raised to equal the value in question. For example, the logarithm of 100 is 2, since $10^2 = 100$. The logarithm of 1/100 is −2, because $10^{-2} = 1/10^2 = 1/100$. Like the Richter scale, the logarithm of the risk provides an order of magnitude of measure.
[c]*Source:* Paulos (1988), p. 95.
[d]Estimated based on approximately 100 such deaths annually divided by the approximate U.S. population of 250 million.
[e]*Source:* Paulos (1988), p. 97.
[f]*Source:* Inman (1964).
[g]Crude death rate based on number of deaths reported by the National Center for Health Statistics [NCHS] (1995, p. 101) divided by the approxiamte U.S. resident population of 250 million.
[h]*Source:* Age-adjusted death rate, NCHS (1995), p. 97.

(This is for people of all ages and, of course, the risk varies with age.) In viewing a specific cause of death, we note that death by homicide in the United States occurs 10 times more frequently than in Britain (1 in 10,000 compared with 1 in 100,000), and more than 10 times *less* frequently than premature death due to smoking (1 in 830). The most common cause of death in the United States is heart disease, which kills approximately 1 in 350 people per year.

Also, from Table 6.1, we surmise that people are more fearful of small risks they cannot control than substantial risks they feel in control of. For example, the fear of (and fascination with) a fatal accident associated with commercial air travel (1 in 2.5 million per year) is out of proportion with the reality, especially if one considers the rate of motor vehicle fatalities by comparison (1 in 5000). It is also said that the risk associated with driving to most surgical procedures outweighs the risks of the operative procedure itself (although I suppose it depends on your current state of health, the skill of the anesthetist and surgeon, and the operative procedure in question). Perhaps the media have played a role in shaping our misconceived notions of risk, or perhaps it is the public's general misunderstanding of numbers (see Paulos, 1988). In any event, as epidemiologists, we must develop a firm understanding of measuring the likelihood of disease and health-related events, and this can only be achieved by studying proportions and rates.

Proportions and Rates

Both proportions and rates are composed of **numerators** and **denominators.** They differ, however, in their mathematical construct.

Proportions are fractions in which the numerator is included in the denominator. As such, they are unitless numbers ranging between 0 and 1.0. Proportions are frequency expressed as a percentage. To get a percentage, you multiply the proportion by 100. For example, if a study has 537 people and 136 of these people have disease X, the proportion of people with disease X is .253 (136/537) or 25.3%.

Rates, too, are composed of a numerator and denominator. The numerator and denominator of rates, however, are measured in different units. For example, a familiar rate is "velocity," in which the numerator is a measure of distance (e.g., miles) and the denominator is a measure of time (e.g., hours). When combined (e.g., miles per hour), these form a rate measured in "distance per time" units. Rates represent an instantaneous potential for change. Therefore, some knowledge of calculus is necessary to fully appreciate (true) rates. To avoid this discussion, however, we will restrict our consideration to average rates, which are easily addressed arithmetically.

The **dimension** of a number refers to its units of measure. Note that proportions are dimensionless, having no units. (Numerator and denominator units cancel, leaving a dimensionless number.) Rates, however, are tied to their initial units of measure. For example, a speed of 60 miles per hour must be expressed in its initial units or converted appropriately. (A speed of 60 miles per hour, for example, is equal to 1 mile per minute or approximately 97 kilometers per hour.) Although a proportion has a limited range of 0 to 1.0, a rate, in theory, has no upper bound.

In epidemiology, average rates can be expressed as the number of new cases per unit time of observation. For example, if a study has 100 people and 10 of these people develop disease X during one year of observation, the rate of disease X is 1 per 100 people per year or .01 per person-year.

6.2 PREVALENCE

Prevalence is a proportion that expresses the relative frequency of a disease or condition at a particular time. As such, it is cross-sectional, involving no real follow-up. **Point prevalence** is the total number of instances of a condition in the population at a particular point in time divided by the total population size. **Period prevalence** is the total number of instances of a condition during a particular period divided by the total population size at the midpoint of the observation period. The formula for prevalence (*P*) is

$$P = \frac{\text{number of cases}}{\text{number of people in the population}} \tag{6.1}$$

As a proportion, prevalence will always fall between zero and one.

Illustration Suppose we examine 1000 people and determine that 100 of them have disease X. The prevalence of disease X is

$$P = \frac{100 \text{ people}}{1000 \text{ people}} = .1$$

By convention, prevalence is often expressed in terms of a population unit multiplier. For example, we might want to express the calculated prevalence "per 100 people" or "per 1000 people." To express prevalence in this fashion, formula 6.1 is modified as follows:

$$P \text{ (per } m) = \frac{x}{n} \cdot m \tag{6.2}$$

where x represents the number of cases, n represents the number of people in the population, and m represents a population unit multiplier (usually 100, 1000, 10,000, or 100,000). For example, to express the previous illustration using a multiplier of 100, we calculate

$$P = \frac{100}{1000} \cdot 100 = 10 \text{ per } 100$$

Although prevalence is cross-sectional, with no real accounting for follow-up time, it still represents a dynamic measure that can change over time. This is because it depends on a constant inflow of new cases and outflow of old cases. The dynamics of prevalence can be represented by the fluid level in a basin (Fig. 6.1). Water is continually flowing into the basin while the basin drains through a conduit. The inflow of water represents **incident** (new) cases, while the outflow of water represents case resolution through recovery or death. The water level represents the prevalence of disease in the population. An increase in prevalence can result from increases in inflow (i.e., increased incidence) or decreases in outflow (i.e., increases in the duration of disease).

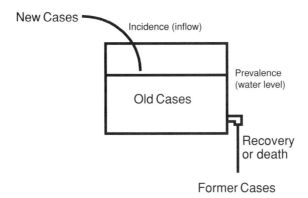

Figure 6.1. *Relationship between incidence, prevalence, recovery, and death.*

6.3 INTRODUCTION TO INCIDENCE

Incidence is used to reflect the probability of developing a disease or condition over a given period of time. As such, it is a measure that must account for time of follow-up. Incidence can be measured as a proportion or rate. Because common usage of the term "rate" has blurred the distinction between proportions and rates (these terms are mistakenly used interchangeably), we use the term **cumulative incidence** to refer to incidence measured by means of a proportion and **incidence density** to refer to incidence measured as a rate.

Moreover, the terms incidence and prevalence are often misused. These are distinct measures that should not be confused. The primary distinction between incidence and prevalences is this: incidence reflects the probability of developing a disease, while prevalence reflects the probability of already having it. Other distinctions between incidence and prevalence are listed in Table 6.2.

6.4 CUMULATIVE INCIDENCE (INCIDENCE PROPORTION)

Cumulative incidence is the proportion of people in a population who develop a disease within a specific interval. Synonyms for cumulative incidence are **incidence proportion, attack rate, incidence risk,** and **average risk of disease.** The term attack rate is especially relevant when dealing with a localized epidemic.

TABLE 6.2. Comparison of Incidence and Prevalence

Incidence	Prevalence
Probability of developing disease	Probability of already having disease
Numerator counts only new cases	Numerator counts both new and old cases
Requires follow-up of individuals in the population	Does not require follow-up
Does not depend on the duration of illness	Depends on duration of disease (long duration will eventually increase the prevalence of a disease)
Preferred measure when studying cause and effect	Preferred measure when estimating the population-based burden of a chronic disease

In estimating cumulative incidence, the candidate population consists of disease-free subjects at the beginning of the study. The follow-up interval for cumulative incidence varies but is usually the same for all members of the study population and is often dictated by the type of disease being studied. For example, for a point-source outbreak, the time at risk is conveniently defined as the duration of the epidemic. Cumulative incidence may also be used to calculate the life-time risk of an event.

Cumulative incidence (*CI*) can be calculated with the formula

$$CI = \frac{\text{no. of new cases that develop during the study period}}{\text{no. of individuals at risk at the beginning of the study period}} \quad (6.3)$$

Note that the denominator includes only disease-free ("at risk") subjects, thus excluding preexisting ("prevalent") cases and people who are unable to get the disease for other reasons (e.g., we would certainly exclude women from a study of prostate cancer).

Illustration   Suppose we start a study with 1000 subjects. One hundred of these subjects have disease X at the beginning of the investigation and 200 new cases develop during the follow-up interval. The cumulative incidence is therefore,

$$CI = \frac{200 \text{ people}}{(1000 - 100) \text{ people}} = .222$$

Notes   The denominator of this cumulative incidence calculation excludes the 100 prevalent cases because they are not at risk of developing the disease. From a practical point of view, removal of nonsusceptibles from the denominator is important only when the prevalence of disease is high (say, affecting at least 5% of the population).

The duration of the investigation is an important determinant of cumulative incidence; longer follow-up of study subjects allows more time for cases to develop. Therefore, when comparing cumulative incidence studies, make certain that the studies were of comparable duration.

Cumulative incidence, like prevalence, is often expressed through a population unit multiplier. To express cumulative incidence with a population multiplier, use formula 6.4:

$$CI \text{ (per } m) = \frac{x}{n'} \cdot m \quad (6.4)$$

where *CI* represents cumulative incidence, *x* represents the number of new cases that develop over the study period, *n'* represents the number of individuals at risk of developing the disease during the same period, and *m* represents a population multiplier (usually 100, 1000, 10,000, or 100,000). To express the cumulative incidence in the above illustration with a multiplier of 100, the cumulative incidence is calculated as

$$CI = \frac{200}{1000 - 100} \cdot 100 = 22.2 \text{ per } 100$$

6.5 INCIDENCE DENSITY (INCIDENCE RATE)

Incidence density (ID) is the rate at which new events occur in population. Synonyms for incidence density include **incidence rate, instantaneous risk, instantaneous probability, hazard rate, person-time incidence rate,** and **the force of morbidity.**

Because incidence density is a rate, its numerator and denominator use different units of measurement. Generally, the numerator of incidence density represents the number of people developing a disease or condition. The denominator generally represents disease-free time of follow-up, although other units of risk are possible (e.g., passenger-miles when measuring risks related to travel, pack-years when measuring risks related to smoking).

The incidence density of an event is calculated as the number of new cases divided by the total person-time at risk:

$$ID = \frac{\text{number of new cases}}{\text{disease-free person-time at risk}} \qquad (6.5)$$

The disease-free person-time (*PT*) is calculated by summing time at risk for all study subjects:

$$PT = \sum_{i=1}^{n'} \Delta t_i \qquad (6.6)$$

where Δt_i is the duration of observation time for the ith individual from entry into the study until disease or withdrawal. Withdrawal, also referred to as **truncation of observation time,** may result from any of the following:

· Migration out of the study area
· Refusal to participate further
· Termination of the study
· Other conditions that remove the study subject from risk (e.g., hysterectomy in a study of uterine disease, discontinuation of oral contraceptive use in a study of oral contraceptive-associated risk)

An example of summing person-time is illustrated in Figure 6.2. In this illustration there are 17 person-years of observation (subject A contributes 1 person-year, subject B contributes 2 person-years, subject C contributes 4 person-years, etc.). During this period, one new case develops (subject B) and the incidence density is

$$ID = \frac{1 \text{ person}}{17 \text{ person-years}} = 0.058 \text{ year}^{-1}$$

By convention, this is reported as 0.058 per **person-year.** Also by convention, incidence densities are reported using a population unit multiplier of 100, 1000, 10,000, or 100,000. The formula incorporating the unit multiplier is

$$ID \text{ (per } m) = \frac{x}{PT} \cdot m \qquad (6.7)$$

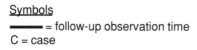

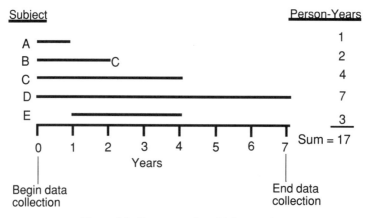

Figure 6.2. Representation of follow-up time.

where x represents the number of new cases that develop during the time of observation, PT represents the disease-free person-time at risk, and m represents the unit multiplier. We recalculate the above illustrative incidence density data incorporating a unit multiplier of 1000 person-years as follows:

$$ID = \frac{1}{17} \cdot 1000 = 58 \text{ per 1000 person-years}$$

Approximate Methods of Calculating Person-Time   If all subjects in a study are followed for the same length of time, person-time can be calculated as follows:

$$PT = (n')(\Delta t) \tag{6.8}$$

where n' represents the number of individuals at risk at the beginning of the study and Δt represents average follow-up time per individual. Note that formula 6.8 does not require knowledge of follow-up times for individual study subjects. It does assume, however, that the population is stable (so that the size and age distribution of the population remains constant over the duration of the study) and the incidence density does not vary over time (so-called **constant hazard**). Furthermore, if the disease under study is rare and hazards are constant, the size of the population at risk (n') is approximately equal to the size of the total population (n), thus permitting us to calculate person-time as the product of total population size and duration of the study. For example, if 600 healthy subjects are studied for 1 year, this would account for 600×1 year = 600 person-years; if 600 subjects were studied for 2 years, this would account for approximately 600×2 years = 1200 person-years, and so on.

Although this chapter presents two mathematically distinct methods for measuring incidences (incidence density and cumulative incidence) this distinction is blurred in practice. This is because *when the cumulative incidence of disease is low* (say, $<.1$),

$$CI \approx ID(\Delta) \tag{6.9}$$

(Kleinbaum et al., 1982, p. 108). For example, a 1-year incidence study that calculates a cumulative incidence of 1 per 1000 would also exhibit an incidence density of approximately 1 per 1000 person-years. This would explain the lack of distinction in utilization of the words "risk" and "rate." In theory, however, the term risk should be reserved for cumulative incidence measures and the term rate should be reserved for incidence density measures.

In practice, the choice of an incidence measure is usually based on pragmatic considerations. Cumulative incidence is well suited for the study of acute diseases with restricted risk periods (i.e., short studies, such as studies of outbreaks), while incidence density seems better suited for studies of chronic diseases with extended risk periods. In addition, incidence density is easily adapted to studies in **dynamic populations** (population in which people frequently leave and enter), while cumulative incidence is well suited for studies of **fixed populations** (populations in which membership is relatively stable). The advantage of using incidence density methods in a dynamic population is related to its ability to adjust follow-up time on a person-by-person basis. Although similar type adjustments are possible with cumulative incidence measures when using **life-table** or **actuarial methods,** life-table methods are more tedious to calculate and are less easily understood than person-time methods.

SUMMARY

1. Epidemiologic measures of disease frequency are used to characterize the occurrence of disease, disability, and death in human populations. They enable us to assess objectively how common a disease or health-related event is in relation to the size of a population. Epidemiologists use two main measures of disease frequency: prevalence and incidence. Prevalence is measured as a proportion; incidence may be measured as a proportion (cumulative incidence) or rate (incidence density) (Table 6.3).

2. Prevalence is a proportion that expresses the probability of having a disease or condition at a particular time. As a proportion, it will always fall between zero and one (inclusive). It is common practice, however, to express prevalence through a unit multiplier, such as "per 1000," "per 1000," and so on. Although prevalence is cross-sectional, involving no real follow-up, it is still a dynamic measure that can change over time. The prevalence of disease depends on the rate of inflow of new (incident) cases and the rate of outflow of old (prevalent) cases through recovery or death.

3. Cumulative incidence is the proportion of people in a population who develop a disease within a specified interval. A cumulative incidence is calculated by counting the number of new cases that develop during the study and dividing this number by the number of disease-free subjects at the beginning of the study. In theory, the denominator includes only disease-free people at risk at the beginning of the study. However, when the disease is rare, this value will be similar to the total population size, thus making adjustment of the denominator unnecessary.

TABLE 6.3. Summary of Disease Frequency Measures

Frequency Measure	Symbol	Mathematical Construct	Units
Prevalence	P	Proportion	None
Cumulative incidence	CI	Proportion	None
Incidence density	ID	Rate	Person-time or other unit of risk (e.g., pack-years)

4. Incidence density is the rate at which new cases develop in the population. It is calculated as the number of new cases divided by the total person-time at risk. Person-time at risk can be calculated in two ways. First, we can sum the individual units of time people are under observation. Second, we can multiply the number of people in the study by the average disease-free time of follow-up.

NOTATION AND FORMULA REFERENCE

x Number of cases (numerator of prevalence and incidence)
m Population multiplier (100, 1000, 10,000, or 100,000)
n Population size
n' Population size adjusted to include only those individuals at risk of the disease
Δt_i Follow-up time, study subject i
Δ Duration of study
P Prevalence (definitional formula: 6.1; calculation formula: 6.2)
CI Cumulative incidence (definitional formula: 6.3; calculation formula: 6.4)
ID Incidence density (definitional formula: 6.5; calculation formula: 6.7)
PT Population person-time (exact formula: 6.6; approximate formula: 6.8)

EXERCISES

1. Consider the schematic in Figure 6.3. Assume the disease in question is an infectious disease that confers lifelong immunity upon recovery. There are no exclusions or withdrawals from the study.

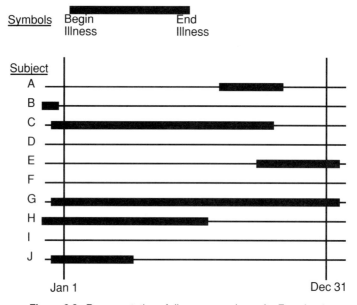

Figure 6.3. *Representation of disease experience for Exercise 1.*

(A) What is the point prevalence on January 1?

(B) What is the point prevalence on December 31?

(C) What is the period prevalence for the interval January 1 to December 31?

(D) What is the cumulative incidence for the period January 1 to December 31?

2. A study of coronary heart disease (CHD) begins with 1000 40- to 45-year-old men. Of these, 50 already have detectable CHD. The remaining 950 are followed for 5 years, during which 64 men develop CHD.

(A) Calculate the prevalence (per 100) of CHD at the beginning of the study.

(B) Calculate the 5-year cumulative incidence (per 100) of CHD.

(C) Calculate the approximate incidence density (per 100 person-years).

3. Formulas for selected public health rates are reported below:

$$\text{Crude birth rate (per } m) = \frac{\text{number of births}}{\text{total population}} \times m \qquad (6.10)$$

$$\text{Crude death rate (per } m) = \frac{\text{number of deaths}}{\text{total population}} \times m \qquad (6.11)$$

$$\text{Infant mortality rate (per } m) = \frac{\text{no. of deaths} <1 \text{ year of age}}{\text{number of live births}} \times m \qquad (6.12)$$

$$\text{Age-specific death rate (per } m) = \frac{\text{no. of deaths in age group}}{\text{no. of people in age group}} \times m \qquad (6.13)$$

$$\text{Cause-specific death rate (per } m) = \frac{\text{no. deaths due to cause}}{\text{total population}} \times m \qquad (6.14)$$

Using the formulas and data presented in Table 6.4, calculate each of the following statistics:

(A) crude birth rate per 100

(B) crude death rate per 100

(C) infant mortality rate per 100

(D) age-specific death rate for people over 65 years of age, per 100

(E) cause-specific death rate for heart disease per 100

(F) cause-specific death rate for cancer per 100

TABLE 6.4. Vital Statistics and Data for Exercise 3

Total midyear population	100,000
Population size, 65 years of age or older	25,000
Number of infants born alive	3,000
Total deaths (all causes)	1,500
Deaths of infants under 1 year of age	50
Deaths of persons 65 years of age and over	1,000
Deaths from heart disease	300
Deaths from cancer	100

TABLE 6.5. Data from an Outbreak of Acute Nausea and Vomiting at a Banquet

Food Item	Ill Ate Food	Ill Did Not Eat Food	Not Ill Ate Food	Not Ill Did Not Eat Food
Macaroni and cheese	20	5	60	15
Ham	25	0	55	20
Cabbage salad	10	15	45	30
Rolls	12	13	38	37
Coffee	20	5	65	10
Milk	3	22	8	67
Ice cream	25	0	75	0

4. Data presented in Table 6.5 are from an outbreak of gastroenteritis among 100 people attending a banquet.

   (A) Using formula 6.15, calculate the attack rate associated with *each* food. (An attack rate is a form of cumulative incidence.)

$$\text{Attack rate, food X} = \frac{\text{no. people eating food X who became ill}}{\text{total no. of people eating food X}} \quad (6.15)$$

   (B) Using formula 6.16, calculate the attack rate associated with *not* eating *each* food.

$$\text{Attack rate, not eating food X} = \frac{\text{no. people not eating food X who became ill}}{\text{total no. of people not eating food X}} \quad (6.16)$$

   (C) Based on these data, what food is the most likely source of the agent?

5. What effect will each of the following have on the prevalence of a disease, assuming the population in question does not otherwise change?

   (A) immigration of cases into the study area
   (B) emigration of cases out of the study area
   (C) emigration of healthy persons out of the study area
   (D) immigration of healthy persons into the study area
   (E) increases in the case fatality rate

6. Based on the vital statistics reported in Table 6.6, compute each of the following:

   (A) crude birth rate (per 100)
   (B) crude death rate (per 100)
   (C) infant mortality rate (per 100)

7. A treatment is developed that prolongs the life of people suffering from a particular chronic disease.

   (A) How does this affect the incidence of disease?
   (B) How does this affect the prevalence?

TABLE 6.6. Vital Statistics for the United States, 1992

Population size[a]	255,078,000
Approximate number of live births[b]	4,065,014
Number of deaths (all ages)[c]	2,175,631
Approximate number of deaths in infants under 1 year of age[d]	34,553

[a]Source: NCHS (1995), p. 63.
[b]Source: NCHS (1995), p. 66.
[c]Source: NCHS (1995), p. 101.
[d]Source: NCHS (1995), p. 104.

8. According to the *Statistical Abstract of the United States* (U.S. Bureau of the Census, 1995), in 1993, there were approximately 40,100 traffic fatalities. During this year, there were approximately 2297 billion miles traveled in vehicles.

(A) What is the incidence density of traffic fatalities per 100 million miles traveled?

(B) The worldwide airline fatality rate in 1993 was 0.05 fatalities per 100 million miles flown on scheduled air transportation flights. How does this compare to the risk of traffic fatalities calculated in part A above?

9. Data on accidents in hospitalized patients are reported in Table 6.7. The article from which data were reported stated: "Statistical analysis by patient age group reveals that patients 62 years and older are most prone to accidents. The next greatest risk occurs among the 6 to 14 age group." Comment on this interpretation.

ANSWERS TO EXERCISES

1. A $\quad P_{\text{Jan.1}} = 4/10 = 40\%$.

B $\quad P_{\text{Dec. 31}} = 2/10 = 20\%$.

C $\quad P_{\text{Jan. 1–Dec. 31}} = 6/10 = 60\%$.

D $\quad CI_{\text{Jan. 1–Dec. 31}} = 2/5 = 40\%$.

TABLE 6.7. Age Distribution of 82 Injured Patients

Age (years)	Number of Accidents
0–2	5
3–5	6
6–14	18
15–21	8
22–31	5
32–41	8
42–51	7
52–61	4
62 and over	21

2. A $P = 5$ per 100.
   B $CI = 6.7$ per 100.
   C $ID = 1.3$ per 100 person-years.

3. A Crude birth rate = 3 per 100.
   B Crude death rate = 1.5 per 100.
   C Infant mortality rate = 1.7 per 100.
   D Age-specific death rate, 65 years of age and above = 4.0 per 100.
   E Heart disease-specific death rate = 0.3 per 100.
   F Cancer-specific death rate = 0.1 per 100.

4. A See Table 6.8, column 2.
   B See Table 6.8, column 3.
   C The food demonstrating the biggest difference in attack rates is the ham (31% versus 0%). This makes ham the prime suspect.

5. A Increase.
   B Decrease.
   C Potential increase (but a lot of healthy people would have to leave the population for one to see an effect).
   D Potential decrease (once again, a lot of healthy people would have to enter the population for one to see an effect).
   E Decrease.

6. A 1.59 per 100.
   B 0.85 per 100.
   C 0.85 per 100.

7. A It has no influence on incidence (incidence only counts new cases).
   B It will increase the prevalence of the disease (prevalence = incidence × duration).

8. A 1.75 fatalities per 100 million passenger-miles.
   B The risk of death per passenger-mile during scheduled air transportation mile is approximately 35 times smaller than the risk of death in a car.

9. This interpretation is incorrect. The reported statistics are based on simple case counts with no reported denominator. Therefore, the data do not represent risk and should not be interpreted as such.

TABLE 6.8. Answers to Exercise 4

Food	(Answers to 4A) Attack Rates in Those Eating the Food Ill/Total (%)	(Answers to 4B) Attack Rates in Those Not Eating the Food Ill/Total (%)
Macaroni and cheese	20/80 (25%)	5/20 (25%)
Ham	25/80 (31%)	0/20 (0%)
Cabbage salad	10/55 (18%)	15/45 (33%)
Rolls	12/50 (24%)	13/50 (26%)
Coffee	20/85 (24%)	5/15 (33%)
Milk	3/11 (27%)	22/89 (25%)
Ice cream	25/100 (25%)	0/0 (undefined)

REFERENCES

Inman, W. H. M. (1964). Risks in medical intervention: balancing therapeutic risks and benefits. *Wolfson College Lecture, University of Southampton Drug Surveillance Research Unit, Prescription Event Monitoring News,* 2, 16–37.

Kleinbaum, D. G., Kupper, L. L., & Morgenstern, H. (1982). *Epidemiologic Research: Principles and Quantitative Methods.* New York: Van Nostrand Reinhold.

National Center for Health Statistics [NCHS]. (1995). *Health, United States, 1994* (DHHS Publication No. (PHS) 95-1232). Washington, DC: U.S. Government Printing Office.

Paulos, J. A. (1988). *Innumeracy. Mathematical Illiteracy and Its Consequences.* New York: Hill and Wang.

U.S. Bureau of the Census. (1995). *Statistical Abstracts of the United States (115th edition): 1995.* Washington, DC: U.S. Government Printing Office.

Wallis, W. A., & Roberts, H. V. (1962). *The Nature of Statistics.* New York: The Free Press.

7

Stratification and Adjustment

In the last chapter we considered incidence and prevalence for an entire population. In this chapter we divide the population into age groups so that comparisons of "like to like" can be made. This chapter introduces two methods for combining age-specific rates to derive a single adjusted rate that compensates for age differences in populations.

7.1 INTRODUCTION

Note: Because methods in this chapter apply equally to prevalence, cumulative incidence, and incidence density, we will use the term **rate** and **risk** to refer to all three. This will allow for the presentation of formulas and ideas without unnecessary redundancy.

Age influences the risk of most diseases. Comparisons of risk must therefore be based on comparably aged populations. Otherwise, observed differences could be **confounded** by age and comparisons will be **biased.** (The term "bias," as used by epidemiologists, implies a systematic error in inference, *not* an imputation of prejudice due to partisanship or other factors—see Table 7.1 for this and other definitions.) The problem of relying on rates for the entire population—**crude rates**—is exemplified by the hypothetical data presented in Table 7.2. This table contains incidence density data for two different populations **stratified** by age. The stratification process divides a population into subgroups based on the extraneous "stratification" factor, in this case age. Each subgroup is called a **stratum** or, more specifically in this instance, an **age stratum.** From the crude data, it appears as if population B in Table 7.2 has a crude rate that is almost 10 times higher than that of population A (991 per 100,000 versus 109 per 100,000, respectively). Yet, when one compares rates within age strata, rates are identical. The explanation for this apparent paradox is that population B is much older than population A. Given that age is a strong predictor of this disease, population B's much higher crude rate is attributable to its difference in age and not to any underlying difference in risk.

TABLE 7.1. Definitions of Selected Terms

Bias: a systematic error in inference
Confounding: the type of bias that comes about because of the effects of extraneous factors
Crude rate: a rate for the entire population
Stratum: a subgroup in a population defined by a specified criterion such as age, sex, or race
Stratum-specific rate: a rate for a population subgroup
Adjusted rate: a rate that has been mathematically or statistically manipulated so that the effects of differences in composition of the populations being compared have been minimized
Study population: the population for which rates are being adjusted
Reference population: an external population that provides an age (or other) distribution for adjustment procedures
Standard million: an age distribution for a million citizens selected at random from the reference population

We have two general options to compensate for this difference in age. First, we can restrict our comparisons to similarly aged subgroups (i.e., age-specific comparisons). This can be confusing, however, especially when many age strata exist and comparisons are made between many different populations. Combining age-specific rates to derive a single adjusted rate is therefore often desirable. The adjusted rate can then be trusted in a head-to-head comparison with other age-adjusted rates.

Age adjustment can be achieved in several ways. The two most common approaches are by direct and indirect weighting of strata-specific rates. We start by considering direct adjustment.

7.2   DIRECT ADJUSTMENT

Direct age adjustment is a statistical procedure used to eliminate the effect of differences in the age distributions of populations being compared. This method uses the age distribution of an external **reference population** as the basis for comparison. The specific reference population used for this purpose is usually unimportant but must be consistent within a given set of comparisons. The age distribution of the U.S. population as a whole is frequently used for this purpose. A **standard million** U.S. age distribution (age distribution for a million citizens picked at random) for the year 1991 is listed in Table 7.3. If a reliable external reference population is unavailable, we may combine the age distributions of the study populations to derive an arbitrary reference distribution. A combined age distribution of this type for the hypothetical data in Table 7.2 is shown in Table 7.4.

TABLE 7.2. Incidence Densities in Two Hypothetical Populations Stratified by Age

| Age (years) | Population A | | | Population B | | |
	Cases	Person-years	Incidence Density (per 100,000 person-years)	Cases	Person-years	Incidence Density (per 100,000 person-years)
0–34	99	99,000	100	1	1,000	100
35+	10	1,000	1,000	990	99,000	1,000
All	109	100,000	109	991	100,000	991

TABLE 7.3. Standard Million Age Distribution for the Year 1991, United States

Age Group	Standard Million
0–4	76,158
5–24	286,501
25–44	325,971
45–64	185,402
65–74	72,494
75+	53,474
Total	1,000,000

Source: U.S. Bureau of the Census (1994), p. 14.

Direct adjustment is a procedure for creating a weighted average of the age-specific rates from a **study population** (the population for which rates are being adjusted) based on the age distribution of a reference population. This gives us the hypothetical rate of disease expected in the reference population if it were to experience those same age-specific rates as the study population. The formula for direct age adjustment is

$$aR(direct) = \frac{\sum_{i=1}^{k} N_i r_i}{\sum_{i=1}^{k} N_i} \tag{7.1}$$

where $aR(direct)$ represents the adjusted rate by the direct method, subscript i represents the stratum counter (there are k strata), N_i represents the number of people in stratum i of the reference population, r_i represents the rate of disease in stratum i of the study population, and Σ denotes the summation operator defined as $\Sigma_{i=1}^{k} N_i = N_1 + N_2 + \cdots + N_k$. Note that capital letters (N_i) denote values that come from the reference population and small letters (r_i) denote values from the study population. Also, be aware that multiplication takes precedence over addition in the order of mathematical operations, so that $\Sigma_{i=1}^{k} N_i r_i = (N_1 r_1) + (N_2 r_2) + \cdots + (N_k r_k)$.

We consider death rates in Alaska and Florida to illustrate the use of this formula. Data are presented in Table 7.5. Note that the crude death rate (cR) per 100,000 Alaska residents is 387 and the crude death rate per 100,000 Floridians is 1026. Based on these crude rates it might appear that Floridians are at much higher risk of death than

TABLE 7.4. Combined Age Distribution of the Hypothetical Populations Presented in Table 7.2

Age (years)	Population A person-years	Population B person-years	Combined person-years
0–34	99,000	1,000	100,000
35+	1,000	99,000	100,000

TABLE 7.5. Vital Statistics for Alaska and Florida, 1991

Age (years)	Alaska		Florida	
	Deaths[a]	Population[b]	Deaths[c]	Population[b]
0–4	122	57,000	2,177	915,000
5–24	144	179,000	2,113	3,285,000
25–44	382	222,000	8,400	4,036,000
45–64	564	88,000	21,108	2,609,000
65–74	406	16,000	30,977	1,395,000
75+	582	7,000	71,483	1,038,000
Totals	2,200	569,000[d]	136,258	13,278,000[d]

[a]*Source:* NCHS (1993), p. 101.
[b]*Source:* Bureau of the Census (1992), p. 26.
[c]*Source:* NCHS (1993), p. 105. Age not stated for 35 decedents (omitted from table).
[d]Total may not sum accurately due to rounding error.
cR_{Alaska} (per 100,000 residents) = 2200/569,000 × 100,000 = 387
$cR_{Florida}$ (per 100,000 residents) = 136,258/13,278,000 × 100,000 = 1026

Alaskans. However, given Florida's proclivity for attracting retirees, we might ask if this difference is entirely due to different age distributions in the two states and, if not, then what is the size of the real difference after the effect of age has been accounted for mathematically.

The first step in adjusting for age by the direct method is to calculate age-specific death rates in both populations. These values are shown in Table 7.6. From these data, we note that age-specific death rates vary only slightly by state. Using the 1991 standard million U.S. population as the reference (Table 7.3), we compute an age-adjusted mortality rate of 843 per 100,000 in Alaska (Table 7.7) and an age-adjusted mortality rate of 784 per 100,000 in Florida (Table 7.8). Thus, the initial excess in Florida disappears and, if anything, Florida has a marginally lower mortality rate.

TABLE 7.6. Age-Specific Death Rates per 100,000 Residents for Alaska and Florida, 1991, Based on Data in Table 7.5

Stratum	Age (years)	Alaska	Florida
1	0–4	214[a]	238
2	5–24	80	64
3	25–44	172	208
4	45–64	640	809
5	65–74	2538	2221
6	75+	8314	6887

[a]Example of calculation: age-specific rate, 0–4 year-olds, Alaska, per 100,000. Data are from Table 7.5.

$$r_{stratum\ 1,\ Alaska} = \frac{deaths}{population} \times multiplier = \frac{122}{57,000} \times 100,000 = 214$$

TABLE 7.7. Calculation of the Age-Adjusted Death Rate for Alaska, 1991, Using the Standard Million from Table 7.3 as the External Reference Population

Stratum (i)	Age (years)	Rate (per 100,000) (r_i)	Standard Million (N_i)	Product ($N_i r_i$)
1	0–4	214	76,158	16,297,812
2	5–24	80	286,501	22,920,080
3	25–44	172	325,971	56,067,012
4	45–64	640	185,402	118,657,280
5	65–74	2,538	72,494	183,989,772
6	75+	8,314	53,474	444,582,836
		Column Sums→	1,000,000	842,514,792

Calculations:

$$\Sigma N_i r_i = N_1 r_1 + N_2 r_2 \cdots + N_6 r_6 = 16,297,812 + 22,920,080 + \cdots + 444,582836 = 842,514,792$$

$$\Sigma N_i = N_1 + N_2 + \cdots + N_6 = 76,158 + 286,501 + \cdots + 53,474 = 1,000,000$$

$$aR(direct) = \frac{\sum\limits_{i=1}^{k} N_i r_i}{\sum\limits_{i=1}^{k} N_i} = \frac{842,514,792}{1,000,000} \approx 843$$

7.3 INDIRECT ADJUSTMENT

The indirect method of age adjustment is used when age-specific rates are unavailable in the study population. The adjusted rate using the indirect method—*aR(indirect)*—is based on multiplying the crude rate (*cR*) in the study population by a ratio known as the standardized mortality ratio (*SMR*):

$$aR(indirect) = (cR)(SMR) \tag{7.2}$$

TABLE 7.8. Calculation of the Age-Adjusted Death Rate for Florida, Using the Standard Million from Table 7.3 as the External Reference Population

Stratum (i)	Age (years)	Rate (per 100,000) (r_i)	Standard Million (N_i)	Product ($N_i r_i$)
1	0–4	238	76,158	18,125,604
2	5–24	64	286,501	18,336,064
3	25–44	208	325,971	67,801,968
4	45–64	809	185,402	149,990,218
5	65–74	2,221	72,494	161,009,174
6	75+	6,887	53,474	368,275,438
		Column Sums→	1,000,000	783,538,466

Notation and calculation of adjusted rate:

$$\Sigma N_i r_i = N_1 r_1 + N_2 r_2 + \cdots + N_6 r_6 = 18,125,604 + 18,336,064 + \cdots + 368,275,438 = 783,538,466$$

$$\Sigma N_i = N_1 + N_2 + \cdots + N_6 = 76,158 + 286,501 + \cdots + 53,474 = 1,000,000$$

$$aR(direct) = \frac{\sum\limits_{i=1}^{k} N_i r_i}{\sum\limits_{i=1}^{k} N_i} = \frac{783,538,466}{1,000,000} \approx 784$$

TABLE 7.9. Vital Statistics for Zimbabwe

Age (years)	Deaths[a]	Population[b]	Rate (No Multiplier)
0–4	?	1,899,204	?
5–24	?	5,537,992	?
25–44	?	2,386,079	?
45–64	?	974,235	?
65–74	?	216,387	?
75+	?	136,109	?
Total	98,808	11,150,006	0.00886

[a]Data are for 1992. *Source:* United Nations (1996), p. 138.
[b]Data are for 1994. *Source:* United Nations (1996), pp. 186–187.
$cR_{Zimbabwe}$ = 98,808/11,150,006 = 0.00886 = 886 per 100,000

The *SMR* is the ratio of the observed number of cases (x) to the expected number (μ):

$$SMR = \frac{x}{\mu} \tag{7.3}$$

The expected number of cases, μ, is calculated according to formula 7.4:

$$\mu = \sum_{i=1}^{k} R_i n_i \tag{7.4}$$

where R_i represents the rate of disease in the *ith* stratum of the external reference population and n_i represents the number of people in the *ith* stratum of the study population. The product $R_i n_i$ is the expected number of cases in the *ith* stratum of the study population (μ_i), assuming the study population has the same underlying risk as the comparable stratum in the reference population. Note, once again, that capital letters (R_i) denote values that come from the reference population and small letters (n_i) denote values from the study population.

To illustrate age adjustment by the indirect method, we compare death rates in Zimbabwe and the United States. The crude death rate in Zimbabwe in the early 1990s was 886 per 100,000 (Table 7.9). The crude death rate in the United States in 1991 was 860 per 100,000 (Table 7.10). On inspection, we determine that Zimbabwe's population is much younger than the United States' (Fig. 7.1). Given the observed difference in age distributions, we might ask what the real difference in death rates is after age has been accounted for.

TABLE 7.10. Vital Statistics for United States, 1991

Age (years)	Deaths[a]	Population[b]	Rate (No Multiplier)
0–4	44,000	19,204,000	0.00229
5–24	45,000	72,244,000	0.00062
25–44	147,700	82,197,000	0.00180
45–64	368,800	46,751,000	0.00789
65–74	478,600	18,280,000	0.02618
75+	1,084,900	13,484,000	0.08046
Total	2,169,000	252,160,000	0.00860

[a]*Source:* NCHS (1993), pp. 101–102.
[b]*Source:* U.S. Bureau of the Census (1992), p. 26.
reference rate (crude U.S. mortality rate = 2,169,000/252,160,000 = 0.00860 = 860 per 100,000.

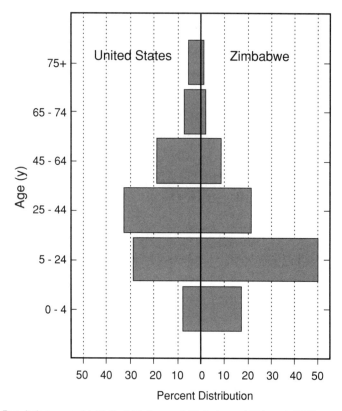

Figure 7.1. *Population pyramid, United States and Zimbabwe, 1991 and 1994, respectively. (Data sources:* U.S. Bureau of the Census, 1992; United Nations, 1996.)

Age-specific death rates in Zimbabwe are unavailable, but the age distribution of the population is known (Table 7.9). To adjust the Zimbabwe death rate using the indirect method, we apply age-specific death rates from the United States to determine the number of expected deaths in Zimbabwe. This value is used to calculate the *SMR* and the indirectly adjusted death rate (Table 7.11). The indirectly adjusted Zimbabwein death rate of 2410 per 100,000 can now be compared directly to the U.S. death rate of 860 per 100,000, showing a 2.8-fold difference in risk.

7.4 CONCLUDING REMARK

The adjustment techniques presented in this chapter apply equally to stratification by factors other than age. For example, data are routinely stratified by sex and race to derive sex-specific and race-specific rates. After stratification, adjustments are done to factor out sex and race differences between populations so that comparison can be made without concern for confounding by these factors. Thus, direct and indirect adjustment techniques provide a basic method to control for potentially biasing effects of many different kinds of extraneous factors. We will have more to say about controlling for confounding in Chapter 11.

TABLE 7.11. Calculation of the Adjusted Rate by the Indirect Method for Zimbabwe, Using the United States, 1991, as the External Reference Population

Stratum (i)	Age (years)	Rate (per 100,000) (r_i)	Standard Million (N_i)	Product ($N_i r_i$)
1	0–4	.00229	1,899,204	4,349
2	5–24	.00062	5,537,992	3,434
3	25–44	.00180	2,386,079	4,295
4	45–64	.00789	974,235	7,687
5	65–74	.02618	216,387	5,665
6	75+	.08046	136,109	10,951
			Column sum→	36,381

$cR_{Zimbabwe} = 0.00886$ (see Table 7.9)

$$\mu = \Sigma R_i n = R_1 n_1 + R_2 n_2 + \cdots + R_6 n_6 = 4349 + 3434 + \cdots + 10{,}951 = 36{,}381$$

$$\text{SMR} = \frac{x}{\mu} = \frac{98{,}808 \text{ (see table 7.9)}}{36{,}381} = 2.72$$

$$aR(indirect) = (cR)(SMR) = (0.00886)(2.72) = 0.02410 = 2410 \text{ per } 100{,}000$$

SUMMARY

1. Statistical adjustment methods are used to eliminate or reduce the confounding effects of extraneous factors (such as age) when comparing disease rates in populations. Before rates can be adjusted, data must be stratified by the extraneous factor. Stratum-specific rates are then combined to derive a single adjusted rate using either direct or indirect adjustment methods.

2. Direct age adjustment methods apply age-specific rates from study populations to an age distribution from a reference population. This provides the expected rate of disease in the reference population if it were to experience the same age-specific rates as the study population. Adjusted rates from different populations can then safely be compared without concern for differences in age.

3. The indirect method of age adjustment uses the age-specific rates from an external reference population to derive the expected number of cases in the study population. The expected count is used to calculate a standardized mortality ratio (SMR), which is then used to adjust the rate in the study population.

NOTATION AND FORMULA REFERENCE

$aR(direct)$	Adjusted rate, direct method (formula 7.1)
$aR(indirect)$	Adjusted rate, indirect method (formula 7.2)
SMR	Standardized mortality ratio (formula 7.3)
μ	Expected number of cases (formula 7.4)
cR	Crude (unadjusted) rate
i	Stratum counter (used as a subscript)
n_i	Number of people, stratum i, study population
N_i	Number of people, stratum i, reference population
r_i	Rate, stratum i, study population
R_i	Rate, stratum i, reference population
x	Observed number of cases

TABLE 7.12. Vital Statistics for California, 1991

Age (years)	Deaths[a]	Population[b]
0–4	5,500	2,651,000
5–24	5,736	8,824,000
25–44	19,178	10,539,000
45–64	38.313	5,179,000
65–74	45,306	1,874,000
75+	102,078	1,314,000
Total	215,111	7,487,000

[a]*Source:* NCHS (1993), p. 102.
[b]*Source:* U.S. Bureau of the Census (1992), p. 26.

EXERCISES

1. Table 7.12 reports vital statistics for the state of California in 1991.
   (A) Calculate the crude death rate for the state. Compare this rate to that of Florida (Table 7.5).
   (B) Calculate age-specific death rates.
   (C) Using the standard million reported in Table 7.3 as the external reference population, directly adjust California's death rate.
   (D) Compare California's adjusted death rate to that of Florida (Table 7.8).

2. Table 7.13 reports vital statistics for the state of Arkansas in 1991.
   (A) Calculate the crude death rate for the state. Compare this rate to that of Florida (Table 7.5).
   (B) Calculate age-specific death rates.
   (C) Using the standard million reported in Table 7.3 as the external reference population, directly adjust Arkansas's death rate.
   (D) Compare Arkansas's adjusted death rate to that of Florida (Table 7.8).

3. Table 7.14 reports vital statistics for Egypt.
   (A) Calculate Egypt's crude death rate. How does this compare to the 1991 U.S. crude death rate of 860 per 100,000.
   (B) Adjust Egypt's death rate using the indirect method, using the U.S. data reported in Table 7.10 as the external reference population. Interpret your results.

TABLE 7.13. Vital Statistics for Arkansas, 1991

Age (years)	Deaths[a]	Population[b]
0–4	449	170,000
5–24	562	697,000
25–44	1,459	694,000
45–64	4,072	458,000
65–74	5,466	196,000
75+	13,037	157,000
Total	25,045	2,372,000

[a]*Source:* NCHS (1993), p. 102.
[b]*Source:* U.S. Bureau of the Census (1992), p. 26.

TABLE 7.14. Vital Statistics for Egypt

Age (years)	Deaths[a]	Population[b]
0–4	?	7,909,000
5–24	?	24,560,000
25–44	?	13,764,000
45–64	?	6,921,000
65–74	?	1,485,000
75+	?	524,000
Total	416,000	55.163,000

[a]Data are for 1994. *Source:* United Nations (1996), p. 136.
[b]Data are for 1992. *Source:* United Nations (1996), pp. 178–179.

ANSWERS TO EXERCISES

1. A cR (per 100,000) = 215,111/30,381,000 × 100,000 = 708 per 100,000. This rate is substantially lower than Florida's crude death rate of 1026 per 100,000.
   B See Table 7.15, column labeled Rate (per 100,000).
   C $aR(direct)$ = 818 per 100,000.
   D California's age-adjusted death rate is slightly higher than Florida's adjusted death rate of 784 per 100,000.

2. A cR (per 100,000) = 25,045/2,372,000 × 100,000 = 1056 per 100,000. This rate is similar to Florida's crude death rate of 1026 per 100,000.
   B See Table 7.16, column labeled Rate (per 100,000).
   C $aR(direct)$ = 923 per 100,000.
   D Arkansas's age-adjusted death rate is substantially higher than Florida's adjusted death rate of 784 per 100,000.

TABLE 7.15. Calculation of the Age-Adjusted Death Rate for California, 1991, Using the Standard Million from Table 7.3 as the External Reference Population

Stratum (i)	Age (years)	Deaths	Population	Rate (per 100,000) (r_i)	Standard Million (N_i)	Product ($N_i r_i$)
1	0–4	5,500	2,651,000	207	76,158	15,800,415
2	5–24	5,736	8,824,000	65	286,501	18,623,864
3	25–44	19,178	10,539,000	182	325,971	59,317,505
4	45–64	37,313	5,179,000	720	185,402	133,576,073
5	65–74	45,306	1,874,000	2,418	72,494	175,262,175
6	75+	102,078	1,314,000	7,768	53,474	415,412,403
Column Sums→		215,111	30,381,000	708	1,000,000	817,992,435

Calculations:

$$\Sigma N_i r_i = N_1 r_1 + N_2 r_2 + \cdots + N_6 r_6 = 15,800,415 + 18,623,864 + \cdots + 415,412,403 = 817,992,435$$

$$\Sigma N_i = N_1 + N_2 + \cdots + N_6 = 76,158 + 286,501 + \cdots + 53,474 = 1,000,000$$

$$aR(direct) = \frac{\sum_{i=1}^{k} N_i r_i}{\sum_{i=1}^{k} N_i} = \frac{817,992,435}{1,000,000} \approx 818$$

TABLE 7.16. Calculation of the Age-Adjusted Death Rate for Arkansas, 1991, Using the Standard Million from Table 7.3 as the External Reference Population

Stratum (i)	Age (years)	Deaths	Population	Rate (per 100,000) (r_i)	Standard Million (N_i)	Product ($N_i r_i$)
1	0–4	449	170,000	264	76,158	20,114,672
2	5–24	562	697,000	81	286,501	23,100,941
3	25–44	1,459	694,000	210	325,971	68,529,062
4	45–64	4,072	458,000	889	185,402	164,837,761
5	65–74	5,466	196,000	2,789	72,494	202,169,492
6	75+	13,037	157,000	8,304	53,474	444,038,559
Column Sums→		25,045	2,372,000	1,056	1,000,000	922,790,487

Calculations:

$$\Sigma\, N_i r_i = N_1 r_1 + N_2 r_2 + \cdots + N_6 r_6 = 20,114,672 + 23,100,941 + \cdots + 444,038,559 = 922,790,487$$

$$\Sigma\, N_i = N_1 + N_2 + \cdots + N_6 = 76,158 + 286,501 + \cdots + 53,474 = 1,000,000$$

$$aR(direct) = \frac{\sum_{i=1}^{k} N_i r_i}{\sum_{i=1}^{k} N_i} = \frac{922,790,487}{1,000,000} \approx 923$$

3. A $cR = 416,000/55,163,000 = 0.00754 = 754$ per 100,000. This rate is substantially lower than that of the United States.

B $aR(indirect) = 1621$ per 100,000 (see Table 7.17 for calculations). As suggested by the SMR, this mortality rate is more than twice that of the United States.

TABLE 7.17. Calculation of Adjusted Rate by the Indirect Method for Egypt, Using the United States, 1991, as the External Reference Population

Age (years)	U.S. Rate (R_i)	Egyptian Population (n_i)	Product ($R_i n_i$)
0–4	.00229	7,909,000	18,112
5–24	.00062	24,560,000	15,227
25–44	.00180	13,764,000	24,775
45–64	.00789	6,921,000	54,607
65–74	.02618	1,485,000	38,877
75+	.08046	524,000	42,161
Total		55,163,000	193,759

$cR = 416,000/55,163,000 = 0.00754 = 754$ per 100,000.

$$\mu = \Sigma R_i n_i = R_1 n_1 + R_2 n_2 + \cdots + R_6 n_6 =$$
$$18112 + 1\,5227 + \cdots + 42161 = 193,759$$

$$SMR = \frac{x}{\mu} = \frac{416,000 \ (\text{see table 7.14})}{193,759} = 2.15$$

$$aR(indirect) = (cR)(SMR) = (0.00754)(2.15) =$$
$$.01621 = 1.621 \text{ per } 100,000$$

REFERENCES

National Center for Health Statistics [NCHS]. (1993). *Vital Statistics of the United States, 1991, Volume II, Mortality, Part B*. Hyattsville, MD: U.S. Department of Health and Human Services, PHS #90-1102.

United Nations Department for Economic and Social Information and Policy Analysis [United Nations]. (1996). *1994 Demographic Yearbook*. New York: United Nations, Publication E/F.96.XIII.1.

U.S. Bureau of the Census. (1992). *Statistical Abstracts of the United States 1992*. Washington, DC: U.S. Government Printing Office.

U.S. Bureau of the Census. (1994). *Statistical Abstracts of the United States 1994*. Washington, DC: U.S. Government Printing Office.

8

Measures of Association and Potential Impact

Measures of association in epidemiologic studies are used to investigate the etiology, treatment, and prevention of disease. Measures of potential impact are used to reflect how much disease is likely to be prevented by removing an etiologic factor from the population. This chapter discusses the two general types of measures of association: ratio measures ("relative risks") and difference measures ("excess risks"). It also discusses two types of potential impact measures: the attributable fraction in the population and the attributable fraction among the exposed.

8.1 INTRODUCTION

Epidemiologic **measures of association** are calculated by categorizing the population into two or more groups. Following this division, the rate of disease in each category is compared with that of a single reference category. Although the selection of a reference category is arbitrary, the reference category should, if possible, represent a natural group by which to establish baseline risk. For example, in studying the health effects of exercise, the group with the lowest level of exercise might serve as the reference category.

Although the etiologic factor under study may represent any agent, host, or environmental factor, traditionally, the explanatory variable in epidemiologic studies has been called the **exposure**. That is, in epidemiologic jargon, an exposure is any variable that could causally explain the outcome under study. An **association** is said to exist if the exposure increases or decreases the risk of disease in one or more groups. A **positive association** is said to exist if the exposure tends to increase risk. A **negative association** is said to exist if the exposure tends to decrease risk.(See Table 8.1.)

Because a difference in risk implies that the exposure might cause or prevent the disease in question, measures of association are also sometimes called measures of effect. We prefer, however, to avoid this term, as *statistical associations are not always causal.*

TABLE 8.1. Definitions of Selected Terms

Exposure: any explanatory variable that could be statistically associated with the outcome under study

Disease: the pathologic or health-related outcome under study

Association: a statistical relationship between the study exposure and disease

Positive association: a statistical relationship in which the explanatory variable predicts an average increase in the outcome

Negative association: a statistical relationship in which the explanatory variable predicts an average decrease in the outcome

Relative risk: a term that, when applied loosely, refers to any of the ratio measures of association discussed in this chapter; a measure that seeks to quantify the likelihood of a disease or cause of death among the exposed relative to the likelihood of the same disease or cause of death among the unexposed

Excess risk: a term that, when applied loosely, refers to any difference measure of association; a measure that seeks to estimate the absolute difference in the likelihood of death or disease among the exposed and unexposed

Attributable fraction: a measure of potential impact that refers to either the expected percentage reduction in the number of cases in the population (attributable fraction in the population) or among exposed cases (attributable fraction among the exposed) if the exposure were entirely eliminated

The distinction between causal and noncausal associations in health and disease was considered by George Bernard Shaw in 1911, when he wrote:

> Comparisons which are really comparisons between two social classes with different standards of nutrition and education are palmed off as comparisons between the results of a certain medical treatment and its neglect. Thus it is easy to prove that the wearing of tall hats and the carrying of umbrellas enlarges the chest, prolongs life, and confers comparative immunity from disease; for the statistics show that the classes which use these articles are bigger, healthier, and live longer than the class which never dreams of possessing such things. It does not take much perspicacity to see that what really makes this difference is not the tall hat and the umbrella, but the wealth and nourishment of which they are evidence, and that a gold watch or membership of a club in Pall Mall might be proved in the same way to have the like sovereign virtues. A university degree, a daily bath, the owning of thirty pairs of trousers, a knowledge of Wagner's music, a pew in church, anything, in short, that implies more means and better nurture than the mass of laborers enjoy, can be statistically palmed off as a magic-spell conferring all sorts of privileges (p. 1xiv)

Therefore, "association" should not be confused with the "causation"—the term causation implies that observed differences have biological meaning whereas the term "association" makes no such assumption. Thus, the discovery of a statistical association between an exposure and disease should *not* immediately be construed as causal. Associations do, however, provide an important link in determining cause and effect.

8.2 RATIO MEASURES OF ASSOCIATION ("RELATIVE RISKS")

Background

Ratio measures of association are calculated by dividing the frequency of disease in an exposed group by the frequency of disease in a reference (unexposed) group. Because there are three distinct measures of disease frequency, there are also three distinct ratio measures of association. These are the **prevalence ratio, cumulative incidence ratio,**

and **incidence density ratio.** In addition, we cover a separate but related measure of association called the **disease odds ratio.** Because epidemiologic frequency measures are almost always calculated to reflect the risk or rate of disease or death, these measures of association are often called **relative risks, risk ratios,** or **rate ratios.**

Prevalence Ratio

A **prevalence ratio** is a ratio comparison of two prevalences. Notation and general data layout for prevalence studies are shown in Table 8.2. The formula for prevalence ratio is

$$PR_i = \frac{P_i}{P_0} = \frac{a_i/n_i}{a_0/n_0} \tag{8.1}$$

where PR_i represents the prevalence ratio associated with exposure level i, P_i represents the prevalence in group i, P_0 represents the prevalence in the reference group, and a_i, n_i, a_0, and n_0 represent the table cell labels listed in Table 8.2A. For situations in which only two exposure categories are present, the formula is

$$PR = \frac{P_1}{P_0} = \frac{a/n_1}{b/n_0} \tag{8.2}$$

(See Table 8.2B for notation.)

The prevalence ratio can range from zero to infinity, with zero indicating a strong negative association and infinity indicating a strong positive association. Under the assumption of no association, the prevalence ratio is one.

Note that prevalence ratios are not true risk ratios because prevalence measures the likelihood of already having a disease or condition and the term risk implies the likelihood that an event *will* occur. Nevertheless, if we assume that the mean durations of disease among exposed and unexposed cases are similar and that the disease does not affect

TABLE 8.2. Notation for Comparative Prevalence and Cumulative Incidence Studies

A. Multiple Exposure Categories

Exposure Category ($i = 0, \ldots, k$)

	E_k	$\ldots$	E_1	E_0	
Disease +	a_k	$\ldots$	a_1	a_0	m_1
Disease −	c_k	$\ldots$	c_1	c_0	m_0
	n_k		n_1	n_0	n

B. Two Exposure Categories

	Exposure + E_1	Exposure − E_0	
Disease +	a	b	m_1
Disease −	c	d	m_0
	n_1	n_0	n

TABLE 8.3. Prevalence Study, Hypothetical Data

	Exposure + E_1	Exposure - E_0	
Disease +	20	10	30
Disease -	80	90	170
	100	100	200

$P_1 = 20/100 = .2$
$P_0 = 10/100 = .1$
$PR = .2/.1 = .2$

exposure status, the prevalence ratio is a reasonable estimate of relative risk (Kleinbaum et al., 1982, pp. 147–148).

A simple example using the hypothetical data in Table 8.3 shows a prevalence ratio of 2. This suggests that the exposed people in the study have twice the prevalence of disease as the unexposed people.

Cumulative Incidence Ratio

A ratio comparison of two cumulative incidences is called a **cumulative incidence ratio.** Using the notation established in Table 8.2A, the cumulative incidence for exposure level i is

$$CIR_i = \frac{CI_i}{CI_0} = \frac{a_i/n_i}{a_0/n_0} \tag{8.3}$$

For situations in which only two exposure categories are present, the formula is

$$CIR = \frac{CI_1}{CI_0} = \frac{a/n_1}{b/n_0} \tag{8.4}$$

Interpretation of the cumulative incidence ratio is roughly the same as interpretation of prevalence ratios (i.e., zero suggests a strong negative association, infinity suggests a strong positive association, and one suggests no association). However, because cumulative incidences reflect true measures of risk, the cumulative incidence ratio is aptly and directly called a risk ratio without the need for further assumptions regarding duration of disease or whether the disease affects exposure status.

Table 8.4 displays an example of cumulative incidence data that considers spontaneous abortions and occupational exposure to video display terminal use. Data include 54 spontaneous abortions in 366 video display terminal-exposed pregnancies and 82 spontaneous occurrences in 516 unexposed pregnancies. The *CIR* associated with occupational video display terminal use is, therefore, 0.93. (Calculations are shown below the table.) This suggests a slight negative or almost no association between video display terminal use and spontaneous abortion.*

---

*Relative risks close to one are generally considered evidence of "nonassociation" because small deviations may result from random and nonrandom measurement error.

TABLE 8.4. Video Display Terminal Use and Spontaneous Abortions, Cumulative Incidence Study

	Video Display Terminal Exposure +	Video Display Terminal Exposure −	
Spontaneous Abortion +	54	82	136
Spontaneous Abortion −	312	434	746
	366	516	882

$CI_1 = 54/366 = .148$
$CI_0 = 82/516 = .159$
$CIR = .148/.159 = 0.93$

Source: Schnorr (1993).

Incidence Density Ratio

The **incidence density ratio,** also called the **rate ratio,** is a ratio comparison of two incidence densities. This statistic is calculated by dividing the incidence density in an exposed group by the incidence density in the reference group. Notation and general data layout for incidence density studies are shown in Table 8.5. Using this notation, the incidence density ratio in group i is

$$IDR_i = \frac{ID_i}{ID_0} = \frac{a_i/L_i}{a_0/L_0} \tag{8.5}$$

In restricting the analysis to two exposure categories, the formula is

$$IDR = \frac{ID_1}{ID_0} = \frac{a/L_1}{b/L_0} \tag{8.6}$$

TABLE 8.5. Notation for Comparative Incidence Density (Person-Time) Studies

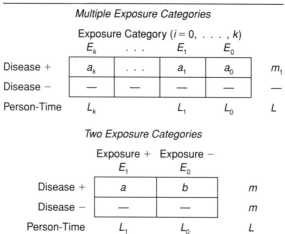

Multiple Exposure Categories

	Exposure Category ($i = 0, \ldots, k$)				
	E_k	$\cdots$	E_1	E_0	
Disease +	a_k	$\cdots$	a_1	a_0	m_1
Disease −	—	—	—	—	—
Person-Time	L_k		L_1	L_0	L

Two Exposure Categories

	Exposure + E_1	Exposure − E_0	
Disease +	a	b	m
Disease −	—	—	m
Person-Time	L_1	L_0	L

TABLE 8.6. Myocardial Infarction Rates in Three Groups of Women

	E_2	E_1	E_0
	OC^a+ SMOKE^b+	OC+ SMOKE−	OC− SMOKE−
Incidence density (per 100,000 woman-years)	30	6	2

Source: Adapted from Stadel (1981), table 4.
^{a}Current oral contraceptive use.
^{b}Based on smoking at least 15 cigarettes per day.
$IDR_1 = ID_1/ID_0 = 6$ per 100,000 woman-years/2 per 100,000 woman-years = 3
$IDR_2 = ID_2/ID_0 = 30$ per 100,000 woman-years/2 per 100,000 woman-years = 15
$IDD_1 = ID_1 - ID_0 = 6$ per 100,000 woman-years − 2 per 100,000 woman-years = 4 per 100,000 woman-years
$IDD_2 = ID_2 - ID_0 = 30$ per 100,000 woman-years − 2 per 100,000 woman-years = 28 per 100,000 woman-years

To illustrate the *IDR*, let us consider myocardial infarction rates in three groups of women (Table 8.6). Group 0 represents women who neither use oral contraceptives nor smoke, group 1 represents women who use oral contraceptives and do not smoke, and group 2 represents women who use oral contraceptives and smoke. Using these data, the incidence density ratio associated with oral contraceptive use (alone) is 3 and the incidence density ratio associated with oral contraceptive use and smoking (combined) is 15. These estimates suggest oral contraceptives triple the risk of myocardial infarction in nonsmokers and increase the risk 15-fold in smokers.*

Disease Odds Ratio

The **disease odds ratio** provides an alternate to the prevalence ratio and cumulative incidence ratio as a ratio measure of association when data represent proportions. Disease odds ratios, however, are not relevant when working with person-time (incidence density) data.

To understand disease odds ratios, we must introduce the idea of **disease odds** (or "odds of disease"). The disease odds is the ratio of the probability of disease to that of nondisease. In keeping with the notation in Table 8.2B, the disease odds in the exposed group (DO_1) is

$$DO_1 = \frac{a}{c} \tag{8.7}$$

The disease odds in the unexposed group (DO_0) is

$$DO_0 = \frac{b}{d} \tag{8.8}$$

The disease odds ratio (*DOR*) is

$$DOR = \frac{DO_1}{DO_0} = \frac{a/c}{b/d} = \frac{ad}{bc} \tag{8.9}$$

*These estimates are based on epidemiologic studies from the 1970s and should not be construed to apply to currently marketed formulations. Today's formulations are much safer.

Disease odds ratios can be interpreted in a way similar to other ratio measures of association: values of one suggest no association, values greater than one suggest a positive association, and values less than one suggest a negative association. Moreover, the disease odds ratio is approximately equal to the cumulative incidence ratio when the disease is uncommon (say, when the cumulative incidence $<.05$):

$$DOR \approx CIR$$

The disease odds ratio, however, will separate from the simple ratio measure when the disease is common and association is strong. So, for example, the data in Table 8.3 demonstrate a prevalence ratio of 2.00 but a (prevalence) disease odds ratio of $(20/80)/(10/90) = 2.25$. The disease odds ratio, nonetheless, remains a valid measure of association in its own right. In fact, the disease odds ratio is superior to the cumulative incidence ratio in several ways:

· The calculation formula in simple, rapid, and foolproof.
· The disease odds ratio is well suited for advanced statistical modeling techniques, such as logistic regression.
· The disease odds ratio demonstrates mathematical symmetry whether one studies death or survival (see Table 8.7).

TABLE 8.7. Symmetry of the Odds Ratio

A study shows two deaths in 100 exposed people and one death in 100 unexposed people (table A, below). The cumulative incidence ratio and disease ratio are, therefore, both 2.0. Now, let us look at the same data but with the outcome defined in terms of survival (table B, below). The cumulative incidence ratio of surviving is approximately 1.0, while the odds ratio is approximately 0.5. Note that use of the cumulative incidence ratio results in apparently contradictory results depending on whether the study outcome is defined in terms of death or survival. Results based on odds ratio calculations, however, remain consistent (i.e., the exposure either doubles the risk of death or halves the risk of survival). Consequently, odds ratios demonstrate symmetry, whereas cumulative incidence ratios are not necessarily so.

A. Risk of Dying

	Exposure +	Exposure −	
Death +	2	1	3
Death −	98	99	197
	100	100	200

$CIR = (2/100)/(1/100) = 2.0$
$DOR = (2)(99)/(1)(98) \approx 2.0$

B. Risk of Surviving

	Exposure +	Exposure −	
Survive +	98	99	
Survive −	2	1	
	100	100	200

$CIR = (98/100)/(99/100) = 1.0$
$DOR = (98)(1)/(99)(2) \approx 0.5$

Source: Kahn & Sempos (1989).

· The odds ratio can be adapted to case-control studies, a type of study we have not yet considered but will introduce in the next chapter.

With this said, disease odds ratios are less intuitively understood than prevalence ratios and cumulative incidence ratios. Consequently, prevalence ratios and cumulative incidence ratios are still encountered in many epidemiologic studies.

Further Remarks on Ratio Measures of Association

· The standardized mortality ratio (*SMR*), discussed in Section 7.3, is also a ratio measure of association. Unlike the studies discussed in this chapter, however, *SMR* studies have no internal comparison group. Instead, the reference rate comes from an external population. In theoretical terms, the *SMR* and *CIR* are highly related (Miettinen, 1972).
· Given a constant incidence density ratio over a short period, the cumulative incidence ratio is equal to the incidence density ratio. Using calculus, it can be proved that the theoretical limit of the cumulative incidence ratio over time period Δ is equal to the incidence density ratio as Δ approaches zero (Kleinbaum et al., 1982, p. 145):

$$\lim_{\Delta \to 0} CIR = IDR$$

Indeed, most epidemiologists take this fact for granted by interchangeably using the terms relative risk, risk ratio, and rate ratio to refer to both the cumulative incidence ratio and incidence density ratio. Nevertheless, the incidence density ratio is better suited for the study of diseases that develop over an extended period of observation, especially if there is a high turnover rate in the population or many people withdraw from the study. The cumulative incidence ratio is generally better suited for studying acute diseases that occur over relatively short periods of observation (e.g., during outbreak investigations).

· The interpretation of all ratio measures of association can be summarized as follows: ratio measures equal to one suggest no association, ratio measures significantly greater than one suggest a positive association, and ratio measures significantly less than one suggest a negative association (Table 8.8). This rule should not be taken too literally, however, because the calculated value of a ratio measure will inevitably suffer from random and nonrandom measurement error. Thus, a deviation from 1 should be construed as suggestive of an effect rather than a definitive indication of risk.
· Ratio measures of association quantify an association's strength. The farther the value is from one, the stronger the association. Factors that double the risks of a disease are considered moderately strong risk factors and factors that quadruple the risks of disease are considered strong risk factors (Table 8.9).

TABLE 8.8. Direction of Association for Ratio Measures of Association ("Relative Risks")

Value of Relative Risk	Direction of Association	Potential Effect of Exposure
Approximately 1	No association	Neutral
Significantly greater than 1	Positive association	Risk
Significantly less than 1	Negative association	Benefit

TABLE 8.9. Strength of Association Rules of Thumb for Positive Relative Risks

Relative Risk	Strength of Association
Greater than 4	Very strong
2–4	Moderate to strong
Greater than 1, but less than 2	Weak

- Mathematically, ratio measures of association are unitless numbers varying from zero to infinity. (Initial units of measure, if any, cancel out in the numerator and denominator.) Moreover, ratio measures of association "travel" on a logarithmic scale. Note that a logarithmic relative risk of one is zero, indicating no association between the exposure and disease. The farther the logarithmic value of the relative risk is from zero, the stronger the association (Fig. 8.1).

- Although ratio measures are adept at determining the strength and direction of an association, they are unable to measure excess risk on an absolute scale. To better understand excess risk, we must study difference measures of association.

8.3 DIFFERENCE MEASURES OF ASSOCIATION ("EXCESS RISKS")

Background

Difference measures of association are calculated by subtracting the frequency of disease in the unexposed group from the frequency of disease in the exposed group. Epidemiologic terms used to refer to difference measures of association include **excess risk, excess rate, risk difference,** and **absolute increase in risk.**

The three difference measures of association are the **prevalence difference, cumulative incidence difference,** and **incidence density difference.** However, *because of their similarities in form, we consider only the incidence density difference, thus avoiding some redundancy.*

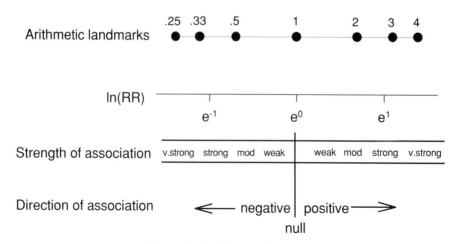

Figure 8.1. Relative risk landmarks.

Incidence Density Difference

Using the previously established notation, the **incidence density difference** in exposure group i (IDD_i) is

$$IDD_i = ID_i - ID_0 \tag{8.10}$$

where ID_i represents the incidence density in exposure groups i and ID_0 represents the incidence density in the reference (unexposed) group. In comparing two groups,

$$IDD = ID_1 - ID_0 \tag{8.11}$$

Interpretation

The null value of no association for the incidence density difference is zero. Positive incidence density differences suggest a positive association; negative incidence density differences suggest a negative association (Table 8.10). The farther the incidence density deviates from zero, the greater is the excess in risk associated with the exposure.

Incidence density differences provide a measure of excess risk on an absolute scale. For example, in calculating the incidence density difference associated with oral contraceptive use (alone) based on the data in Table 8.6, the incidence density difference is 6 per 100,000 woman-years $-$ 2 per 100,000 woman-years = 4 per 100,000 woman-years. The incidence density difference associated with oral contraceptive use and smoking (combined) is 28 per 100,000 woman-years. This suggests an excess of 4 cases per 100,000 woman-years of oral contraceptive use and an excess of 28 cases per 100,000 woman-years of oral contraceptive use with smoking, thus quantifying risk on an absolute scale.*

Alternative Method of Calculation

The incidence density difference can also be calculated as follows:

$$IDD = (ID_0)(IDR - 1) \tag{8.12}$$

where ID_0 represents the incidence density in the unexposed group and IDR represents the incidence density ratio associated with the exposure. In applying this formula to oral contraceptive use and myocardial infarction rates, the incidence density difference is (2 per 100,000 woman-years)(3 $-$ 1) = 4 per 100,000 woman-years.

TABLE 8.10. Direction of Association for Difference Measures of Association ("Excess Risks")

Value of Excess Risk	Direction	Potential Effect of Exposure
Approximately 0	No association	Neutral
Significantly greater than 0	Positive association	Risk
Significantly less than 0	Negative association	Benefit

*Recall that the data apply to older oral contraceptive formulations that are no longer marketed.

TABLE 8.11. Mortality Rates for Lung Cancer and Cardiovascular Disease in All People and in Smokers (Group 1) and Nonsmokers (Group 0)

Disease	ID_1 per 1000 person-years (Smokers)	ID_0 per 1000 person-years (Nonsmokers)	IDR	IDD per 1000 person-years
Lung cancer	1.30	0.07	18.5	1.23
Cardiovascular disease	9.51	7.32	1.3	2.19

Source: Center for Disease Control and Prevention (1992), p. 7.

Comparison of Ratio Measures of Association and Difference Measures of Association

Table 8.11 shows incidence density ratios (*IDR*s) and incidence density differences (*IDD*s) for smoking and lung cancer mortality and smoking and cardiovascular disease mortality. Although the *IDR* of smoking for lung cancer mortality far exceeds the *IDR* of smoking for cardiovascular disease mortality (18.5 versus 1.3), the *IDD* for cardiovascular disease is greater than the *IDD* for lung cancer (1.23 per 1000 versus 2.19 per 1000). This is because cardiovascular disease is a much more common outcome than lung cancer. Thus, even a relatively small increase in its occurrence can create a large excess on an absolute scale. It is clear, therefore, that ratio measures and difference measures quantify different aspects of an association. It is said that ratio measures of association are preferred when attempting to determine cause and effect and difference measures of association do a better job reflecting the potential public health consequences of an exposure.

8.4 MEASURES OF POTENTIAL IMPACT ("ATTRIBUTABLE FRACTIONS")

Background

Measures of potential impact are used to reflect the expected reduction in a disease when eliminating a risk factor from a group and, thus, are useful in evaluating the potential benefits of a proposed intervention. The two types of measures of potential impact are the **attributable fraction in the population** (AF_p) and the **attributable fraction among the exposed** (AF_e). Distinguishing between these two types of attributable fractions is important because they represent measures of impact in different groups. Synonyms for attributable fraction are **attributable proportion** and **etiologic fraction.**

Attributable Fraction in the Population (AF_p)

The **attributable fraction in the population** represents the expected proportional reduction in new cases in the population that would occur if the risk factor were removed. This is equivalent to the probability that a randomly selected case from the population developed the disease because of the risk factor.

In its simplest form, the attributable fraction in the population (AF_p) is calculated by taking the difference between the incidence density of the disease in the population as a whole (called the crude incidence density, cID) and the incidence density in the unexposed population (ID_0) and dividing this difference by the crude incidence density:

$$AF_p = \frac{cID - ID_0}{cID} \tag{8.13}$$

This formula assumes the exposure causes the disease, so that $cID > ID_0$.

A frequently cited attributable fraction included as part of an epidemiologic review for the U.S. Congress attributed 80% of all human cancers to environmental factors (Doll & Peto, 1981). This statistic suggests that if we rid the environment of all carcinogens, 80% of all human cancers would be averted. In other words, the current cancer-specific death rate of approximately 200 per 100,000 person-years would be reduced to approximately 40 per 100,000 person-years. Application of formula 8.12 provides

$$AF_p = \frac{cID - ID_0}{cID}$$
$$= \frac{200 \text{ per } 100{,}000 \text{ person-years} - 40 \text{ per } 100{,}000 \text{ person-years}}{200 \text{ per } 100{,}000 \text{ person-years}} = .8$$

An alternative formula for the attributable fraction in the population is

$$AF_p = \frac{(p)(IDR - 1)}{1 + (p)(IDR - 1)} \tag{8.14}$$

where IDR represents the incidence density ratio and p denotes the proportion of the population that is exposed, calculated as

$$p = \frac{L_1}{L} \tag{8.15}$$

where L_1 represents the person-time characterized by exposure and L represents the total person-time in the population. For example, assuming that the IDR for cigarette smoking-related lung cancer is 15 and the prevalence of smoking was .4 in the 1970s (use of this value assumes a 25-year latent period for lung cancer), the population fraction of lung cancer attributable to cigarette smoking is

$$AF_p = \frac{(.4)(15 - 1)}{1 + (.4)(15 - 1)} = .848$$

Consequently, approximately 85% of the lung cancers are due to cigarette smoking. Attributable fractions for other known contributors to lung cancer are listed in Table 8.12. Note that attributable fractions for a particular disease need not total 100%. This is because removing one component in the causal pathway is often sufficient to prevent disease, making it possible to prevent a disease in multiple ways. Selected attributable fractions for cancer death are noted in Table 8.13.

TABLE 8.12. Attributable Fractions in the U.S. Population for Lung Cancer Associated with Modifiable Risk Factors

Risk Factor	Attributable Fraction (Population) Best Estimate[a] (%)	Attributable Fraction (Population) Range (%)
Cigarette smoking	87	84–90
Occupation[b]	13	10–20
Residential radon	10	7–25
Low vegetable diet	5	—[c]
Environmental tobacco smoke	2	1–6

Source: Brownson et al. (1993), p. 145.
[a]Attributable risks need not add up to 100% because of the overlapping effects of contributing factors.
[b]Includes occupational exposure to asbestos, polycyclic hydrocarbons, arsenic, and radon gas.
[c]Unavailable.

Note that the population attributable fraction is a function of two values:

• The strength of association between the exposure and disease (as measured by the *IDR*)
• The prevalence of the exposure in the population (p)

Although the *IDR* is a constant function of the exposure and disease, the prevalence of exposure in the population may vary. This makes attributable fractions in the population specific to a particular place and time—declines in the prevalence of exposure will show a resultant decrease in the population attributable fraction. For example, as the prevalence of smoking declines in a country, the attributable fraction of lung cancer will also decline (allowing for the latent period of disease to follow).

TABLE 8.13. Approximate Attributable Fractions in the U.S. Population for Overall Cancer Mortality, Various Risk Factors

Risk Factor	Attributable Fraction (Population) (%) Doll and Peto (1981) Estimates	Attributable Fraction (Population) (%) Miller (1992) Estimates
Tobacco	30	29
Diet	35	20
Occupation	4	9
Family history	—	8
Reproductive and sexual history	7	7[a]
Geophysical[b]	3	1[c]
Alcohol[d]	3	6
Pollution	2	—
Medication and medical procedures	1	2[e]
Industrial and consumer products	<1	—
Infective processes	10	—

Source: Brownson et al. (1993), p. 142.
[a]Attributed to parity (4%) and sexual activity (3%).
[b]Mainly natural background radiation and sunlight.
[c]Attributed to sunlight.
[d]With the exception of liver cancer, most alcohol-related cancers result from the combination of alcohol consumption and cigarette smoking (Thomas, 1992).
[e]Attributed to drugs (1%) and radiation (1%).

Attributable Fraction Among the Exposed (*AF$_e$*)

The prior consideration of attributable fraction addressed the preventable fraction for the entire population. This second form of the attributable fraction, the **attributable fraction among the exposed (*AF$_e$*)**, restricts its consideration to exposed cases. The attributable fraction in exposed cases can be interpreted as the probability that an exposed case developed the disease as a result of the risk factor in question. Consequently, this form of the attributable fraction is useful in assigning liability. It does *not*, however, address whether a case chosen at random from the population is due to the exposure.

The definitional formula for the attributable fraction in the exposed population (*AF$_e$*) is

$$AF_e = \frac{ID_1 - ID_0}{ID_1} \tag{8.16}$$

where ID_1 represents the incidence density of disease in the exposed population and ID_0 represents the incidence density of disease in the unexposed population. This is equivalent to

$$AF_e = \frac{IDR - 1}{IDR} \tag{8.17}$$

Note that the attributable fraction among the exposed is a function of the *IDR* alone. For example, an exposure associated with an *IDR* of 2 yields an attributable fraction among the exposed of .5, suggesting that half of the exposed cases were caused by the exposure and that the other half would have occurred anyway.

SUMMARY

1. Measures of association are used to study the etiology, treatment, and prevention of disease. Measures of potential impact are used to reflect the proportion of a disease attributable to a particular exposure. The measures of association and potential impact considered in the chapter are listed in Table 8.14.

2. Ratio measures of association ("relative risks") provide an index of the strength and direction of an association. Relative risks of approximately one suggest no association, relative risks significantly greater than one suggest a positive association, and relative

TABLE 8.14. Measures of Association and Potential Impact Covered in This Chapter

Type of Measure	Statistics	Measurement Component
Ratio measure	Prevalence ratio (*PR*) Cumulative incidence ratio (*CIR*) Incidence density ratio (*IDR*) Disease odds ratio (*DOR*)	"Relative Risk" Strength and direction of association
Difference measure	Incidence density difference (*IDD*)	"Excess Risk" Absolute difference in risk
Potential impact	Attributable fraction in the population (*AF$_p$*) Attributable fraction among the exposed (*AF$_e$*)	"Attributable Fraction" Proportional reduction in the number of cases following removal of the exposure

risks significantly less than one suggest a negative association. The farther away the relative risk is from one, the stronger the association.

3. Difference measures of association ("excess risks") provide an index of the excess in risk associated with an exposure. Difference measures of approximately zero suggest no association, difference measures significantly greater than zero suggest a positive association, and difference measures significantly less than zero suggest a negative association.

4. Measures of potential impact ("attributable fractions") are used to reflect the expected reduction in a disease when eliminating a risk factor from the population. The two types of measures of potential impact are the attributable fraction in the population and the attributable fraction among the exposed. The attributable fraction in the population represents the probability that a randomly selected case from the population developed the disease because of the risk factor. The attributable fraction among the exposed represents the likelihood that a randomly selected exposed case developed the disease because of the exposure.

NOTATION AND FORMULA REFERENCE

See Tables 8.2 and 8.5 for cell references.

P_i	Prevalence in exposure group i
P_0	Prevalence in the reference (unexposed) group
PR_i	Prevalence ratio, exposure group i (formula 8.1)
PR	Prevalence ratio, study restricted to two groups (formula 8.2)
CI_i	Cumulative incidence in exposure group i
CI_0	Cumulative incidence in the reference (unexposed) group
CIR_i	Cumulative incidence ratio, exposure group i (formula 8.3)
CIR	Cumulative incidence ratio, study restricted to two groups (formula 8.4)
ID_i	Incidence density in exposure group i
ID_0	Incidence density in the reference (unexposed) group
IDR_i	Incidence density ratio, exposure group i (formula 8.5)
IDR	Incidence density ratio, study restricted to two groups (formula 8.6)
DO_1	Disease odds, exposed group (formula 8.7)
DO_0	Disease odds, unexposed group (formula 8.8)
DOR	Disease odds ratio (formula 8.9)
IDD	Incidence density difference (formulas 8.10, 8.11, and 8.12)
AF_p	Attributable fraction in the population (formulas 8.13 and 8.14)
p	Prevalence of exposure in the population (formula 8.15)
AF_e	Attributable fraction among the exposed (formulas 8.16 and 8.17)

EXERCISES

1. Data from a cross-sectional study of human immunodeficiency virus (HIV) infection and intravenous drug use (IVDU) in women entering the New York State Prison system are presented in Table 8.15. Based on these data, calculate:

   (A) the prevalence of HIV infection in intravenous drug users

   (B) the prevalence of HIV infection in women not using intravenous drugs

   (C) the prevalence ratio

TABLE 8.15. Human Immunodeficiency Virus (HIV) Infection and Intravenous Drug Use (IVDU) in Women Entering the New York State Prison System

	IVDU +	IVDU −	
HIV +	61	27	88
HIV −	75	312	387
	136	339	475

Source: Smith et al. (1991).

(D) the prevalence difference

(E) the attributable fraction in the population

(F) the attributable fraction among the exposed

2. Since 1948, the Framingham Study has followed 2336 males and 2873 females in order to investigate the relationship between risk factors and the development of cardiovascular disease. Data from the Framingham Study on serum cholesterol levels and coronary heart disease (CHD) in men and women are shown in Table 8.16. Calculate the values for boxes labeled A through N in this table. Briefly interpret your findings.

3. Each year, cardiologists surgically open clogged arteries only to have the arteries undergo resterosis in about half of their patients. Until now, no one has been able to predict which patients will experience this adverse outcome. A study by Zhou et al. (1996) was conducted to determine whether there is an association between infection with cytomegalovirus and regrowth of arterial plaque. Researchers found that out of 49 patients infected with cytomegalovirus, 21 had regrowth of arterial plaque following surgery to open the clogged artery. In contrast, only 2 of the 26 patients without cytomegalovirus had regrowth of plaque. (Data are also reported in Table 8.17.)

(A) What is the cumulative incidence ratio of restenosis associated with cytomegalovirus infection?

TABLE 8.16. Six-Year Cumulative Incidences of Coronary Heart Disease (CHD), Ages 40–59, Framingham Study

Serum Cholesterol (mg/100 mL)	New CHD Cases	Population at Risk	Cumulative Incidence (per 1000)	Cumulative Incidence Ratio	Cumulative Incidence Difference (per 1000)
Men					
Less than 210	16	454	A	1 (Reference)	0 (Reference)
210–244	29	455	B	D	F
245 or more	51	424	C	E	G
Women					
Less than 210	8	445	H	1 (Reference)	0 (Reference)
210–244	16	527	I	K	M
245 or more	30	689	J	L	N

Source: Adapted from Kannel et al. (1961), p. 38.

TABLE 8.17. Cytomegalovirus Infection and Restenosis Following Surgery

	Cytomegalovirus +	Cytomegalovirus −	
Restenosis +	21	2	23
Restenosis −	28	24	52
	49	26	75

Source: Zhou et al. (1996).

(B) What is the cumulative incidence difference of restenosis associated with cytomegalovirus infection?

(C) What percentage of the restenoses in the population are due to cytomegalovirus?

4. Determine the direction (positive or negative) and strength of association (weak, moderate to strong, or very strong) for each of the following relative risks:

   (A) 1.5

   (B) 0.73

   (C) 18.0

   (D) 0.31

5. In Chapter 6, Exercise 4, you calculated attack rates of gastroenteritis in people who ate and did not eat particular foods served at a banquet. These results are displayed in Table 8.18. Calculate the cumulative incidence ratios associated with each of the following items:

   (A) macaroni and cheese

   (B) ham

   (C) cabbage salad

   (D) rolls

   (E) coffee

   (F) milk

   (G) ice cream

TABLE 8.18. Attack Rates of Gastroenteritis in People Attending a Banquet

Food	Attack Rates in Those Eating the Food Ill/Total (%)	Attack Rates in Those Not Eating the Food Ill/Total (%)
Macaroni and cheese	20/80 (25%)	5/20 (25%)
Ham	25/80 (31%)	0/20 (0%)
Cabbage salad	10/55 (18%)	15/45 (33%)
Rolls	12/50 (24%)	13/50 (26%)
Coffee	20/85 (24%)	5/15 (33%)
Milk	3/11 (27%)	22/89 (25%)
Ice cream	25/100 (25%)	0/0 (undefined)

ANSWERS TO EXERCISES

1. A $P_1 = 61/136 = .449$.
   B $P_0 = 27/339 = .080$.
   C $PR = .449/.080 = 5.63$.
   D   Prevalence Difference $= .449 - .080 = .369$.
   E $AF_p = (.185 - .080)/.185 = .568$.
   F $AF_e = (5.63 - 1)/5.63 = .822$.

2. A   35.2 (per 1000).
   B   63.7 (per 1000).
   C   120.3 (per 1000).
   D   1.81.
   E   3.41.
   F   28.5 (per 1000).
   G   85.0 (per 1000).
   H   18.0 (per 1000).
   I   30.4 (per 1000).
   J   43.5 (per 1000).
   K   1.69.
   L   2.42.
   M   12.4 (per 1000).
   N   25.6 (per 1000).

3. A $CIR = 42.9\%/7.7\% = 5.57$.
   B   Cumulative incidence difference $= 42.9\% - 7.7\% = 35.2\%$.
   C $EF = .749$ (almost 75% of the restenosis cases in the population are attributed to cytomegalovirus infection).

4. A   Weak positive association.
   B   Weak negative association.
   C   Very strong positive association.
   D   Moderate to strong negative association.

5. A   1.00.
   B   Undefined (zero denominator); limit $\rightarrow +\infty$.
   C   0.55.
   D   0.92.
   E   0.71.
   F   1.10.
   G   Undefined (undefined denominator); limit $\rightarrow 1$.

REFERENCES

Brownson, R. C., Reif, J. S., Alavanja, M. C. R., & Bal, D. G. (1993). Cancer. In R. C. Brownson, P. L. Remington, & J. R. Davis (Eds.), *Chronic Disease Epidemiology and Control* (pp. 137–167). Washington, DC: American Public Health Association.

Centers for Disease Control and Prevention. (1992). *Cigarette Smoking and Lung Cancer. 1992 EIS Course.* (Available from the Association of Teachers of Preventive Medicine, 1015 15th Street, N.W., Suite 405, Washington, DC, 20005.)

Doll, R., & Peto, R. (1981). *The Causes of Cancer.* New York: Oxford University Press.

Kahn, K. A., & Sempos, C. T. (1989). *Statistical Methods in Epidemiology.* New York: Oxford University Press.

Kannel, W. B., Dawber, T. R., Kagan, A., Revotskie, N., & Stokes, J. (1961). Factors of risk in the development of coronary heart disease—six year follow-up experience. *Annals of Internal Medicine,* 55, 33–50.

Kleinbaum, D. G., Kupper, L. L., & Morgenstern, H. (1982). *Epidemiologic Research. Principles and Quantitative Methods.* New York: Van Nostrand Reinhold.

Miettinen, O. (1972). Components of the crude risk ratio. *American Journal of Epidemiology,* 96, 168–172.

Miller, A. B. (1992). Planning cancer control strategies. In *Chronic Diseases in Canada. Volume 13, No. 1.* Ontario: Health and Welfare.

Schnorr, T. (1993). Video display terminals and adverse pregnancy outcomes. In K. Steenland (Ed.), *Case Studies in Occupational Epidemiology* (pp. 7–20). New York: Oxford University Press.

Shaw, G. B. (1911). *The Doctor's Dilemma, with a Preface on Doctors.* New York: Brentano's.

Smith, P. F., Mikl, J., Truman, B. I., et al. (1991). HIV infection among women entering the N.Y. State correctional system. *American Journal of Public Health,* 81 (Supplement), 35–40.

Stadel, B. V. (1981). Oral contraceptives and cardiovascular disease. *New England Journal of Medicine,* 305, 612–618, 672–677.

Thomas, D. B. (1992). Cancer. In J. M. Last and R. B. Wallace (Eds.), *Maxcy–Rosenau–Last Textbook of Public Health and Preventive Medicine* (pp. 811–826). Norwalk, CT: Appleton & Lange.

Zhou, Y. F., Leon, M. B., Waclawiw, M. A., Popma, J. J., Yu, Z. X., Finkel, T., & Epstein, S. E. (1996). Association between prior cytomegalovirus infection and the risk of restenosis after coronary atherectomy. *New England Journal of Medicine,* 335, 624–630.

9

Analytic Study Designs

Analytic epidemiologic studies are used to draw inferences about the etiology, treatment, and prevention of a disease. Study designs may be either observational or experimental. Observational studies are either cross-sectional, cohort, or case-control. Types of experimental studies include clinical trials and community trials.

9.1 ANATOMY OF STUDY DESIGN

Descriptive and Analytic Studies

Descriptive epidemiologic studies are used to explore and describe the general patterns of disease in populations. Studies of this type are usually done early in the phase of an investigation, when little is known about the frequency, natural history, or determinants of the disease. Results from descriptive studies are used to generate hypotheses about the cause, transmission, prevention, and prognosis of the disease in question. In describing the epidemiology of the disease, specific groups with higher than expected rates of disease might be identified, thus suggesting hypotheses to be tested in future studies.

    Analytic epidemiologic studies are done for the primary purpose of testing hypotheses derived from descriptive epidemiologic studies and other sources. Analytic epidemiology has these objectives:

- To understand the biology and natural history of disease by explaining the etiology in terms of risk factors and modes of transmission
- To predict the number of cases and distribution of cases, health patterns, and determinants of disease in populations and subgroups
- To control disease in populations by preventing new occurrences, curing old occurrences, prolonging life, improving the quality of life, and testing interventions aimed at improving health in individuals and groups

Although epidemiologists frequently distinguish between descriptive and analytic studies, the difference is not absolute. Both descriptive and analytic epidemiologic research represent a continuum of design and intent, with most epidemiologic studies serving both hypothesis-generating and hypothesis-testing purposes.

Study Design Dimensions

Epidemiologists have at their disposal an array of study design options. Although a comprehensive consideration of every conceivable experimental and observational study design feature is beyond the scope of this book, a fundamental understanding of key study design dimensions is crucial if one hopes to interpret the results of analytic research. The most important facets of study design are (Kramer & Baivin, 1987):

- Whether the study is **observational or experimental**
- The **directionality** of the study (cross-sectional, cohort, case-control)
- The **timing** of data collection (concurrent, historical, or mixed)
- The **sample selection criteria** (fixed-exposure, fixed-disease, nonfixed)

Observational Studies Versus Experimental Studies   The most fundamental study design consideration is whether the study is observational or experimental. **Observational studies** take a "come as you are" approach, allowing nature to take its course. In its simplest form, an observational study considers two groups of people—one group characterized by an exposure and the other by its absence. The investigator searches for a difference in incidence or prevalence of disease by group to infer a possible etiologic link between the exposure and disease. Indeed, this has been the method we have discussed to date. **Experimental studies,** on the other hand, allow the investigator to control a treatment or intervention through **random allocation.** Epidemiologic experiments may be used to test vaccines, medical practices, and behavioral programs intended to reduce disease or disability. In the simplest form of an experiment, one group is given an experimental treatment while another group is given either a sham or alternative treatment. After a period of follow-up, groups are measured with respect to a change in disease status or difference in response. Noted differences allow the investigator to infer whether the experimental treatment had an effect. Thus, the defining element of experimental epidemiology is the investigator's ability to allocate individuals or groups of individuals to experimental or control groups, ideally through randomization.

Two types of epidemiologic experiments are possible: clinical trials and community trials. In **clinical trials,** the treatment or intervention is randomized on an individual basis, so that the unit of analysis is the person. In **community trials,** the treatment or intervention is randomized on a group basis, so that the unit of analysis is the community. Clinical and community trials may also afford control over environmental factors other than the main study factor. Consequently, experimental designs enable the investigator to isolate the effects of the factor under study. However, experimentation is often unethical and impractical in humans, thus limiting its application to the study of relatively few human health problems.

Directionality   The **directionality** of a study refers to the order in which the exposure and disease are investigated. Although there are many dimensions to observational studies, directionality is perhaps the most important in helping to orient an analysis. Investigations in which the exposure and disease are measured with respect to approximately the same point in time are adirectional or **cross-sectional studies.** Investigations that take a forward-looking approach from exposure to disease are **cohort studies.** Investigations that take a backward-looking approach from disease to exposure are **case-control studies.** It is this scheme that determines our three basic observational designs (Fig. 9.1). Figure 9.2 shows how observational dimensions combine with experimental control to determine our five primary study designs as:

- Cross-sectional (observational)
- Case-control (observational)
- Cohort (observational)
- Clinical trial (experimental)
- Community trial (experimental)

Timing **Timing** refers to the chronological relationship between the time data are collected and when the primary phenomenon actually occurred. When the exposure and disease actually occurred prior to the beginning of the study proper, the timing of the study is said to be **historical.** Historical information might be obtained from preexisting records (e.g., birth and death certificates, medical records, census information, employment history) or from the recall of prior events by study subjects, their friends, or relatives. When the exposure and disease information actually occur during the investigation, the study is said to be **concurrent.** When some of the study information is collected historically and other information is collected concurrently, the study is said to have **mixed timing.*** Unlike directionality, timing does not determine our basic observational study

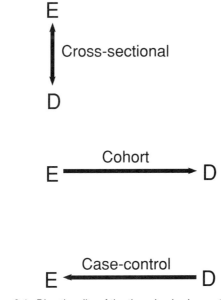

Figure 9.1. *Directionality of the three basic observational designs.*

*Note that the now outdated terms "prospective" and "retrospective" have been avoided in this discussion. These ambiguous terms have historically been used to refer to both the directionality, timing, and sample selection criteria of studies and should, therefore, be avoided.

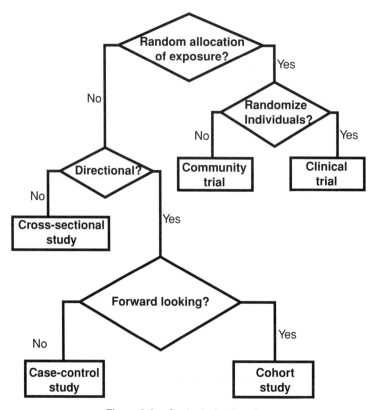

Figure 9.2. Study design flowchart.

design classification scheme. Timing, however, does play an important role in determining data quality (concurrent data are generally more reliable than historical data).

Sampling the Target Population   In analyzing the relationship between exposure E and disease D, researchers rarely get the opportunity to study the entire population. Instead, a sample of the population is studied. Sampling offers the following advantages (Cochran, 1977):

Reduced Cost. If data are collected from only a small fraction of the aggregate, expenditures are smaller than if a complete census is attempted.

Greater Speed. Data can be collected and summarized more quickly with a sample than with a complete census.

Greater Scope. Studies that rely on sampling can collect information about more factors and have greater flexibility in the type of information that can be collected.

Greater Accuracy. Better-trained personnel and higher-quality equipment can be employed to collect data because of the reduced volume of work.

In effect, sampling provides a practical, timely, and economical way to derive the information we seek.

Before selecting a sample, the investigator must clearly define the population to which inferences will be made. We call this population the **target population, internal population,** or **study base.** Choice of a target population is determined by the nature of the research question and sources of data available to the researcher. A distinction is made between this (internal) target population and the larger **external population,** about which additional generalizations may be made. The extent to which the sample reflects the target population is called the study's **internal validity.** The extent to which the target population reflects the external population is called the study's **external validity** (Fig. 9.3). For example, in studying the effects of smoking on health, we may start with a sample of smokers and nonsmokers from a specific community. The extent to which the sample reflects what is going on in the community is referred to as the study's internal validity. The extent to which the goings on in the community reflect the health effects of smoking in general is referred to as the study's external validity.

The prime motive in sampling is to select a group of people who represent the target population. From a validity standpoint, it is always preferable to use impartial chance (random) mechanisms to select your sample. Otherwise, human choice may adversely influence the representativeness of the sample. Although the only statistically reliable way to achieve representativeness is through a random sample, many epidemiologic studies are unable to achieve this ideal, using, instead, a sample of convenience ("nonprobability" sample). This can pose a threat to the representativeness of a sample and, hence, potentially degrade a study's internal validity.

The most fundamental chance mechanism for random sampling is called **simple random sampling.** A simple random sample is a sample in which each population member has an equal and independent probability of entering the sample. To select a simple random sample of size n from a target population of size N, we sequentially number the population members with identifying numbers 1 through N. (This of course assumes a census is available.) Then, a corresponding sample size n is determined using an appropriate statistical formula. (Sample size calculation methods are covered in most introductory

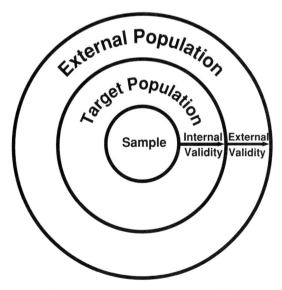

Figure 9.3. *Internal and external validity.*

texts on statistics.) Finally, a random number table or generator is used to determine which population members enter the sample.

More sophisticated random sampling techniques are also available. Examples of more sophisticated random sampling techniques are **stratified random sampling** (based on dividing the population into strata before taking a random sampling) and **cluster random sampling** (random sampling natural groups or clusters, as opposed to individuals). These variants offer advantages in efficiency under certain conditions. For example, in using a stratified random sample based on age strata, we can ensure a sufficient number of elderly people enter the sample. However, in using these more advanced random sampling techniques, specialized computational formulas must be used. Otherwise, inaccuracies will result. By this I mean to say that most of the statistical techniques presented in this and other introductory texts assume data are derived by a simple random sample. Violations in this assumption (or the extent to which samples do not represent a simple random sample) invalidate statistical inferences that follow.

Sample Selection Criteria

A study may choose to select subjects from the target population based on their exposure status, disease status, or other criteria. When the exposure is rare, a sampling procedure based on the exposure status of population members ensures that a sufficient number of exposed and unexposed subjects reach the sample (i.e., the investigator can sample a set number of subjects from each category). We call this **fixed-exposure sampling** because the exposure status of subjects is fixed, but the disease status of subjects is left free to vary. Fixed-exposure sampling is most common in (but not exclusive to) cohort studies.

When the disease is rare, a sampling procedure based on the disease status of population members ensures that a sufficient number of cases and noncases ("controls") will be in the sample. We call this **fixed-disease sampling** because the disease status of subjects is fixed, but the exposure status of subjects is left free to vary. Fixed-disease sampling is most common in (but not exclusive to) case-control studies.

When neither the exposure nor the disease is rare, the investigator may choose a sampling procedure based on other criteria (e.g., a fully random sample of the population). We call this **nonfixed sampling** because both the exposure and disease status of subjects are left free to vary. Use of nonfixed sampling criteria is most common in (but not exclusive to) cross-sectional studies.

The criteria used to sample the target population is related to, but not entirely determined by, the study's directionality. The fixed-exposure sampling model is available to cohort studies and cross-sectional studies, but not to case-control studies. The fixed-disease sampling model is available to case-control studies and cross-sectional studies, but not to cohort studies. The nonfixed sampling model is available to all observational study designs. In all, seven possible directionality/sampling model combinations are possible (Table 9.1).

TABLE 9.1. Combinations of Directionality and Sampling Selection Criteria for Observational Studies; ✔ = Possible, ✗ = Impossible

Sample Selection Criteria	Directionality		
	Cohort	Case-control	Cross-sectional
Fixed-exposure	✔	✗	✔
Fixed-disease	✗	✔	✔
Nonfixed	✔	✔	✔

Source: Adapted from Kramer (1988), p. 42; used with permission of Springer-Verlag.

The criteria used to sample the target population is seen as separate from the timing of a study. Thus, many combinations of study timing, sample selection criteria, and study directionality are possible. For example:

- A cohort study recruits a non-fixed, sample from the target population and then follows subjects forward to complete a *concurrent, nonfixed, cohort study* (timing = concurrent, sample selection criteria = nonfixed, directionality = cohort).
- A case-control study recruits a fixed-disease sample of cases and controls from the target population, concurrently determines disease status, and determines exposure status historically to complete a *mixed-timing, fixed-disease, case-control study*.
- A cross-sectional study recruits a sample from the target population according to exposure criteria (e.g., a set number of exposed workers and nonexposed workers) and concurrently classifies study subjects according to their disease status to complete a *concurrent, fixed-exposure, cross-sectional study*.

By combining all possible directionality, timing, and sample selection criteria dimensions, 21 unique study designs are possible (Fig. 9.4). Note that case-control studies cannot utilize a fixed-exposure sample and cohort studies cannot utilize a fixed-disease sample. All other combinations, however, are possible.

9.2 CROSS-SECTIONAL STUDIES

Directionality, Timing, and Sampling Criteria

Cross-sectional studies are adirectional studies in which the exposure and disease are measured with respect to approximately the same point in time. Consequently, cross-sectional studies are also called **prevalence studies** or simply **surveys**. The timing of data collection in cross-sectional studies can be concurrent, historical, or mixed. Study subjects can be sampled using fixed-exposure, fixed-disease, or nonfixed samples.

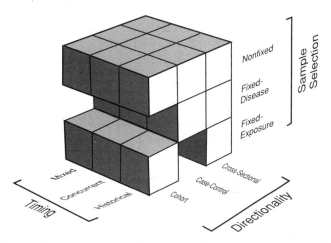

Figure 9.4 *Directionality, timing, and sampling criteria. The two tunnels represent the six impossible combinations. (Source: Kramer, M. S. (1988).* Clinical Epidemiology and Biostatistics. A Primer for Clinical Investigators and Decision Makers. *Berlin: Springer-Verlag, p. 44, sample selection axis labels (on the right-hand aspect of the cube) have been modified to conform with the terminology in this book; used with permission from the publisher.)*

Data Analysis

The analysis of data from cross-sectional studies depends on the sampling model used to recruit subjects. If data are collected using a fixed-exposure or nonfixed sample, the prevalence of disease in the exposed group is compared with that of the unexposed group to form a prevalence ratio (see Section 8.2). If the mean duration of the disease is identical in exposed and unexposed cases, and if the disease does not affect exposure status, the prevalence ratio will approximate the cumulative incidence ratio (Kleinbaum et al., 1982, pp. 148–149). Note, however, that these preconditions do not often hold. For this and other reasons discussed below, cross-sectional studies are seldom the design of choice when investigation disease etiology.

If data are collected using a fixed-disease sample, the prevalence of exposure in the diseased group is compared with that of the nondiseased group in the form of a prevalence odds ratio (formula 8.9). When the overall prevalence of disease is small (prevalence < .05), the prevalence odds ratio will approximate the prevalence ratio. Once again, if the mean duration of the disease is identical in exposed and unexposed cases and if the disease does not affect exposure status, this value will approximate the cumulative incidence ratio.

Strengths and Limitations

Cross-sectional studies are particularly useful for describing the characteristics of a population, especially when data are collected using a nonfixed sample. Consequently, prevalence studies are often done to assess the extent of chronic problems in a population. As an example of cross-sectional data, let us consider the prevalence of disabilities in the United States. A 1989 Institute of Medicine report (as cited in Shaar and McCarthy, 1994) estimated age-adjusted prevalences of limitations in daily activities of 12.9% and 13.2% in women and men, respectively. However, a 1988 article by Russo and Jansen (as cited in Shaar and McCarthy, 1994) estimated that 24% of women with work-related disabilities participated in the workforce in 1982 compared with 42% of men with work-related disabilities. Therefore, men and women have comparable rates of limitations in physical activities, but women with disabilities are less likely to participate in the workforce than disabled men.

In using a cross-sectional design, a problem called **reverse causality bias** can occur. Reverse causality bias, also called **cart before the horse bias,** refers to the detection of an association that is temporally reversed so that the disease precedes the exposure in time. For example, we might observe a cross-sectional association between lean body mass and certain forms of cancer. Without knowing whether the lean body mass preceded the cancer, a likely explanation is that the cancer caused a loss of body weight (through the disease process, chemotherapy, cachexia, etc.) The time sequence necessary to establish lean body mass as a risk factor for these forms of cancer is therefore lacking. With exposure factors that are present at birth (e.g., sex, blood type), reverse causality bias is not a problem. However, for other factors that might change over time, it may be difficult to be sure whether the exposure preceded or followed the disease when using a cross-sectional design.

9.3 COHORT STUDIES

Directionality, Timing, and Sampling Criteria

Cohort studies are forward directional studies in which the incidence of disease is compared in groups defined by exposure status. The exposure-defined groups are followed through periodic reexamination or surveillance for new occurrence of the disease. Cohort studies also called **follow-up studies** or **incidence studies.**

The timing of data collection in cohort studies can be concurrent, historical, or mixed. Concurrent data collection might not be feasible, however, for studying rare diseases or diseases that develop after long latency. Use of historical or mixed data can remedy this limitation, assuming study factor information is available for the population. Historical data for cohort studies may come from health-care, occupational, and vital statistics sources. A potential problem in follow-up studies of long duration is the loss of subjects because of withdrawal or death. This problem is can often be remedied by using incidence density procedures that adjust for person-time of follow-up on an individual basis (see Section 6.5).

Study subjects in cohort studies can be sampled using fixed-exposure or nonfixed selection criteria. Use of a fixed-disease sample invalidates the cohort design.

Data Analysis

The analysis of cohort data was covered in Chapter 8 and will, therefore, only be briefly reviewed. Recall the measures of association are calculated by categorizing the population into two or more exposure groups. The incidence of disease in each category is compared with that of an unexposed (or least exposed) reference category, with the unexposed group serving to establish a **baseline rate.** Measures of association can be based on ratios (cumulative incidence ratios or incidence density ratio) or differences (cumulative incidence difference or incidence density difference). Measures of potential impact are the attributable fraction in the population and attributable fraction among the exposed.

Doll and Hill's 1970 cohort study of lung cancer in British physicians provides a classic example of the cohort design. The target population represents a homogeneous group ("cohort") of highly educated men. All physicians in the study were lung cancer free at the beginning of follow-up. Data represent age-adjusted incidence densities of lung cancer death, with incidence densities in the exposed groups compared with the baseline rate in nonsmokers (Table 9.2). Data suggest an increase in risk with each successive increase in smoking level.

Cohort studies can also be done by using a reference rate from outside the target population (i.e., the baseline rate is provided by a "reference population"). External reference rates can come from other studies or from the National Center of Health Statistics. Studies of this type are called **standardized mortality (morbidity) studies** and, as such, were discussed in Chapter 7.

TABLE 9.2. Smoking and Lung Cancer in British Physicians

Smoking Status	Person-Years of Follow-up	Lung Cancer Cases	Age-Adjusted Incidence Density (per 1000 person-years)	Incidence Density Ratio	Incidence Density (per 1000 person-years)
Nonsmokers	15,107	1	0.07	Reference	Reference
Light smokers[a]	38,586	22	0.47	6.7	0.40
Moderate smokers[b]	36,089	24	0.86	12.3	0.79
Heavy smokers[c]	23,415	34	1.66	23.7	1.59

Source: Doll & Hill (1970).

[a]Light smokers = 1–14 grams of tobacco per day.
[b]Moderate smokers = 15–24 grams of tobacco per day.
[c]Heavy smokers = greater than 25 grams of tobacco per day.

Strengths and Limitations

Cohort studies have a major methodological advantage over cross-sectional studies in their ability to discern the onset of disease. As a result, the researcher can be certain that the exposure preceded the disease and reverse causality bias is absent. Moreover, cohort studies can study the natural history of disease in an inartificial setting like no other design, can adjust for subjects lost to follow-up, and are statistically efficient when studying rare exposures and common diseases.

The cohort study design also exhibits several limitations and disadvantages. For example, they are statistically inefficient when studying rare diseases and can be costly to complete. Concurrent cohort studies are also inefficient when studying diseases with long latency. Moreover, if exposure groups differ with respect to the distribution of extraneous risk factors at baseline, differences in incidence at the end of the study may reflect differences due to extraneous factors, rather than to the study exposure. This phenomenon, called confounding, was introduced in Chapter 7 and is further considered in Chapter 11.

Cohort study design strengths and weaknesses are summarized as part of Table 9.5.

9.4 CASE-CONTROL STUDIES

Directionality, Timing, and Sampling Criteria

Case-control studies are backward directional studies that compare a group of people with disease ("cases") with one or more groups of noncases ("controls"). The exposure histories of cases and controls are compared to make causal inferences. When considering the directionality of case-control studies, remember that "time goes backwards from present to past." Case-control studies are also called **case-referent studies** and **trohoc** ("cohort" spelled backward) **studies.**

The timing of data collection in case-control studies can be concurrent, historical, or mixed. The timing of data collection for the disease status of subjects can be concurrent (based on current status) or historical (derived from preexisting records). The timing of data collection for most exposure data must be historical, allowing for a latent period to pass between the exposure and disease. However, the timing of data for the exposure of "permanent" factors (e.g., sex, blood type, race) can be concurrent, because these factors do not change.

Sample selection criteria can be fixed-disease or nonfixed. The latter option negates the efficiency advantages of the case-control approach, however, and is, consequently, rarely used.

The main requirement when selecting cases and controls is that they typify their respective counterparts in the target population. That is, cases must be typical of incident cases in the target population and controls must be typical of nondiseased people in the target population. Selection of cases is usually straightforward: a complete listing of population cases is often available from death certificates, hospital and clinical patient data, special reporting systems (e.g., cancer registries), or other surveillance sources, thus allowing a random sampling or complete enumeration of cases. However, the selection of controls is not as straight forward and has, therefore, been an issue of ongoing epidemiologic concern (Feinstein and Horwitz, 1983; Lasky & Stolley, 1994; Miettinen, 1985; Pearce and Checkoway, 1988; Savitz and Pearce, 1988; Schlesselman, 1985; Smith, 1983; Wacholder et al., 1992a,b,c) In theory, controls are selected to be typical of healthy people in the target population. Defining this target population, however, is not always an easy task. In practice, controls might be selected from the following sources:

- Hospitals or clinics
- Disease registries, representing people with similar diseases as cases (e.g., in studying cancer X, controls may have cancer Y)
- Death certificates, representing people who had died of other diseases (e.g., in studying fatal disease X, controls may have had fatal disease Y)
- The population giving rise to the cases
- A cohort giving rise to cases (so-called **nested case-control design**)

Miettinen's (1976) conceptualization of the case-control method suggests we sample disease-free person-time from a "study base" of noncases and future cases to describe the distribution of exposure time in the healthy population. This distribution of exposure time is compared to that of incident cases to provide an estimate of the incidence density ratio.

Another approach suggests using multiple control groups from different sources (e.g., hospital-based controls and community controls). If comparisons based on the different control groups provide similar results, increased confidence in the analysis is gained. If the results differ, however, neither analysis can be trusted.

For further discussion of principles, types, and design options for selecting controls in case-control studies, the interested reader is referred to Wacholder et al. (1992a,b,c).

Data Analysis

The analysis of data from case-control studies requires methods different from anything discussed so far. As with other analytic studies, the purpose of case-control studies is to measure the statistical association between an exposure and disease. To accomplish this objective, each study subject's history is examined to determine the level to which they have been exposed. Such information may be provided by the study subjects themselves, a proxy, or through preexisting health-care or occupational records. For a dichotomous study factor, data are parsed into a two-by-two table with conventional cells labeled (Table 9.3).

For descriptive purpose, exposure proportions in cases and controls are compared. The exposure proportions in cases (EP_1) is

$$EP_1 = \frac{a}{m_1} \tag{9.1}$$

TABLE 9.3. Notation and Data Layout for Case-Control Studies

	Exposure + E_1	Exposure − E_0	
Disease +(Cases)	a	b	m_1
Disease −(Controls)	c	d	m_0
	n_1	n_0	n

The exposure proportion in controls (EP_0) is

$$EP_0 = \frac{c}{m_0} \tag{9.2}$$

If the cases and controls have similar exposure proportions, we might infer no effect of the study factor on the disease. If, on the other hand, cases are significantly more likely than noncases to have been exposed, we might infer a deleterious effect of the exposure. We have essentially reasoned that if cases are more likely than noncases to have been exposed, the exposure is likely to have caused the disease. The measure of association to address this relationship is called the **exposure odds ratio,** often referred to simply as the **odds ratio.** As the name implies, the exposure odds ratio is the ratio of two odds. The exposure odds in cases (EO_1) is

$$EO_1 = \frac{a}{b} \tag{9.3}$$

The exposure odds in controls (EO_0) is

$$EO_0 = \frac{c}{d} \tag{9.4}$$

The exposure odds ratio (EOR) is

$$EOR = \frac{EO_1}{EO_0} = \frac{a/b}{c/d} = \frac{ad}{bc} \tag{9.5}$$

Note that the exposure odds ratio is the same cross-product (ad/bc) as the disease odds ratio presented in formula 8.9. Moreover, under Bayes's theorem, the exposure odds ratio has the same probabilistic interpretation as the disease odds ratio (Neutra & Drolette, 1978). *Thus, the exposure odds ratio provides yet another way to estimate relative risk.* Consequently, exposure odds ratios of approximately one suggest no association between the exposure and disease, exposure odds ratios significantly greater than one suggest a positive association, and exposure odds ratios significantly less than one suggest a negative association.

Attributable fractions can also be inferred from case-control studies. The **attributable fraction for the population** (AF_p) can be calculated from case-control data by applying the formula

$$AF_p = \frac{(EP_0)(EOR - 1)}{(EP_0)(EOR - 1) + 1} \tag{9.6}$$

where EOR represents the exposure odds ratio and EP_0 represents the exposure proportion in controls (see formula 9.2).

The **attributable fraction among the exposed** (AF_e) can be calculated as

$$AF_e = \frac{EOR - 1}{EOR} \tag{9.7}$$

TABLE 9.4. Smoking and Lung Cancer, Case-Control Data

	Smoke +	Smoke −	
Lung Cancer +(Cases)	647	2	649
Lung Cancer −(Controls)	622	27	649
	1269	29	1298

$$EP_1 = 647/649 = .997$$

$$EP_0 = 622/649 = .958$$

$$EO_1 = 647/2 = 323.5$$

$$EO_0 = 622/27 = 23.0$$

$$EOR = \frac{(647)(27)}{(2)(622)} = 14.0$$

$$AF_p = \frac{(.958)(14.0 - 1)}{(.958)(14.0 - 1) + 1} = .926$$

$$AF_e = \frac{14.0 - 1}{14} = .929$$

Source: Doll & Hill (1950).

Illustration   Data from Doll and Hill's 1950 case-control study of smoking and lung cancer are presented in Table 9.4. Case-control statistics are reported at the bottom of the table. The calculated exposure odds ratio of 14 suggests that smokers have 14 times the risk of lung cancer as nonsmokers. The attributable fraction in the population suggests that slightly less than 93% of the lung cancer cases in British men at that time were attributable to cigarette smoking. The etiologic fraction among the exposed is also approximately 93%.

Strengths and Limitations

Case-control studies offer several practical advantages over other study design options. First, their convenient and efficient sampling strategy avoids the large sample size requirements of cohort studies. Second, their inherently backward directionality avoids the lengthy follow-up times that are necessary when studying diseases that occur only after long latent periods. Third, case-control studies are often less expensive and less time consuming than comparable cohort studies. Fourth, case-control methodology allows for the study of multiple exposures in relation to a single disease. Thus, it is well suited for generating and testing etiologic hypotheses.

Case-control studies also have major limitations. First, selecting an appropriate control group is often difficult and controversial. Second, the accuracy of historically derived exposure information is prone to error, especially when the information relies on subjective memory and recall. Third, because of their backward directionality and reliance on recall, accurately placing exposure- and disease-related events in time may be difficult. Fourth, case-control studies are statistically inefficient when studying rare exposures. Fifth, case-control studies cannot directly determine disease frequency or difference measures of association. Sixth, case-control studies cannot study the multiple health effects of a single exposure. Because of these potential pitfalls, case-control studies have been called "the

TABLE 9.5. Selected Strengths and Limitations of Clinical Trials, Cohort Studies, and Case-Control Studies

	Clinical Trials	Cohort Studies	Case-Control Studies
Strengths	1. Randomization creates groups that are similar at the beginning of the study (minimizes confounding) 2. Application of admissibility criteria creates homogeneity within groups 3. Conducive to blinding	1. Statistically efficient when studying rare exposures 2. Can adjust for withdrawals 3. Can study the natural history of disease	1. Statistically efficient when studying rare disease 2. Results can be derived in a short period of time, even if the disease is characterized by long latency 3. Can evaluate multiple exposures with a single study 4. Less expensive and quicker to complete than comparable cohort studies
Limitations	1. Often unethical outside the realm of clinical medicine 2. Expensive 3. Impractical (especially when studying behavioral risk factors) 4. May have limited generalizability	1. Poor statistical efficiency when studying rare disease 2. Can be costly and resource intensive 3. Concurrent cohort studies are ill-suited for studies with long latency 4. Groups may differ at beginning of study (problem with confounding)	1. Difficult in determining appropriate control group 2. Prone to recall bias 3. Difficult to precisely place events in time 4. Statistically inefficient for the study of rare exposures 5. Cannot determine the frequency of disease 6. Cannot study the multiple effects of single exposure

whipping-boy of epidemiologic research" (Rothman, 1986, p. 69). As Rothman points out, however, insufficiencies of case-control studies often stem from their inept conduct rather than from an inherent weakness in the design itself.

Case-control study design strengths and weaknesses are summarized as part of Table 9.5.

9.5 EXPERIMENTAL STUDIES

Directionality, Timing, Sampling Criteria, and Other Concepts

Experimental epidemiology uses randomization to allocate subjects to treatment or intervention groups. The two forms of experimental epidemiology are clinical trials and community trials. In **clinical trials,** the study factor is randomly assigned at the individual level. In **community trials,** the unit of random assignment is the group. Other than in their ability to randomize the study factor, experimental designs are similar to cohort studies in directionality and analysis (Fig. 9.5). Consequently, they are also called **experimental cohort studies** or **cohort studies with randomization.**

Because of the need to assemble subjects for randomization, the timing of true experimental studies is always concurrent. Quasi-experiments may use historical controls, however (see below).

Experimental Studies

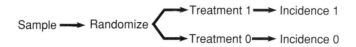

Cohort Studies

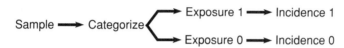

Figure 9.5. *Experimental studies and cohort studies.*

Also, because of the need to randomize, selection of study subjects is based on neither exposure nor disease status. Instead, recruitment of subjects is based on other criteria. For example, when studying the efficacy of a new arthritis drug, the investigator would have to specify that the subjects have arthritis of a certain type, severity, and duration. In addition, the age and sex of subjects might be restricted. For example, we may admit only 50- to 59-year-old men with osteoarthritis of the knee that is severe enough to limit daily activities. Inclusion and exclusion criteria of this type are called **study admissibility criteria.** Thus, study admissibility criteria are used to define the target population. Once the study's admissibility criteria are defined, subjects may be recruited either during the study (accrual method) or before the study begins (nonaccrual method). The number of subjects selected for participation should be dictated by sample size calculations completed before the study begins.

Recruited subjects are randomly allocated to the treatment group (group 1) or control group (group 0). Randomization can be achieved in different ways. For example, in the case of evaluating a single treatment, we could flip a coin as each new subject enters the study. If the coin turns heads up, the subject is assigned to group 1. If the coin turns heads down, the subject is assigned to group 0. By using the "luck of the draw," factors extraneous to the analysis (i.e., everything other than the treatment) will tend to distribute equally among the groups. Consequently, all other things are made equal at the beginning of the study and differences noted at the end of the study can be attributed directly to the treatment.

Several types of control groups are employed in clinical and community trials. **Active controls** are study subjects who have been allocated to a treatment or control group. Active controls may receive an alternative therapy, true placebo, or no treatment. **Passive controls** are subjects from outside the domain of the study. Passive controls may be observed concurrently with the study or historically. In fact, use of passive controls does not fully comply with our definition of an experiment because they were not randomly assigned a treatment or placebo. Therefore, we call clinical trials that use passive controls

quasi-experiments, rather than true experiments. The final type of control group consists of **self-controls.** Self-controls are subjects who cross over from one study treatment to another. Studies that use self-controls are, therefore, called **crossover trials.** Usually, a **washout period** during which the current treatment is metabolized and leaves the body is necessary if self-controls are to be used.

Improvements Unrelated to Treatment

When analyzing the results from a clinical trial or community trial, investigators must be aware of the tendency of study participants to improve in response to being studied, *per se*. Two related phenomena apply: The placebo effect and the Hawthorne effect. The **placebo effect** refers to the improvement of a patient following treatment with a pharma-cologically inert substance (placebo). Placebo-associated improvements are attributable to the patient's mistaken belief that he/she is receiving an effective treatment. A related phenomenon, the **Hawthorne effect,** refers to the tendency of subjects to alter their be-havior simply because they are being studied. This term grew out of a 1920s study at the Hawthorne Works of the Western Electric Company in Chicago in which investigators no-ticed improvements in worker performance no matter the quality of an intervention. For example, worker output improved whether the lighting intensity at plants was increased or decreased. This suggests that the knowledge of being observed has an influence on the behavior and state of mind of study participants. To neutralize both the placebo effect and Hawthorne effect, the investigator compares the improvement rate in the treatment group to that of a similarly observed control group. The improvement rate in the control group then serves as a standard by which to make comparisons.

Blinding

To decrease the opportunity for biased ascertainment of the study outcome, clinical trials em-ploy a technique called blinding. **Blinding** (also called **masking**) refers to a study technique in which the subjects, observers, or investigators are kept ignorant of the group to which subjects are assigned. For example, when studying the pharmacologic treatment of chronic pain, we might randomly assign treatments to two groups. Group 1 receives a new anti-inflammatory medicine and group 0 receives a placebo. Subjects agree to participate in a blind study in which they are kept unaware of the medicine they received until after the study is completed. Blinding can occur at different levels in a study. **Single blind** refers to a study that does not reveal to subjects their treatment group until after the completion of the study. **Double blind** refers to a study that does not reveal subjects' group assignments to subjects and clinical observers until after the completion of the study. **Triple blinding** (also called **blind evaluation**) refers to a study that does not reveal subjects' group assignments to sub-jects, clinical evaluators, and statistical analysts until after the completion of the study. The intent of triple blinding is to prevent ascertainment bias from entering the study at all stages.

Data Analysis

The analyses of experimental epidemiologic data and cohort data are similar. In both, the incidence of an outcome in an exposed (treated) group is compared with the incidence of an outcome in an unexposed (control) group. Consequently, the analysis of clinical trial and community trial need not be considered separately from cohort data. Measures of association may take the form of ratios (Section 8.2) and differences (Section 8.3).

Effectiveness Versus Efficacy

Two types of clinical trial analyses exist on top of this background. One considers the effectiveness of a treatment, while the other considers the efficacy of a treatment. **Effectiveness** refers to the extent to which a specific treatment produces its intended effect when employed in a "real world" setting. **Efficacy** refers to the potential effect of the treatment under optimal conditions. Accordingly, **effectiveness analysis** (also called **intention to treat analysis**) considers the results of all subjects according to their originally assigned treatment groups, irrespective of failures in compliance, discontinuation, or other reasons for withdrawal. In contrast, **efficacy analysis** includes only participants who completed the clinical trial protocol and received their intended treatment. Effectiveness analysis is generally preferred when evaluating a treatment in the "real world," in which poor compliance, switching of therapies, and withdrawal from therapy are commonplace. From a physiological perspective, however, efficacy analysis is more pertinent.

Strengths and Limitations

The strengths of experimental studies come from their ability to randomize the factor under study. This creates groups that are similar at the beginning of the study. Thus, extraneous factors that might influence the likelihood of the study outcome (so-called **confounders**) will balance out, leaving any observed difference at the end of the study directly attributable to the study factor. Moreover, application of study admissibility criteria can create groups that are homogeneous with respect to potential predictors of the outcome, thus reducing "background noise" in detecting differences due to the study factor. Finally, clinical trials are conducive to blinding, thus decreasing bias in the detection of the study outcome.

Clinical trials are not without limitations, however. First, ethical concerns are such that potentially hazardous exposures cannot randomly be assigned and exposures that are widely believed to be beneficial cannot ethically be withheld. Thus, a true void in knowledge about risks and benefits of a study factor must exist before a clinical or community trial can be considered. Consequently, ethical concerns limit the use of experimental designs outside the realm of clinical medicine. Second, the expense of clinical and community trials may further limit their use. Because of the careful controls required by clinical trials, they are often much more expensive than comparable observational studies. Third, clinical and community trials assume the study factor can be effectively assigned to subjects and subjects will be compliant with this allocation. This may not be realistic when studying behavioral and life-style determinants of health. Fourth, because experiments often take place in an artificial setting in a self-selected sample of volunteers, observed effects in the sample may not be generalizable to the larger population. Thus, one of the main strengths of the experimental design—its control over the study situation—is also the source of one of its weaknesses.

Strengths and limitations of the cohort, case-control, and clinical trial study designs are summarized in Table 9.5.

SUMMARY

1. Descriptive epidemiologic studies are used to describe and explore the general patterns of disease in a population. Studies of this type are typically done early in the phase of an investigation to generate hypotheses about the cause, transmission, prevention, and prognosis of the disease in question. Analytic epidemiologic studies are used to test causal hypotheses generated by descriptive epidemiologic studies and other sources.

2. The most important facets of analytic study design are (a) whether they are experimental or observational, (b) the directionality of the study, (c) the timing of data collection, and (d) the criteria used to sample the target population.

(a) *Experimental epidemiologic studies* randomize the study factor, whereas *observational studies* take a "come as you are approach," studying people without intervention.

(b) The *directionality* of a study refers to the order in which the exposure and disease are investigated. This is perhaps the most important study design dimension in helping to orient an observational analysis. The three study directionalities are *cross-sectional* (adirectional), *cohort* (forward), and *case-control* (backward).

(c) The *timing* of a study refers to the chronological relationship between the time data are collected and when the primary phenomenon occurred. The three study timings are *concurrent* (events occur during the study proper), *historical* (events occurred before the study began), and *mixed* (partially historical and partially concurrent).

(d) *Sample selection criteria* refers to the way in which subjects are selected for study. A study may choose to select subjects from the target population based on their exposure status, disease status, or other criteria. *Fixed-exposure sampling* refers to a sampling procedure that selects a fixed number of people from each exposure category. This is done to ensure that a sufficient number of exposed and unexposed subjects reach the sample. Fixed-exposure sampling is available to cross-sectional and cohort studies, but not to case-control studies. *Fixed-disease sampling* refers to a sampling procedure that selects a fixed number of people with the disease under study ("cases") and fixed number of people without the disease under study ("controls"). This is done to ensure that enough cases and controls reach the sample. Fixed-disease sampling is available to cross-sectional and case-control studies, but not to cohort studies. *Nonfixed sampling* refers to a sampling procedure that is neither fixed-exposure nor fixed-disease. Nonfixed sampling is available to studies of all three directionalities.

3. Sampling involves selecting a subset of a target population for study. Advantages of sampling include reduced costs, greater speed, greater scope, and greater accuracy. The extent to which the sample reflects the study's target population is called its internal validity. The extent to which the target population reflects a larger ("external") population to which further inference might be made is called the study's external validity. From a validity standpoint, using impartial random mechanisms to select your sample is always preferable. However, due to pragmatic concerns, this ideal is not always achieved.

4. Cross-sectional studies are adirectional observational studies in which the exposure and disease are measured with respect to approximately the same point in time. This type of study is particularly useful for describing the extent of chronic problems. Their utility for causal inference, however, is limited.

5. Cohort studies are forward directional observational studies in which the population is classified into various exposure categories. Groups are then followed forward to determine the incidence of various study outcomes. Cohort studies are particularly useful for studying the incidence, etiology, prognosis, and history of diseases in a natural setting.

6. Case-control studies are backward directional studies that compare exposure histories in a group of people with disease ("cases") with one or more groups of noncases ("controls"). Cases and controls should be selected so that they reflect exposure histories of their respective counterparts in the target population. The selection of controls is one of the thorniest issues in case-control methodology and has been an issue of ongoing concern. The analysis of data from case-control studies is different from anything discussed prior to this chapter. Briefly, exposure odds are compared in cases and controls to calculate an exposure odds ratio. The exposure odds ratio is an estimate of relative risk assuming incident cases are used and the controls adequately represent the distribution of exposure levels in the nondiseased population. Case-control methods offer sampling efficiencies that make them a popular study design choice. Most notably, case-control methods are efficient for studying rare diseases that occur after long latency.

7. Clinical trials and community trials are experimental epidemiologic study designs that use randomization to allocate subjects to treatment and control groups. In clinical trials, the investigator randomly assigns the treatment at the individual level. In community trials, the investigator randomly assigns the treatment at the group level. Because of randomization, extraneous factors (confounders) that might otherwise influence the likelihood of the study outcome will be equally distributed among groups. Thus, observed differences at the end of the study can be directly attributable to the study factor. However, clinical and community trials are not commonly encountered outside the realm of clinical medicine because of ethical and pragmatic concerns.

NOTATION AND FORMULA REFERENCE

See Table 9.3 for cell references.

EP_i	Exposure proportion, group i (formulas 9.1 and 9.2)
EO_i	Exposure odds, group i (formulas 9.3 and 9.4)
EOR	Odds ratio (formula 9.5)
AF_p	Attributable fraction for the population (formula 9.6)
AF_e	Attributable fraction among the exposed (formula 9.7)

EXERCISES

For each of the brief study descriptions 1–8 presented below, identify whether the study is experimental or observational and, if observational, its directionality (cross-sectional, cohort, case-control) and timing (concurrent, historical, mixed).

1. Avian adeno-associated virus is suspected of resulting from exposure to poultry. Serum samples from poultry workers and from a general adult population sample are tested to determine the proportion of individuals with positive avian A-Av antibody.

2. A behavior pattern identified as Type A (characterized by a hard-driving time urgency) is thought to be associated with coronary heart disease. Type A behavior is assessed for a group of men in a post coronary rehabilitation program. All men not falling into the Type A group are denoted Type B. Type A and Type B men are followed for 5 years to assess recurrence rates.

3. Investigators are studying employees at a bus company to test their hypothesis that occupational stress causes high blood pressure. Two major groups of employees are of interest: bus drivers and office workers in the same salary range. The investigators measure the blood pressure of all bus drivers and of a group of office workers matched to the bus drivers on age, sex, race, and length of employment. The mean blood pressure of the drivers is higher than that of the office workers and the investigators conclude that stress causes high blood pressure.

4. One hundred newly diagnosed breast cancer patients are interviewed to determine their lifelong dietary history for the consumption of fat. Healthy first-degree female relatives (mothers or sisters) of cases are interviewed in a similar manner. We compare the proportion of women reporting a history of high dietary fat consumption in breast cancer patients and the control group.

5. Fifteen hundred adult males working for Locheed Aircraft are recruited to participate in a study of coronary heart disease. Every 3 years they are examined for new occurrences of this disease. Coronary heart disease rates are compared among groups defined by personal characteristics as they were recorded at the beginning of the study.

6. A random sample of middle-age sedentary males was selected from four census tracts, and each man was examined for coronary heart disease. All those having the disease were excluded from the study. All others were randomly assigned to either an exercise group, which followed a 2-year program of systematic exercise, or a control group, which had no exercise program. Both groups were observed semiannually for any differences in the incidence of coronary heart disease.

7. One hundred persons with infectious hepatitis and 100 healthy neighbors were questioned regarding their history of eating raw clams or oysters within the preceding 3 months.

8. Questionnaires were mailed to every tenth person listed in the city telephone directory. Each person was asked to list their age, sex, smoking habits, and respiratory symptoms during the preceding 7 days. Over 90% of the questionnaires were completed and returned. The prevalence of upper respiratory symptoms was determined from the responses.

9. The following data come from a hypothetical case-control study of coronary heart disease (CHD) and diet:

	High Fat	Low Fat	
CHD+	50	50	100
CHD−	25	75	100
	75	125	200

(A) Calculate the exposure proportion in cases.

(B) Calculate the exposure proportion in controls.

(C) Calculate the exposure odds in cases.

(D) Calculate the exposure odds in controls.

(E) Calculate the exposure odds ratio.

(F) Calculate the attributable fraction in the population.

(G) Calculate the attributable fraction among the exposed.

ANSWERS TO EXERCISES

1. Observational, cross-sectional, concurrent.

2. Observational, cohort, concurrent.

3. Observational, cross-sectional, concurrent.

4. Observational, case-control, mixed timing (disease status is concurrent, exposure status is historical).

5. Observational, cohort, concurrent.

6. Experimental (clinical trial).

7. Observational, case-control, mixed timing (disease status is concurrent, exposure status is historical).

8. Observational, cross-sectional, concurrent (based on the wording "during the preceding 7 days").

9. A $EP_1 = 50 / 100 = .5$
B $EP_0 = 25 / 100 = .25$
C $EO_1 = 50 / 50 = 1$
D $EO_0 = 25 / 75 = .3333$
E $EOR = 1 / .3333 = 3.00$

F $AF_p = \dfrac{(EP_0)(EOR - 1)}{1 + (EP_0)(EOR - 1)} = \dfrac{(.25)(3 - 1)}{1 + (.25)(3 - 1)} = .333$

G $AF_e = \dfrac{EOR - 1}{EOR} = \dfrac{3 - 1}{3} = .667$

REFERENCES

Cochran, W. G. (1977). *Sampling Techniques* (3rd ed.). New York: John Wiley & Sons.

Doll, R., & Hill, A. B. (1950). Smoking and carcinoma of the lung: preliminary report. *British Medical Journal, 2*, 739–748.

Doll, R., & Hill, A. B. (1970). Mortality in relation to smoking: 20 years' observations on male British doctors. *British Medical Journal, 2*, 1525–1536.

Feinstein, A. R., & Horwitz, R. I. (1983). On choosing the control group in case-control studies. *Journal of Chronic Diseases, 36*, 311–313.

Kleinbaum, D. G., Kupper, L. L., & Morgenstern, H. (1982). *Epidemiologic Research. Principles and Quantitative Methods.* New York: Van Nostrand Reinhold.

Kramer, M. S. (1988). *Clinical Epidemiology and Biostatistics. A Primer for Clinical Investigators and Decision-Makers.* Berlin: Springer-Verlag.

Kramer, M. S., & Boivin, J. F. (1987). Toward an "unconfounded" classification of epidemiologic research design. *Journal of Chronic Diseases, 40,* 683–688.

Lasky, T., & Stolley, P. D. (1994). Selection of cases and controls. *Epidemiologic Reviews, 16,* 6–17.

Miettinen, O. S. (1976). Estimability and estimation in case-referent studies. *American Journal of Epidemiology, 103,* 226–235.

Miettinen, O. S. (1985). The "case-control" study: valid selection of subjects. *Journal of Chronic Disease, 38,* 543–548.

Neutra, R. R., & Drolette, M. E. (1978). Estimating exposure-specific disease rates from case-control studies using Bayes' Theorem. *American Journal of Epidemiology, 108,* 241–222.

Pearce, H., & Checkoway, H. (1988). Case-control studies using other diseases as controls: problems of excluding exposure-related diseases. *American Journal of Epidemiology, 127,* 851–856.

Rothman, K. J. (1986). *Modern Epidemiology.* Boston: Little, Brown and Company.

Savitz, D. A., & Pearce, N. (1988). Control selection with incomplete case ascertainment. *American Journal of Epidemiology, 127,* 1109–1117.

Schlesselman, J. J. (1985). Valid selection of subjects in case-control studies. *Journal of Chronic Disease, 38,* 549–550.

Shaar, K., & McCarthy, M. (1994). Definitions and determinants of handicap in people with disabilities. *Epidemiologic Reviews, 16,* 228–242.

Smith, A. H. (1983). Factors in the selection of control groups. In L. Chiazze, Jr., F. E. Lundin, & D. Watkins (Eds.), *Methods and Issues in Occupational and Environmental Epidemiology* (pp. 107–116). Ann Arbor, MI: Ann Arbor Science.

Wacholder, S., McLaughlin, J. K., Silverman, D. T., et al. (1992a). Selection of controls in case-control studies. I. Principles. *American Journal of Epidemiology, 135,* 1019–1028.

Wacholder, S., McLaughlin, J. K., Silverman, D. T., et al. (1992b). Selection of controls in case-control studies. II. Types of controls. *American Journal of Epidemiology, 135,* 1029–1041.

Wacholder, S., Silverman, D. T., McLaughlin, J. K., et al. (1992c). Selection of controls in case-control studies. III. Design options. *American Journal of Epidemiology, 135,* 1042–1050.

10

Inaccuracy in Epidemiologic Studies, Part I (Imprecision)

This chapter introduces fundamental notions of measurement error, statistical inference, confidence interval estimation, and hypothesis testing. Ninety-five percent confidence interval formulas for measures of disease frequency and association are presented and illustrated. A chi-square statistic for testing measures of association is discussed.

10.1 INTRODUCTION TO MEASUREMENT ERROR

Epidemiologic measures of disease frequency and association are inevitably and adversely affected by both random and systematic sources of error. The difference between random and systematic error is fundamental: **random error (imprecision)** is governed by chance and **systematic error (bias)** is determined by other factors. As a result, they represent two distinct problems.

We can further understand the difference between random and systematic error with the help of an analogy. Imagine a sharpshooter shooting at a target in which the bull's-eye represents the true value of interest. The skilled sharpshooter consistently delivers bullets to the bull's-eye center (Fig. 10.1A). Shots are thus free from both random and systematic error. If the sighting device of the gun is true, but the sharpshooter is forced to shoot from a vibrating surface, random error is introduced and shots are scattered about the target (Fig. 10.1B). If the sighting device of the gun is askew, a form of systematic error is introduced that causes shots to be delivered consistently off-center (Fig. 10.1C). Finally, use of an improperly calibrated sighting device on a vibrating surface results in both random and systematic error (Fig. 10.1D).

Instead of considering sharpshooters and targets, now consider epidemiologic measures of disease frequency and association. For illustrative purposes, consider a study that has as its objective the measurement of an incidence density ratio. The *population's true* incidence density ratio that is free from random and systematic error is called the incidence density ratio **parameter** (denoted *IDR*). The *sample's calculated* incidence density ratio that is prone to random and systematic error is referred to as the incidence density

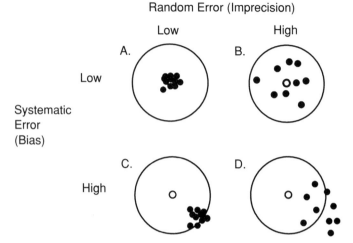

Figure 10.1. *Random and systematic error.*

ratio **estimate** (denoted $\widehat{IDR}$; pronounced "IDR hat"). The parameter and estimate are comparable to the bull's-eye and a single shot, respectively, in our target shooting analogy. To carry this analogy one step further, the study is repeated in the same population using indepdendent samples of equal size, thus deriving independent incidence density ratio estimates $\widehat{IDR}_1$, $\widehat{IDR}_2$, . . . , $\widehat{IDR}_k$. (Each calculated $\widehat{IDR}_i$ represents a separate "shot" at the "target": Fig. 10.2.) If estimates are free from systematic error, they will center on the parameter. If they are free from random error, they will cluster tightly.

Let us briefly consider a different illustration of measurement error. Suppose scales A, B, and C are used to repeatedly measure the weight of an object. Scale A consistently underestimates the weight of the object, scale B consistently overestimates the weight of the object, and scale C averages the correct weight. By that, we can say that scale A exhibits a negative bias, scale B exhibits a positive bias, and scale C exhibits no bias. Now con-

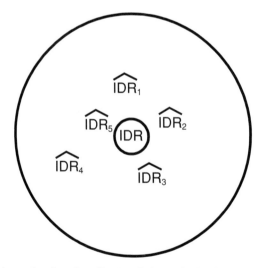

Figure 10.2. *Incidence density ratio estimates aiming at the incidence density ratio parameter.*

sider scales C and D. Both scales average the correct weight, but scale C demonstrates a relatively narrow range of values and scale D demonstrates a wide range of values. By that, both scales are unbiased, but scale C is more precise (i.e., exhibits less random error) than scale D. As with these hypothetical scales, incidence density ratio studies may tend to underestimate (Fig. 10.3A), overestimate (Fig. 10.3B), or accurately estimate (Fig. 10.3C) the parameter it is supposed to estimate. If the study design tends to reproduce similar results upon repetition, the study is said to be precise (Figs. 10.3A, B, and C). If the study design tends to calculate widely different results upon repetition, the study is said to be imprecise (Fig. 10.3D).

Statistical inference is the process used to address random measurement error in epidemiologic research. In learning about statistical inference, differentiating between estimates and parameters is important. As previously noted, different symbols are used for each—"hats" are placed on estimates, while parameters remain "hatless." For example, the symbol $\hat{\theta}$ ("theta hat") is used to represent a generic estimate and the symbol θ (theta) is used to represent a generic parameter. Due to sampling variation and other sources of random error, statistical estimate $\hat{\theta}$ varies from sample to sample. The degree to which this estimate varies determines its statistical precision (freedom from random error). The degree to which this estimate tends to center on the parameter it is trying to estimate determines its validity (freedom from bias). The goal of statistical inference is to infer the location of the parameter based on the calculated value of the estimate. The two main inferential tools used for this purpose are **estimation** and **hypothesis testing.**

10.2 ESTIMATION

Introduction to Confidence Intervals

Estimation is the process of using calculated sample values to determine the probable value of a population parameter. There are two forms of estimation: **point estimation** and **interval estimation.**

Point estimation provides a single estimate of the parameter. For example, let us say we want to know the prevalence of disease X in the population. Rather than sampling the entire population, we take a random sample of, say 1000 individuals. If 100 of these individuals have disease X, the **point estimate** of the population prevalence is .1. This calculated prevalence estimate $\hat{P}$ predicts the probable value of prevalence parameter P. Note, however, that point estimates provide no insight into the precision of the estimate. To address precision, a confidence interval must be calculated.

Confidence interval estimation provides a range of values that has known probability of capturing the parameter. It accomplishes this objective by surrounding the point estimate with a margin of error (Fig. 10.4). We can calculate confidence intervals at almost any level of confidence, but by convention, we almost always use a 95% level of confidence. A **95% confidence interval** is constructed to have a 95% chance of capturing the parameter. That is, 95% of the confidence intervals will capture the parameter and 5% will not. By that, the location of the parameter is estimated with 95% certainty.

Figure 10.5 displays confidence intervals and point estimates from three different studies, each estimating a different relative risk (cumulative incidence ratio, incidence density ratio, or odds ratio). The point estimate is indicated by a dot. The lower extent of each interval is called the **lower confidence limit** (*LCL*). The upper extent is called the **upper confidence limit** (*UCL*).

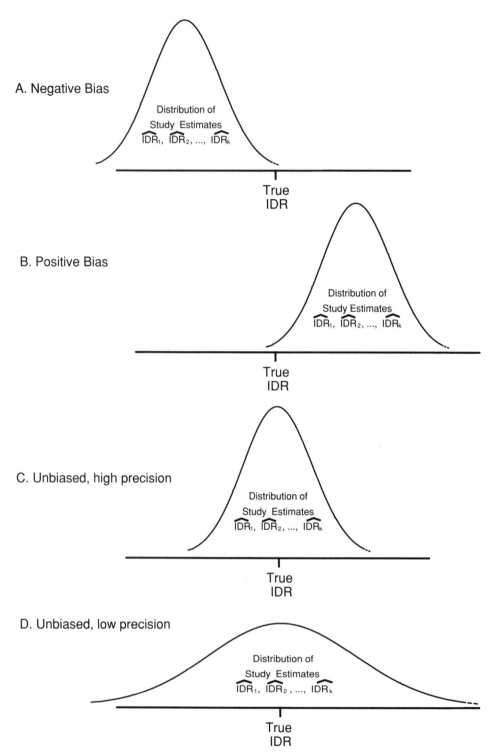

Figure 10.3. *Distribution of incidence density ratio estimates: A = negative bias, B = positive bias, C = no bias, D = no bias with low precision.*

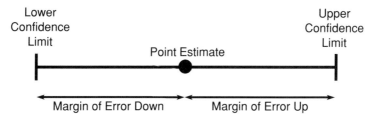

Figure 10.4. *Representations of a confidence interval.*

Confidence interval length is a measure of a study's precision. Wide confidence intervals indicate low precision; narrow confidence intervals indicate high precision. (Precision, of course, is a relative term.) In Figure 10.5, study 2 has the widest confidence interval and hence the least precision. Studies 1 and 3 appear to be of approximately equal precision. All other things being equal, the precision of a study is inversely related to the square root of its sample size. Studies based on large samples will have relatively high precision (narrow confidence intervals); studies based on small samples will have relatively low precision (wide confidence intervals).

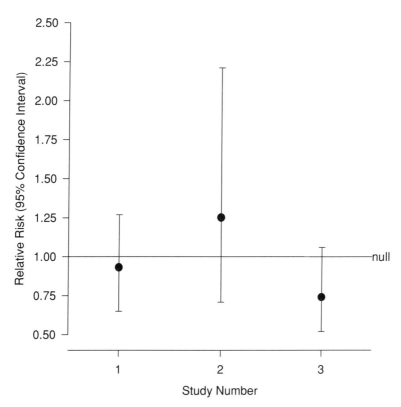

Figure 10.5. *Confidence intervals, illustrative data sets in this chapter.*

95% Confidence Intervals for Measures of Disease Frequency

We presently focus on calculating confidence intervals for the three main measures of disease frequency: prevalence, cumulative incidence, and incidence density.

Prevalence   The point estimate for prevalence is

$$\hat{P} = \frac{c}{n} \tag{10.1}$$

where $\hat{P}$ represents the prevalance estimate, c represents the number of prevalent cases in the sample, and n represents the sample size.

The 95% confidence interval for prevalance parameter P is

$$\hat{P} \pm (1.96) \sqrt{\frac{\hat{P}(1 - \hat{P})}{n}} \tag{10.2}$$

For example, if $c = 10$ and $n = 100$, then $\hat{P} = .1$ and the 95% confidence interval for P is

$$\hat{P} \pm (1.96) \sqrt{\frac{\hat{P}(1 - \hat{P})}{n}} = .1 \pm (1.96) \sqrt{\frac{(.1)(1 - .1)}{100}}$$

$$= .1 \pm .0588 = (.0412, .1588)$$

Formula 10.2 is accurate when $c \geq 5$. When $c < 5$, more exact formulas based on the binomial distribution are needed.*

Cumulative Incidence   The point estimate for cumulative incidence is

$$\widehat{CI} = \frac{i}{n} \tag{10.3}$$

where $\widehat{CI}$ represents the cumulative incidence estimate, i represents the number of new ("incident") cases in the sample, and n represents the number of people at risk at the beginning of the study.

A 95% confidence interval for cumulative incidence parameter CI is

$$\widehat{CI} \pm (1.96) \sqrt{\frac{\widehat{CI}(1 - \widehat{CI})}{n}} \tag{10.4}$$

For example, if $i = 15$ and $n = 100$, then $\widehat{CI} = .15$ and the 95% confidence interval for CI is

$$.15 \pm (1.96) \sqrt{\frac{(.15)(1 - .15)}{100}} = .15 \pm .0700 = (.0800, .2200)$$

---

*For exact binomial methods, see Rosner (1995), pp. 176–178.

Formulas 10.2 and 10.4 are both based on the normal approximation to the binomial distribution. Hence, their accuracy is suspect when the estimates are based on fewer than 5 cases. When fewer than 5 cases are encountered, more exact formulas based on the binomial distribution are needed. Such exact binomial calculations are beyond the scope of this book but are available in Rosner (1995), pp. 176–178.

Incidence Density   The point estimate for incidence density is

$$\widehat{ID} = \frac{i}{L} \tag{10.5}$$

where $\widehat{ID}$ represents the incidence density point estimate, i represents the number of incidence cases in the sample and L represents the length of follow-up time.

The 95% confidence interval for incidence density parameter ID is calculated in two steps. First, the confidence limits for the number of incident cases are determined. Table 10.1 contains 95% confidence limits for up to 40 incident cases. (*Note:* These limits are based on calculating a 95% confidence interval for a Poisson parameter according to the method of Pearson and Hartley, 1966 (Zar, 1996, p. 572).) Second, the following formula is applied:

$$\left(\frac{i_{LCL}}{L}, \frac{i_{UCL}}{L} \right) \tag{10.6}$$

where i_{LCL} represents the lower confidence limit for the number of incident cases based on the values in Table 10.1, i_{UCL} represents the upper confidence limit for the number of incident cases based on the values in Table 10.1, and L represents the length of follow-up.

For example, if we observe 10 cases during 100 person-years of follow-up, $i_{LCL} =$ 4.7955, $i_{UCL} = 18.3905$, and the 95% confidence interval for ID is

$$\frac{i_{LCL}}{L}, \frac{i_{UCL}}{L} = \frac{4.80 \text{ persons}}{100 \text{ persons-year}}, \frac{18.39 \text{ persons}}{100 \text{ person-years}}$$

$$= (0.0480 \text{ year}^{-1}, 0.1839 \text{ year}^{-1})$$

95% Confidence Intervals for Measures of Association

Confidence interval formulas for the three main epidemiologic measures of association are presented. These are the cumulative incidence ratio, incidence density ratio, and odds ratio. Formulas for odds ratios apply to both disease odds ratios (from cohort studies) and exposure odds ratios (from case-control studies).

Cumulative Incidence Ratio   Notation and data layout are presented in Table 10.2. Using this notation, the point estimate for the cumulative incidence ratio is

$$\widehat{CIR} = \frac{\widehat{CI}_1}{\widehat{CI}_0} = \frac{a/n_1}{b/n_0} \tag{10.7}$$

TABLE 10.1. 95% Confidence Limits for Number of Incident Cases Based on Incidence Density Data

i (Observed Number of Cases)	i_{LCL}	i_{UCL}
0	0.0000	3.69
1	0.0253	5.57
2	0.242	7.22
3	0.619	8.77
4	1.09	10.24
5	1.62	11.67
6	2.20	13.06
7	2.81	14.42
8	3.45	15.76
9	4.12	17.08
10	4.80	18.39
11	5.49	19.68
12	6.20	20.96
13	6.92	22.23
14	7.65	23.49
15	8.40	24.74
16	9.15	25.98
17	9.90	27.22
18	10.67	28.45
19	11.44	29.67
20	12.22	30.89
21	13.00	32.10
22	13.79	33.31
23	14.58	34.51
24	15.38	35.71
25	16.18	36.90
26	16.98	38.10
27	17.79	39.28
28	18.61	40.47
29	19.42	41.65
30	20.24	42.83
31	21.06	44.00
32	21.89	45.17
33	22.72	46.34
34	23.55	47.51
35	24.38	48.68
36	25.21	49.84
37	26.06	51.00
38	28.46	52.15
39	27.73	53.31
40	28.58	54.47

TABLE 10.2. Notation for Prevalence, Cumulative incidence, and Case-Control Studies

	Exposure +	Exposure −	
Disease +	a	b	m_1
Disease −	c	d	m_0
	n_1	n_0	n

A 95% confidence interval for cumulative incidence ratio parameter CIR is

$$(\widehat{CIR})\exp\left(\pm 1.96 \sqrt{\frac{1 - \widehat{CI}_1}{n_1 \widehat{CI}_1} + \frac{1 - \widehat{CI}_0}{n_0 \widehat{CI}_0}}\right) \qquad (10.8)$$

This formula is called the **Taylor series confidence interval** formula. To illustrate its use, let us consider the data previously introduced in Chapter 8 that addresses video display terminal use and spontaneous abortions. Data are from a cohort study comparing the cumulative incidence of spontaneous abortion in telephone operators who are exposed and unexposed to video display terminals (Schnorr, 1993). Data and calculations appear in Table 10.3. The cumulative incidence ratio estimate is 0.92 (95% confidence interval for CIR: 0.68, 1.27). This suggests that we are 95% confident the cumulative incidence ratio parameter lies between 0.68 and 1.27.

Incidence Density Ratio   Notation for incidence density ratio studies is presented in Table 10.4. Using this notation, the point estimate for the incidence density ratio is

$$\widehat{IDR} = \frac{\widehat{ID}_1}{\widehat{ID}_0} = \frac{a/L_1}{b/L_0} \qquad (10.9)$$

A 95% confidence interval for the IDR is

$$(\widehat{IDR})\exp\left(\pm 1.96 \sqrt{\frac{1}{a} + \frac{1}{b}}\right) \qquad (10.10)$$

TABLE 10.3. Illustrative Data Set 1: Video Display Terminal Use and Spontaneous Abortions, Cumulative Incidence Study

	VDT+	VDT−	
Spontaneous Abortion +	54	82	136
Spontaneous Abortion −	312	434	746
	366	516	882

$$\widehat{CIR} = \frac{\widehat{CI}_1}{\widehat{CI}_0} = \frac{54/366}{82/516} = 0.9282$$

95% confidence interval for $CIR = (\widehat{CIR})\exp\left(\pm 1.96 \sqrt{\frac{1 - \widehat{CI}_1}{n_1 \widehat{CI}_1} + \frac{1 - \widehat{CI}_0}{n_0 \widehat{CI}_0}}\right)$

$$= (.9282)\exp\left(\pm 1.96 \sqrt{\frac{1 - .1475}{(366)(.1475)} + \frac{1 - .1589}{(516)(.1589)}}\right)$$

$$= (0.68, 1.27)$$

$$\chi^2_{M-H} = \frac{(n-1)(ad - bc)^2}{n_1 n_0 m_1 m_0} = \frac{(882 - 1)[(54)(434) - (82)(312)]^2}{(366)(5126)(136)(746)} = .21$$

$$p > .10 \quad \text{(based on converting the chi-square statistic using Table 10.8)}$$

Source: Schnorr (1993).

TABLE 10.4. Notation for Incidence Density Ratio (Person-Time) Studies

	Exposure +	Exposure −	
Disease +	a	b	m
Disease −	—	—	—
Person-Time	L_1	L_0	L

To illustrate this formula, we use data from a study on breast cancer and oral contraceptive use (Colditz et al, 1990). In this study, 22 new cases of breast cancer occurred during 14,044 woman-years in 45- to 49-year-old current oral contraceptive users. Twenty-six cases occurred during 20,812 woman-years in 45- to 49-year-old women who never used oral contraceptives. Data and calculations are shown in Table 10.5. The incidence density ratio estimate is 1.25 (95% confidence interval for IDR: 0.71, 2.21). This suggests that we are 95% confident the incidence density ratio parameter lies between 0.71 and 2.21.

Odds Ratio   The notation presented in Table 10.2 also applies to disease odds ratio and exposure odds ratio studies. Using this notation, the point estimate for the odds ratio is

$$\widehat{OR} = \frac{ad}{bc} \tag{10.11}$$

TABLE 10.5. Illustrative Data Set 2: Oral Contraceptive Use and Breast Cancer in 45- to 49-year-old Women, The Nurses Health Study, Incidence Density Data

	Current Oral Contraceptive Use	Never Any Oral Contraceptive Use	
Breast Cancer +	22	26	48
Breast Cancer −	—	—	—
Women-Years	14,044	20,812	34,856

$$\widehat{IDR} = \frac{\widehat{ID_1}}{\widehat{ID_0}} = \frac{22/14{,}044}{26/20{,}812} = 1.25$$

$$95\% \text{ confidence interval for } IDR = (\widehat{IDR})\exp\left(\sqrt{\frac{1}{a} + \frac{1}{b}}\right)$$

$$= (1.2546)\exp\left(\pm 1.96\sqrt{\frac{1}{22} + \frac{1}{26}}\right)$$

$$= (0.71, 2.21)$$

$$\chi^2_{M-H} = \frac{(a - mL_1/L)^2}{(mL_1L_0)/L^2} = \frac{(22 - (48)(14{,}044)/34{,}856)^2}{(48)(14{,}044)(20{,}812)/(34{,}856)^2} = .61$$

$p > .10$ (based on converting the chi-square statistic using Table 10.8)

Source: Colditz et al. (1990).

TABLE 10.6. Illustrative Data Set 3: Electric Blanket Use and Brain Tumors in Children, Case-Control Data

	Electric Blanket Use+	Electric Blanket Use−	
Case	53	485	538
Control	102	693	795
	155	1178	1333

$$\widehat{OR} = \frac{ad}{bc} = \frac{(53)(693)}{(102)(485)} \approx 0.74$$

$$\text{95\% confidence interval for } EOR = (\widehat{EOR})\exp\left(\pm 1.96 \sqrt{\frac{1}{a} + \frac{1}{b} + \frac{1}{c} + \frac{1}{d}}\right)$$

$$= (.7424)\exp\left(\pm 1.96 \sqrt{\frac{1}{53} + \frac{1}{102} + \frac{1}{485} + \frac{1}{693}}\right)$$

$$= (0.52, 1.06)$$

$$\chi^2_{M-H} = \frac{(n-1)(ad-bc)^2}{n_1 n_0 m_1 m_0} = \frac{(1333-1)[(53)(693)-(485)(102)]^2}{(155)(1178)(538)(795)} = 2.76$$

$.05 < p$ .value $< .10$ (based on converting the chi-square statistic using Table 10.8)

Source: Preston-Martin et al. (1996).

A 95% confidence interval for the odds ratio parameter is

$$(\widehat{OR}) \exp\left(\pm 1.96 \sqrt{\frac{1}{a} + \frac{1}{b} + \frac{1}{c} + \frac{1}{d}}\right) \qquad (10.12)$$

To illustrate this formula, let us consider data from a case-control study on electric blanket use and brain tumors in children (Preston-Martin et al., 1996). This study included 538 children with brain tumors and 795 comparably aged nondiseased children used as controls. Data and calculations are displayed in Table 10.6. The odds ratio associated with *in utero* electric blanket exposure is 0.74 (95% confidence interval for *OR*: 0.52, 10.06). Consequently, we are 95% certain that the population odds ratio lies between 0.52 and 1.06.

10.3 HYPOTHESIS TESTING

Setting Up the Hypotheses

Hypothesis testing is the traditional approach used to assess the statistical significance of a study. It involves comparing the observed sample findings with a theoretically expected finding of no association. This comparison allows us to compute the probability that the observed association could have resulted from chance, thus providing an objective and consistent framework for making decisions about the parameter. Within this framework, we set up a **null hypothesis** (H_0) that declares no association between the exposure and disease and an **alternative hypothesis** (H_1) that declares an association. Accordingly, the null and alternative hypotheses for testing the cumulative incidence ratio are

$$H_0: CIR = 1$$
$$H_1: CIR \neq 1$$

The null and alternative hypotheses for testing the incidence density ratio are

$$H_0: IDR = 1$$
$$H_1: IDR \neq 1$$

In testing the odds ratio, the null and alternative hypotheses are

$$H_0: OR = 1$$
$$H_1: OR \neq 1$$

Note that, in each case, the null hypothesis references a value of one. (The so-called **null value**.)

The objective of hypothesis testing is to find evidence that will allow us to reject the null hypothesis. In making a decision to either reject or retain the null hypothesis, two possible errors can occur. We can either falsely reject the null hypothesis—this is called a **Type I error**—or falsely retain the null hypothesis—this is called a **Type II error.** In other words, a Type I error is made by wrongly rejecting a true null hypothesis, and a Type II error is made by wrongly accepting a false null hypothesis. The possible consequences of hypothesis testing decisions are depicted in Table 10.7.

TABLE 10.7. Hypothesis-Testing Framework: Probabilities are Denoted in Parentheses

	Truth	
	H_0	H_1
H_0	OK ☺ $(1 - \alpha)$	Type II error ☹ (β)
H_1	Type I error ☹ (α)	OK ☺ $(1 - \beta)$

Hypothesis-Testing Decision

From a classical hypothesis testing perspective, Type I errors are to be avoided with more rigor than are Type II errors. This is because scientists do not want to say that an association exists when in fact it does not. On the other hand, the risk of Type I and Type II errors are inversely related: the smaller the risk of one, the greater the risk of the other. As a result, overcaution in the avoidance of a Type I error increases the likelihood of a Type II error.

We use the Greek letter **alpha** (α) to denote the probability of making a Type I error. The alpha level of a test represents the probability of rejecting a null hypothesis that is true. It is also called the **Type I error rate** and the **significance levels of the test.** The smaller the alpha level, the more significant the findings (i.e., the smaller the chance that the finding is due to chance). By convention, we usually limit the alpha level of a test to .05 or less.

We use the Greek letter **beta** (β) to denote the probability of making a Type II error. The beta level of a test represents the probability of a retaining a null hypothesis that is false. This involves claiming that no association exists when in fact it does. The beta level of a test is also called its **Type II error rate.** Beta can be viewed as the inability of a hypothesis test to detect a statistical relationship. The opposite of beta—the ability of a statistical test to detect a relationship—is called the **power of a test.** Specifically, the power of a test is the probability of rejecting a null hypothesis when it is false. The power of a test is calculated by subtracting the probability of a Type II error (beta) from 1.0 (power = $1 - \beta$). The maximum power a test can have is one; the minimum is zero. All other things being equal, the power of a test is inversely related to the square root of sample size; large studies have high power; small studies have low power. By convention, we design studies to have statistical power of at least .80.

Hypothesis Testing Using the 95% Confidence Interval

Hypotheses can be tested at the .05 alpha level with a 95% confidence interval. If the 95% confidence interval includes the null value of one, the null hypothesis is **retained.** If the confidence interval excludes one, the null hypothesis is **rejected.** Data that retain null hypotheses are said to be **nonsignificant.** Data that reject null hypotheses are said to be **significant.**

Let us return to the three illustrative examples shown in Tables 10.3, 10.5, and 10.6. All three of these 95% confidence intervals include the null value of one. Consequently, all three null hypotheses are retained and all three studies are declared nonsignificant.

p Values

p Values are probability statements that quantify the likelihood that the null hypothesis is correct. If the *p* value is more than the specified alpha level (normally .05), the null hypothesis is retained. If the calculated *p* value is less than alpha, the null hypothesis is rejected. *p* Values are frequently found in expressions such as $p < .05$. This means "the probability that this association is produced by chance is less than 5%." Consequently, the smaller the *p* value, the greater the likelihood that the result was not merely a fluke.

p Value calculations in this section are based on a chi-square statistic with one degree of freedom. Although there are several options for calculating the chi-square statistic, we presently consider the **Mantel–Haenszel chi-square statistic** (Mantel & Haenszel, 1959; Mantel, 1974). In testing cumulative incidence ratios and odds ratios, the Mantel–Haenszel chi-square statistic is

$$\chi^2_{M \cdot H} = \frac{(n - 1)(ad - bc)^2}{n_1 n_0 m_1 m_0} \qquad (10.13)$$

**TABLE 10.8. Abbreviated Chi-Square Table
for Chi-Square Values with One Degree of Freedom**

Chi-Square Value	p Value	Significance Jargon
$\chi^2 < 2.71$	p value $> .10$	Insignificant
$\chi^2 > 2.71$	p value $< .10$	Marginally significant
$\chi^2 > 3.84$	p value $< .05$	Significant
$\chi^2 > 5.02$	p value $< .025$	Significant
$\chi^2 > 6.63$	p value $< .01$	Highly significant
$\chi^2 > 7.88$	p value $< .005$	Highly significant
$\chi^2 > 10.83$	p value $< .001$	Highly significant

Cautionary note: Chi-square tests are unreliable when used on tables expecting five or fewer counts in any one table cell.

For incidence density ratio data, the formula is

$$\chi^2_{M\text{-}H} = \frac{(a - mL_1/L)^2}{(mL_1L_0)/L^2} \qquad (10.14)$$

The calculated chi-square statistic is translated into a p value by comparing it to a chi-square random variable with one degree of freedom. This can be done with a computer program or a chi-square table. An abbreviated chi-square table for chi-square values with one degree of freedom is presented in Table 10.8. Note that large chi-square values translate into small p values. Chi-square statistics and their associated p values for the illustrative data sets in this chapter appear in their respective tables. All three studies show $p > .05$.

p Values are used to judge the significance of a test. In statistical jargon, tests are deemed either highly significant, significant, marginally significant, or insignificant according to the criteria set forth in Table 10.8. Using these benchmarks, illustration data sets 1 and 2 show insignificant test results and illustration data set 3 shows a marginally significant results.

Limitations of Hypothesis Testing

Before concluding this section, it is worth noting some of the limitations of p values and hypothesis testing in general. First, the p value associated with a test of significance is only a statement of the likelihood that an observed association could have arisen due to chance. By itself, it says very little about the size or clinical importance of a finding. Because a calculated p value is closely related to sample size, nonmeaningful associations can be represented by significant p values and important associations may appear "insignificant."

Second, hypothesis testing does little to establish a particular association as causal. The transference from statistical significance to biologic causation is a separate process that goes beyond statistical reasoning and, as such, is addressed in Chapter 12.

Third, the hypothesis-testing framework was developed to account for random error in preplanned experiments. It is not well suited for identifying previously unknown problems or conducting multiple hypothesis tests, as is the custom of most epidemiologic studies. Note that in testing a single hypothesis at the .05 alpha level, we accept a 1-in-20 chance of erroneously rejecting the null hypothesis. In completing multiple tests, the likelihood of making at least one false rejection increases. For example, in completing x hypothesis tests at the .05 alpha level, there is a $1 - .95^x$ chance of making at least one false rejection. In completing three tests, the probability of making at least one false rejection is $1 - .95^3 = .14$. In completing 15 hypothesis tests, the probability of making at least one false rejection is $1 - .95^{15} = .54$. In completing 50 tests, the likelihood is .92. Thus, the pursuit of multiple hypothesis tests will inevitably lead to many false rejections of the null hypothesis, invalidating the theoretical basis for identifying nonrandom associations. (Readers who have completed a course in analysis of variance will recognize this as the "multiple comparisons problem.") With this said, epidemiology is an empirical science in which recognizing previously unrecognized risks is important. This compels epidemiologists to "look under every rock," testing all possible risk factors. Therefore, the classic hypothesis-testing model is *not* the *sine qua non* of epidemiologic research. In its place is a reliance on confidence interval estimation and the use of p values as a supplement for quantifying Type I error potential (*Note*: Epidemiologists have engaged in interesting discussions and debates about the relative merits of p values versus confidence intervals in epidemiologic research: for example, see Rothman, 1986; Walker, 1986; and Fleiss, 1986a,b.)

Last, the classic hypothesis-testing paradigm does little to address Type II error potential (false retention of the null hypothesis). This topic is addressed separately through a process called power and sample size analysis. Although we do not address these topics here (it is beyond the scope of this book), power and sample size analysis is essential when accepting the null hypothesis of no association. Power and sample size calculation is covered in standard statistical texts (e.g., see Rosner, 1995, Sections 7.6, 7.7, 10.7, 10.11, and 13.4).

10.4 AVAILABILITY OF COMPUTER PROGRAM

The statistics in this chapter can be calculated quickly and accurately with the public domain computer program Epi Info (Dean et al., 1994). Epi Info, a general database and statistical program for epidemiology, includes two statistical calculators useful for direct calculations. The main epidemiologic calculator, StatCalc, calculates point and interval estimates for odds ratios and cumulative incidence ratios. It also calculates three different chi-square statistics and their associated p values. A supplementary calculator called EpiTable calculates incidence density ratio statistics as well. Epi Info can be downloaded from the CDC site http://www.cdc.gov/epo/epi/epiinfo.htm.

SUMMARY

1. This chapter introduces fundamental notions of measurement error as they apply to epidemiologic research. Two essentially different forms of measurement error exist: random error and systematic error. Random error (imprecision) refers to the nonreproducibility of a finding due to chance. Systematic error (bias) refers to anything that produces a nonrandom deviation from the truth. Conceptualization and correction of these problems require different approaches. This chapter considers random error. The next chapter (Chapter 11) considers systematic error.

2. Statistical inference is used to deal with random measurement error in epidemiologic research. This first step in understanding statistical inference requires that we distinguish between population parameters and sample estimates. Population parame-

ters represent hypothetical values that are free from random and systematic error. Sample estimates represent calculated values that are susceptible to random and systematic inaccuracies and, hence, may suffer from positive biases, negative biases, and imprecision.

3. The two main forms of statistical inference are estimation and hypothesis testing. Estimation uses a sample statistic to determine the probable value of a population parameter. Two main forms of estimation exist: point estimation and interval estimation. Point estimation provides a single estimate of the parameter. For example, the sample incidence density (represented by the symbol $\widehat{ID}$) is the point estimate of the incidence density parameter (represented by the symbol ID). The second form of estimation, interval estimation, uses formulas to calculate a range of values that has a known likelihood of capturing the parameter. For example, the 95% confidence interval for ID has a 95% likelihood of capturing the true incidence density. Formulas for 95% confidence intervals for the various measures of disease frequency and measures of association are presented throughout this chapter.

4. The second form of statistical inference, hypothesis testing, is the traditional approach used to assess the statistical significance of a study. Null and alternative hypotheses are declared. We then try to find evidence that will allow us to reject the null hypothesis. In making a decision to reject or retain the null hypothesis, only two possible errors can occur. A Type I error occurs if we falsely reject the null hypothesis. A Type II error occurs if we falsely retain the null hypothesis. By convention, we try to limit the Type I error potential of a test to no more than .05, thus giving us at least 95% confidence in a concluded rejection of the null hypothesis.

5. Two methods for making decisions about hypotheses concerning ratio measures of association are presented. First, 95% confidence intervals can be used to reject or retain the null hypothesis at the alpha .05 level. If the confidence includes the null value of one, the null hypothesis is retained. If the confidence interval excludes the null value of one, the null hypothesis is rejected. Second, p values can be calculated to determine the significance of the findings. The smaller the p value, the greater the likelihood that the result expressed by a study is not merely due to chance. By convention, p values less than .05 are considered significant and p values greater than .05 are considered insignificant.

6. The Mantel–Haenszel chi-square statistic can be used to calculate a p value for cumulative incidence ratios, incidence density ratios, and odds ratios. The calculated chi-square statistic is translated into a p value using a chi-square table with one degree of freedom (e.g., Table 10.8). Generally, Mantel–Haenszel chi-square statistics greater than 3.84 are considered significant.

7. In today's digital age, most epidemiologic calculations are done with the aid of a computer. The public domain program *Epi Info* can be downloaded from http://www.cdc.gov/ for this purpose.

NOTATION AND FORMULA REFERENCE

$\hat{P}$	Prevalence point estimate (formulas 10.1 and 10.2)
P	Prevalence parameter
$\widehat{CI}$	Cumulative incidence point estimate (formulas 10.3 and 10.4)

CI	cumulative incidence parameter
$\widehat{ID}$	incidence density estimate (formulas 10.5 and 10.6)
ID	incidence density parameter
i_{LCL}	95% Lower confidence limit for the number of new cases, incidence density calculation (see Table 10.1)
i_{UCL}	95% Upper confidence limit for the number of new cases, incidence density calculation (see Table 10.1)
$\widehat{CIR}$	Cumulative incidence ratio point estimate (formulas 10.7 and 10.8)
CIR	Cumulative incidence ratio parameter
$\widehat{IDR}$	Incidence density ratio point estimate (formulas 10.9 and 10.10)
IDR	Incidence density ratio parameter
$\widehat{OR}$	Odds ratio point estimate (formulas 10.11 and 10.12)
OR	Odds ratio parameter
H_0	Null hypothesis
H_1	Alternative hypothesis
α	Alpha (Type I error rate, significance level)
$1 - \alpha$	Confidence level
β	Beta (Type II error rate)
$1 - \beta$	Power
$\chi^2_{M\text{-}H}$	Mantel–Haenszel chi-square statistics (formulas 10.13 and 10.14)

EXERCISES

1. Figure 10.6 shows 95% confidence intervals from 10 cohort studies on total fat intake and the relative risk of breast cancer. For most studies, the relative risk of high versus low quartiles of fat intake are shown. In some, quartiles or tertiles are used. (Information is from Table 1 in Hunter & Willet, 1993, p. 113. Original studies are: 1 = Jones et al., 1987; 2 = Willett et al., 1987; 3 = Mills et al., 1989; 4 = Knekt et al., 1990; 5 = Howe et al., 1991; 6 = Kushi et al., 1992; 7 = Willett et al., 1992; 8 = Graham et al., 1992; 9 = Byrne et al., 1992, 10 = van den Brandt et al., 1993.)

   (A) Which of theses studies is most precise?

   (B) Which is least precise?

   (C) Which studies are statistically significant at a 95% level of confidence?

   (D) When data are taken as a whole, do these studies support or refute the proposed association between dietary fat and breast cancer?

2. In 1997, Nathanson and co-workers published a comparison of bovine spongiform encephalopathy (BSE or "mad cow disease") incidence in the United Kingdom and Switzerland (Table 10.9). Based on these data, calculate the point estimate for cumulative incidence ratio and a 95% confidence interval for CIR. Also calculate the Mantel–Haenszel chi-square statistic and the approximate p value. Interpret your results.

3. Oral contraceptives are known to increase the risk of deep venous thromboembolic (DVT) disease. Data comparing DVT disease rates in users of high- and low-dose oral contraceptives are presented in Table 10.10. Based on these data, calculate the incidence density ratio, 95% confidence interval, Mantel–Haenszel chi-square statistic, and approximate p value.

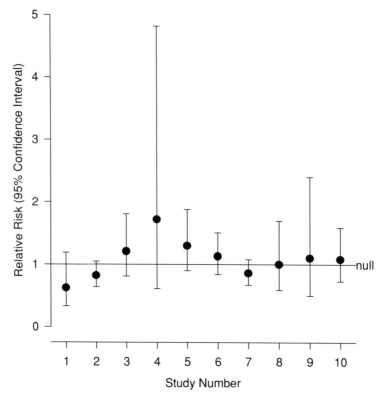

Figure 10.6. *Estimated relative risks of breast cancer associated with high total fat intake, 10 separate cohort studies. (Data source: Hunter & Willet, 1993, p. 113.)*

4. Smoking cessation programs usually have only modest success in helping their clients stop smoking. A study conducted among 234 people who had expressed a desire to stop smoking but have not yet quit finds 201 of its participants returned to smoking within a year of the program. Calculate the point estimate and 95% confidence interval for the cumulative incidence of recidivism.

5. We find 17 smokers in a random sample of 57 people. Calculate the point estimate and 95% confidence interval for the prevalence of smoking in the population.

TABLE 10.9. Bovine Spongiform Encephalopathy (BSE) in the United Kingdom and Switzerland Through May 1996. Numbers Are Approximate

	United Kingdom	Switzerland	Total
BSE +	160,000	213	160,213
BSE −	11,840,000	1,699,787	13,539,787
Total	12,000,000	1,700,000	13,700,000

Source: Nathanson et al. (1997), Table 4.

TABLE 10.10. Deep Venous Thromboembolic (DVT)
Disease Associated with High-Dose (Greater than 50 μg
Estrogen) and Low-Dose (Less than 50 μg Estrogen)
Oral Contraceptives, Michigan Medicaid, 1980–1986

	High Dose	Low Dose	
No. of Cases	20	53	73
—	—	—	—
Person-Years ($\times$ 10,000)	2.0	12.7	14.7

Source: Gerstman et al. (1991).

6. Figure 10.7 shows 95% confidence intervals from clinical trials, community trials, and cohort studies on mammography as a preventative for breast cancer death. The first 10 confidence intervals are for women less than 50 years of age at entry to the study. The second series of confidence intervals (labeled 12–16) are for women aged 50–59 years of age at entry to the study. (Information is from Table 5 in Hurley & Kaldor, 1992,

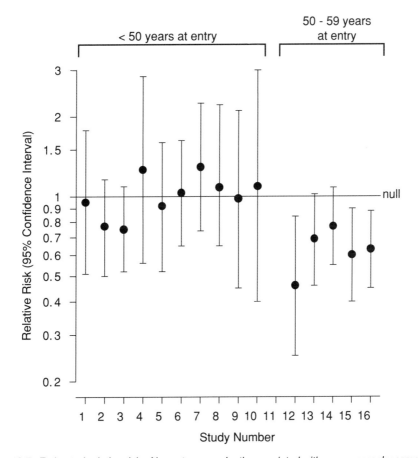

Figure 10.7. *Estimated relative risk of breast cancer death associated with mammography screening, cohort studies with internal comparison groups. (Data source: Hurley & Kaldor, 1992, p. 111.)*

p. 111. Original studies are: 1 = Shapiro et al., 1988, 5-year follow-up; 2 = Shapiro et al., 1988, 10-year follow-up; 3 = Shapiro et al., 1988, 18-year follow-up; 4 = Tabár et al., 1985, 6-year follow-up; 5 = Tabár et al., 1989, 8-year follow-up; 6 = Tabár et al., 1992, 11-year follow-up; 7 = Andersson et al., 1989, 8.8-year follow-up; 8 = Janzon & Andersson, 1991; 11-year follow-up; 9 = Roberts et al., 1990; 10 = Frisell et al., 1991; 12 = Shapiro et al., 1988, 5-year follow-up; 13 = Shapiro et al., 1988, 10-year follow-up; 14 = Shapiro et al., 1988, 18-year follow-up; 15 = Tabár et al., 1989, 8-year follow-up; 16 = Tabár et al., 1992, 11-year follow-up.) Based on these data, does there appear to be an association between decreased breast cancer mortality and mammographic screening for women in their forties? Does there appear to be an association between decreased breast cancer mortality and mammographic screening for women in their fifties?

ANSWERS TO EXERCISES

1. A   Study 2 and 7 appear to be (equally) the most precise.
   B   Study 4 is the least precise.
   C   None of the studies is statistically significant.

2. $\widehat{CIR}$ = 106.4 (95% confidence interval for CIR: 93.0, 121.7); $\chi^2_{M\text{-}H}$ = 22746, $p < .001$; British cows are significantly more likely to have experience BSE than Swiss cows.

3. $\widehat{IDR}$ = 2.4 (95% confidence interval for CIR: 1.4, 4.0); $\chi^2_{M\text{-}H}$ = 11.8, $p < .001$

4. $\widehat{CI}$ = 201/234 = .8590;

$$95\% \text{ confidence interval for } CI = 8590 \pm 1.96 \sqrt{\frac{(.8590)(1 - .8590)}{234}}$$

$$= (.8144, .9036)$$

5. P = 17/57 = .2982;

$$95\% \text{ } CI \text{ for } P = .2982 \pm 1.96 \sqrt{\frac{(.2982)(1 - .2982)}{57}} = (.1794, .4170)$$

6. There does not appear to be significant association between decreased breast cancer mortality and mammographic screening for women in their forties. There does, however, appear to be some benefit for women in their fifties.

REFERENCES

Andersson, I., Aspegren, K., Janzon, L., et al. (1989). Mammographic screening and mortality from breast cancer: the Malmö mammographic screening trial. *British Medical Journal, 297,* 943–948.

Byrne, C., Ursin, G., & Ziegler, R. (1992). Dietary fat and breast cancer in continued follow-up of the First National Health and Nutrition Examination Survey (NHANES I). *American Journal of Epidemiology, 136,* 1024–1025 (abstract).

Colditz, G. A., Stampfer, M. J., Willett, W. C., Hennekens, D. H., Rosner, B., & Speizer, F. E. (1990). Prospective study of estrogen replacement therapy and risk of breast cancer in post-menopausal women. *JAMA, 264,* 2648–2653.

Cornfield, J. (1956). A statistical problem arising from retrospective studies. In J. Neyman (Ed.), *Proceedings of the 3rd Berkeley Symposium on Mathematical Statistics and Probability* (pp. 135–148). Berkeley: University of California Press.

Dean, A. G., Dean, J. A., Coulombier, D., Brendel, K. A., Smith, D. C., Burton, A. H., Dicker, R. C., Sullivan, K., Fagan, R. F., & Arner, T. G. (1994) *Epi Info, Version 6: A Word Processing, Database, and Statistical Program for Epidemiology on Microcomputers.* Atlanta: Centers for Disease Control and Prevention.

Fleiss, J. L. (1986a). Significance tests have a role in epidemiologic research: reactions to A. M. Walker. *American Journal of Public Health, 76,* 559–560.

Fleiss, J. L. (1986b). Confidence intervals vs. significance tests: quantitative interpretations. *American Journal of Public Health, 76,* 587–588 (letter).

Frisell, J., Eklund, G., Hellström, L., et al. (1991). Randomized study of mammographic screening—preliminary report on mortality in the Stockholm trial. *Breast Cancer Research and Treatment, 18,* 49–56.

Gerstman, B. B., Piper, J. M., Tomita, D. K., Ferguson, W. J., Stadel, B. V., & Lundin, F. E. (1991). Oral contraceptive estrogen dose and the risk of deep venous thromboembolic disease. *American Journal of Epidemiology, 133,* 32–37.

Graham, S., Zielezny, M., Marshall, J., et al. (1992). Diet in the epidemiology of postmenopausal breast cancer in the New York State cohort. *American Journal of Epidemiology, 136,* 1327–1337.

Howe, G. R., Friedenreich, C. M., Jain, M., et al. (1991). A cohort study of fat intake and risk of breast cancer. *Journal of the National Cancer Institute, 83,* 336–340.

Hunter, D. J., & Willett, W. C. (1993). Diet, body size, and breast cancer. *Epidemiologic Reviews, 15,* 110–132.

Hurley, S. F., & Kaldor, J. M. (1992). The benefits and risks of mammographic screening for breast cancer. *Epidemiologic Reviews, 14,* 101–130.

Janzon, L., & Andersson, I. (1991). The Malmö mammographic screening trial. In A. B. Miller, J. Chamberlain, N. E. Day, et al. (Eds.), *Cancer Screening* (pp. 37–44). Cambridge: Cambridge University Press.

Jones, D. Y. Schatzkin, A., Green, S. B., et al. (1987). Dietary fat and breast cancer in the National Health and Nutrition Examination Survey. I. Epidemiologic Follow-up Study. *Journal of the National Cancer Institute, 79,* 465–471.

Knekt, P., Albanes, D., Seppanen, R., et al. (1990). Dietary fat and risk of breast cancer. *American Journal of Clinical Nutrition, 52,* 903–908.

Kushi, L. H., Sellers, T. A., Potter, J. D., et al. (1992). Dietary fat and postmenopausal breast cancer. *Journal of the National Cancer Institute, 84,* 1092–1099.

Mantel, N. (1974). Some reasons for not using the Yates continuity correction on 2×2 contingency tables: comments and suggestions. *Journal of the American Statistics Association, 69,* 378–380.

Mantel, N., & Haenszel W. (1959). Statistical aspects of the analysis of data from retrospective studies of disease. *Journal of the National Cancer Institute, 22,* 719–748.

Mills, P. K., Beeson, W. L., Phillips, R. L., et al. (1989). Dietary habits and breast cancer incidence among Seventh Day Adventists. *Cancer, 64,* 582–590.

Nathanson, N., Wilesmith, J., & Griot, C. (1997). Bovine spongiform encephalopathy (BSE): causes and consequences of a common source epidemic. *American Journal of Epidemiology, 145,* 959–969.

Pearson, E. S., & Hartley, H. O. (Eds.). (1966). *Biometrika Tables for Statisticians* (3rd ed., Vol. 1). Cambridge: Cambridge University Press.

Preston-Martin, S., Gurney, J. G., Pogoda, J. M., Holly, E. A., & Mueller, B. A. (1996). Brain tumor risk in children in relation to use of electric blankets and water bed heaters. *American Journal of Epidemiology, 143,* 1116–1122.

Roberts, M. M., Alexander, F. E., Anderson, T. J., et al. (1990). Edinburgh trial of screening for breast cancer: mortality at seven years. *Lancet, 335,* 241–246.

Rosner, B. (1995). *Fundamentals of Biostatistics* (4th ed.). Belmont, CA: Duxbury Press.

Rothman, K. J. (1986). Significance questing. *Annals of Internal Medicine, 105,* 445–447.

Schnorr, T. (1993) Video display terminals and adverse pregnancy outcomes. In K. Steenland (Ed.), *Case Studies in Occupational Epidemiology* (pp. 7–20). New York: Oxford University Press.

Shapiro, S., Venet, W., Strax, P., et al. (1988). *Periodic Screening for Breast Cancer. The Health Insurance Plan Project and Its Sequelae, 1963–1986.* Baltimore, MD: The Johns Hopkins University Press.

Tabár, L, Fagerberg, G., Duffy, S. W., et al. (1989). The Swedish two-county trial of mammographic screening for breast cancer: recent results and calculation of benefit. *Journal of Epidemiology and Community Health, 43,* 107–114.

Tabár, L., Fagerberg, G., Gad, A., et al. (1985). Reduction in mortality from breast cancer after mass screening with mammography. Randomised trial from the Breast Cancer Screening Working Groups of Swedish National Board of Health and Welfare. *Lancet, 1,* 829–832.

Tabár, L., Fagerberg, G., Duffy, S. W., et al. (1992). Update of the Swedish two-county program of mammographic screening for breast cancer. *Radiologic Clinics of North America, 30,* 187–210.

van den Brandt, P. A., van't Veer, P., Goldbohm, R. A., et al. (1993). A prospective cohort study on dietary fat and breast cancer risk. *Cancer Research, 53,* 75–82.

Walker, A. M. (1986). Reporting the results of epidemiologic studies. *American Journal of Public Health, 76,* 556–558.

Willet, W. C., Hunter, D. J., Stampfer, M. J., et al. (1992). Dietary fat and fiber in relation to risk of breast cancer. *JAMA, 268,* 2037–2044.

Willett, W. C., Stampfer, M. J., Colditz, G. A., et al. (1987). Dietary fat and risk of breast cancer. *New England Journal of Medicine, 316,* 22–28.

Zar, J. H. (1996). *Biostatistical Analysis* (3rd ed.). Upper Saddle River, NJ: Prentice Hall.

11

Inaccuracy in Epidemiologic Studies, Part II (Bias)

Bias (systematic error) damages epidemiologic research. This chapter examines the three types of bias found in epidemiologic studies: selection bias, information bias, and confounding. In addition, interaction (effect modification) is discussed.

11.1 INTRODUCTION TO BIAS

Fundamental notions of measurement error were introduced in the previous chapter. To review briefly, two essentially different forms of measurement error exist in epidemiologic research. These are random error (imprecision) and systematic error (bias). Random error, the chance nonreproducibility of study findings, was covered in the prior chapter. This chapter considers systematic error. Systematic error in analytic research refers to any element of study design, data collection, or data analysis that onesidedly distorts study accuracy. Bias, in a statistical sense, is the difference between the expected value of an estimate and the population parameter it purports to estimate. Thus, the technical definition of bias is

$$E(\hat{\theta}) \neq \theta$$

where θ represents the parameter of interest (e.g., prevalence, incidence density, incidence density ratio), $\hat{\theta}$ represents the sample estimate of the parameter, and $E(\hat{\theta})$ represents the expected (average) value of the estimate. Note, therefore, that the term does not carry an imputation of prejudice or other subjective factors, as it might in a racial bias lawsuit, for example. Also note that whereas random error is essentially an attribute of sampling variation, systematic error is attributable to methodologic aspects of the study design and analysis, particularly the quality of information, comparability of the groups at baseline, and unrepresentative nature of the sample. For example, if we conduct a telephone survey at 10 o'clock on a Monday morning and take responses of the first 100 people who answer the phone, surely responders would be more likely to be unemployed (or work at home) compared with other people in the population, and certain groups would systematically be excluded from the sample (e.g., students, hospitalized people). We would be very lucky if these and other factors were not at work to bias the results of our survey by making the 100 responders unrepresentative of the general population.

Bias can be characterized as to its direction (i.e., positive or negative bias) and degree (i.e., a lot or a little). Bias can also be characterized as to its tendency to overestimate (exaggerate) or underestimate an association. A bias that tends to overestimate an association is **bias away from the null.** A bias that tends to underestimate an association is **bias toward the null.** The consideration of bias in epidemiologic studies is central to modern epidemiologic practice, so much so, that a joke traveling the Internet goes as follows:

Question: How many epidemiologists does it take to change a light bulb?
Answer: Six
Explanation: One to change the bulb and five to address potential biases.

Potential biases must be avoided or taken into account in conducting and interpreting epidemiologic research. According to modern epidemiologic theory, three forms of bias exist:

- Selection bias (due to nonrepresentativeness of the sample)
- Information bias (due to the misclassification of study factors)
- Confounding (due to the influence of extraneous factors)

Let us begin by considering selection bias.

11.2   SELECTION BIAS

Selection bias refers to a distortion in a measure of disease frequency or association resulting from the manner in which subjects are selected for the study. This type of bias occurs when the sample is not representative of the target population and can often be traced to faulty sampling mechanisms. Selection bias can also occur when a large percentage of subjects refuse to participate in the study, withdraw from the study, or are lost to follow-up.

Many well-documented cases of selection bias have occurred throughout history. Some of the more colorful examples of selection bias occurred as a result of the faulty political polls of the 1930s and 1940s. Darrell Huff, in his lucid booklet *How to Live with Statistics* (1954), tells the tale of how pre-election polls routinely had Franklin Delano Roosevelt's opponent Alf Landon winning the presidency by landslide electoral margins. These mistaken predictions were based on telephone polls at a time when many people did not have phones. Telephone samples, therefore, were not representative of the general electorate: phone owners were economically better off than nonowners and were thus more likely to vote Republican. In effect, the sample elected the Republican, but the people elected Roosevelt.

A similar mishap occurred during the 1948 reelection bid by President Harry S. Truman. All the major polling organizations of the time had Truman's Republican rival, Thomas E.

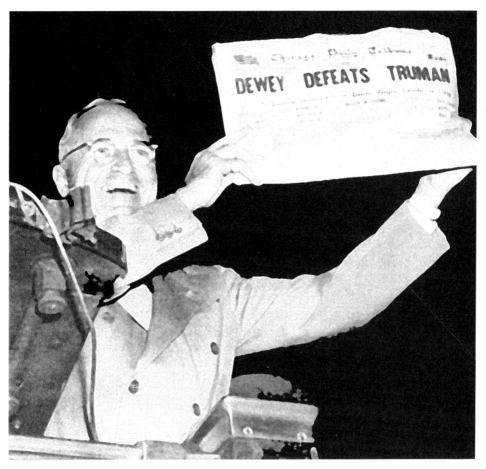

Figure 11.1. Polls mistakenly thought Truman would not win reelection (used with permission of VPI/Corbis-Bettmann).

Dewey, slated to win the election (Fig. 11.1). Apparently, data collectors for these polls had some freedom to choose whom they interviewed, and Republicans were typically easier and more appealing to interview from Democrats (Freedman et al., 1991; Mosteller, 1949). Thus, once again, Republicans were oversampled, thus biasing survey results.

These two historical examples of selection bias illustrate the most important tenets of modern survey methodology:

- Always try to avoid human choice in the selection of a sample.
- Whenever possible, use random sampling mechanisms.

Examples of common forms of epidemiologic selection bias follow.

Berkson's bias (1946), also called **hospital admission rate bias,** is an important form of selection bias that afflicts hospital-based epidemiologic studies. Because hospitalized people are more likely to suffer from multiple illnesses, have more severe illness, and engage in unhealthy behaviors (e.g., smoking), they are often atypical of the target population they are supposed to represent. Berkson's bias may bias a study toward or away from the null, depending on the circumstances of the study.

Prevalence-incidence bias refers to the type of bias that occurs when prevalent cases are used to study disease etiology. Once a person is diagnosed with a disease, they tend to change the habits that may have contributed to their disease. Moreover, prevalent cases are more likely to be long-term survivors and, therefore, may represent a relatively mild form of the illness in question. In studying disease etiology, it is almost always advisable to use incident cases, when possible.

Nonresponse bias, withdrawal bias, and **lost to follow-up bias** are forms of selection bias that occur when potential study subjects refuse or discontinue participation once the study is in progress. A discontinuing subject is often less healthy and more likely to engage in unhealthy behaviors than subjects that fully participate in studies.

Publicity bias occurs when media attention increases awareness of a real or perceived health problem. This stimulates case reporting, resulting in artifactual spikes in occurrence. To avoid this bias, data should be restricted to the period prior to the publicity event.

The **healthy worker effect** is a form of selection bias attributable to the fact that ill and chronically disabled people are, for the most part, excluded from the workforce. This type of bias expresses itself in lower-than-expected morbidity and morality rates among workers, so that, even if a problem were occurring, it could be hidden from epidemiologic measures of association. Similar types of bias may be seen when studying other self-selected groups (so-called **memberships bias**). For example, exercisers may, in part, be healthier on average because unfit people are precluded from regular exercise. Use of incidence measures, rather than prevalence measures, will help avoid this type of bias.

11.3 INFORMATION BIAS

Information bias refers to a distortion due to measurement error or misclassification of subjects on one or more study factors. Consequently, information bias is also called **misclassification bias,** especially when data are dichotomous. Sources of information bias include measurement device defects, questionnaires and interviews that do not measure what they purport to, inaccurate diagnostic procedures, and incomplete or erroneous data sources.

The indices of diagnostic test accuracy considered in Chapter 4 (sensitivity and specificity) can be used to measure the misclassification inherent in a dichotomous variable. Lacking misclassification, both the sensitivity and specificity have a value of one. However, this ideal is seldom achieved; epidemiologists often work with less than perfect data.

Given known sensitivity and specificity, mathematical adjustments for information bias are possible (see Kleinbaum et al., 1982, Chapter 12). Nevertheless, this type of correction is seldom pursued in practice because of the difficulty in accurately determining sensitivity and specificity on an *ad hoc* basis. As a result, efforts are better directed toward correcting underlying misclassifications. From a practical standpoint, however, epidemiologists often do consider whether the misclassification of information in a study is evenly or unevenly distributed among study groups. **Nondifferential misclassification** refers to misclassification that occurs with the same frequency in all study groups. **Differential misclassification** refers to misclassification that varies between study groups. The distinction between nondifferential and differential misclassification has practical implications: nondifferential misclassification biases measures of association toward the null, whereas differential misclassification does not take a uniform direction (Bross, 1954). Thus, from an applied point of view, nondifferential misclassification is preferred because associations so affected still exist in reality (although the study will understate them). In contrast, associations muddied by differential misclassification may, in fact, be entirely artifactual.

Examples of common forms of epidemiologic information bias follow.

Recall bias refers to the form of bias that ensues when self-reported, historical information is inaccurate. This is especially problematic when, in case-control studies, cases scrutinize their history with more rigor than controls. More thorough recall (and false reporting) of risk factors in cases will bias the estimated odds ratio away from the null.

Diagnostic suspicion bias refers to the type of information bias that occurs when one study group undergoes greater diagnostic scrutiny than the other. Horwitz and Feinstein (1978) illustrated this type of bias in a series of case-control studies of estrogen and endometrial cancer in which increased diagnostic attention was received by women who were taking estrogen. After eliminating this bias, the initial odds ratio of 12.0 decreased to 1.7. This suggested that estrogen-induced bleeding may have invoked referral for diagnosis, whereas asymptomatic endometrial cancer cases may have gone undetected. That is, estrogen use might have led to increased detection of endometrial cancer, but not necessarily to its cause.

The **Clever Hans effect (obsequiousness bias)** occurs when subjects systematically alter their responses in the direction they perceive to be desired by the investigator. It is named after a trained horse who could apparently do simple math. Although never proved, Hans's ability stemmed from nonverbal clues from his trainer that helped him to determine when to stop stomping his hoof in response to a question. Like Hans's trainer, interviewers may send nonverbal clues to study objects, thereby influencing the subjects' responses.

11.4 CONFOUNDING AND INTERACTION

Introduction to Confounding and Interaction

Confounding is a distortion of an association between exposure E and disease D brought about by an extraneous factor F (or extraneous factors F_1, F_2, etc.). This form of bias will occur if and only if:

- F and E are associated, and
- F and D are associated in both the exposed (E+) and unexposed (E−) groups.

The latter condition implies that F is an independent risk factor for D (Fig. 11.2).

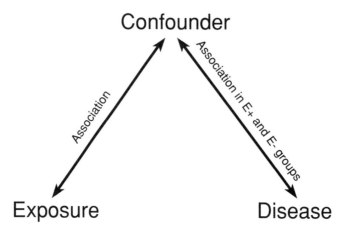

Figure 11.2. *Conditions necessary for confounding.*

An example of confounding is seen in the association between lung cancer (D) and alcohol consumption (E). The association between these two factors is confounded by cigarette smoking (F). F and E are associated (daily alcohol consumers are more likely to smoke than nonconsumers), and F and D are associated (smoking is an independent risk factor for lung cancer). The preconditions for confounding are, therefore, fulfilled and, without adjustment, the association between E and D is confounded. For example, the unadjusted relative risk of lung cancer associated with daily consumption of alcohol in Japanese women is 2.5 (Hirayama, 1990). However, if one holds the smoking habits of people constant, lung cancer risk is unaffected by alcohol consumption.

Separate from confounding, extraneous factors can also modify the effect of an exposure. This biological phenomenon, called **effect modification,** is related to a statistical phenomenon called **interaction.** Interaction refers to a difference in effect of one factor according to the level of another factor. Like confounding, interaction is due to the influence of an extraneous factor. However, unlike confounding, interaction can have direct biological and public health relevance. Effect modification and interaction can be compared to the biological concept of **synergy.** Synergy among factors implies that the combined effect of individual factors has an impact that is not entirely predicted by the sum of their parts. An important example of effect modification is seen with oral contraceptives (E), cardiovascular disease (D), and smoking (F). In the presence of smoking (F+), oral contraceptive use presents a substantial hazard. In the absence of smoking (F−), oral contraceptive use is safe (Fig. 11.3). Thus, without knowledge of the smoking status of an individual, the risk of oral contraceptives cannot be generalized.

A numerical illustration will serve to clarify ways in which extraneous factor F may confound or interact in the association between exposure E and disease D (Table 11.1). Assume data come from three different cohort (cumulative incidence) studies. Data are stratified by extraneous factor F. Pooled ("crude," "unstratified") data are presented at the far right in each instance. The crude cumulative incidence ratio ($\widehat{cCIR}$) is 4.00 for each scenario.

Scenario A represents a situation in which neither confounding nor interaction is present. Note that strata-specific cumulative incidence ratio estimates ($\widehat{CIR}_1$ and $\widehat{CIR}_2$) and

Warnings

Cigarette-smoking increases the risk of serious cardiovascular side effects from oral contraceptive use. This risk increases with age and heavy smoking (15 or more cigarettes per day) and is quite marked in women over 35 years of age. Women who use oral contraceptives should be strongly advised not to smoke.

Figure 11.3. Warning from an oral contraceptive package insert.

TABLE 11.1. Examples of Confounding and Interaction

A. Neither Confounding Nor Interaction

	Stratum 1 (F+)		Stratum 2 (F−)		Pooled	
	E+	E−	E+	E−	E+	E−
D+	160	40	40	10	200	50
D−	240	360	560	590	800	950
	400	400	600	600	1,000	1,000
	$\widehat{CIR_1} = 4.0$		$\widehat{CIR_2} = 4.0$		$\widehat{cCIR} = 4.0$	

B. Confounding

	Stratum 1 (F+)		Stratum 2 (F−)		Pooled	
	E+	E−	E+	E−	E+	E−
D+	194	24	6	26	200	50
D−	606	76	194	874	800	950
	800	100	200	900	1000	1000
	$\widehat{CIR_1} = 1.0$		$\widehat{CIR_2} = 1.0$		$\widehat{cCIR} = 4.0$	

C. Interaction

	Stratum 1 (F+)		Stratum 2 (F−)		Pooled	
	E+	E−	E+	E−	E+	E−
D+	12	45	188	5	200	50
D−	188	775	612	195	800	950
	200	800	800	200	1000	1000
	$\widehat{CIR_1} = 1.1$		$\widehat{CIR_2} = 9.4$		$\widehat{cCIR} = 4.0$	

Source: Jewell (1984), handout #32; reproduced with permission from the author.

the crude cumulative estimate $(\widehat{cCIR})$ are identical. Thus, stratification and adjustment are unnecessary and extraneous factor F may safely be ignored.

Scenario B illustrates confounding. Strata-specific estimates are equal $(\widehat{CIR}_1 = \widehat{CIR}_2 = 1.0)$ but differ from the crude estimate of 4.0. The crude estimate is, therefore, confounded and should be ignored. A single estimate of association is still possible, however, by combining strata-specific estimates to derive an **adjusted (summary) measure of association.** There are many statistical methods by which to achieve this adjustment. One such method, based on using a weighted average of strata-specific estimates, is presented later in this chapter.

Scenario C illustrates interaction. Note that stratum 1 and stratum 2 show dissimilar cumulative incidence ratio estimates $(\widehat{CIR}_1 = 1.1; \widehat{CIR}_2 = 9.4)$. This suggests that F modifies the effect of E on D. When interaction is present, separate measures of association by levels of F must be reported.

Note that confounding and interaction are different phenomena. A variable may manifest itself as a confounder and interactive factor, neither, or both a confounder and interactive factor. Also note that there is a subtle distinction between synergism and statistical interaction. Synergism is a description of a biological mechanism. Interaction, on the other hand, concerns a statistical interrelationship among factors but does not necessarily relate to underlying biological mechanisms. Moreover, the quantification and assessment of interaction is risk-model dependent, dependent upon whether an additive or multiplicative model of risk is used (Kupper & Hogan, 1978; Miettinen, 1974).

Ideally, decisions about the potential importance of extraneous factors are reached before data are collected. This allows the researcher to collect the pertinent information to check for both confounding and interaction. Suspicion about which extraneous factors might be important comes from biological and statistical knowledge about interrelationship between study factors, previous research, an accumulation of clinical experience, small-scale pilot work, and the data itself. Confirmation of confounding requires consideration of both the biological relationships the investigators believes to be operative and the statistical relationships in the data.

Epidemiologists use different strategies to identify confounding and interaction. We will use the following strategy. Initially, data are stratified to calculate intrastrata measures of association. If intrastrata measures of association differ significantly, interaction is present. If intrastrata measures of association are not significantly different, interaction is absent and the researcher searches for confounding. To check for confounding, an appropriate statistical adjustment is made. If the adjustment changes the interpretation of the E–D relationship, confounding is present. If the adjustment does not change the interpretation of the E–D relationship, confounding is small or absent and the extraneous factors can safely be ignored. This analytic strategy is depicted schematically in Figure 11.4.

Chi-Square Tests for Interaction (Heterogeneity)

When interaction is present, we can expect different measures of association among strata. To help determine whether observed differences in strata-specific measures of association are due to chance, the researcher can conduct a chi-square test for interaction.

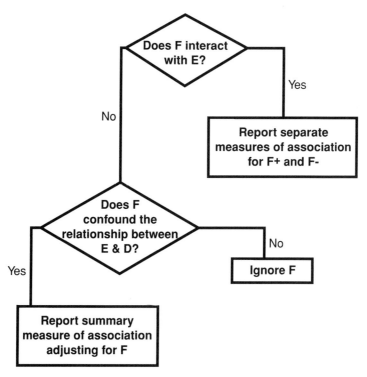

Figure 11.4 *Strategy for addressing interaction and confounding.*

Regardless of the particular measure of association (*MA*), the chi-square test for interaction addresses the following hypotheses:

$$H_0\colon MA_1 = MA_2 = \cdots = MA_k$$

$$H_1\colon \text{at least one strata-specific } MA \text{ differs}$$

where MA_g represents the strata-specific measure of association (e.g., odds ratio) in stratum g. Note that the null hypotheses is a declaration of homogeneity and, hence, *no* interaction. The alternative hypothesis is a declaration of heterogeneity of effect (interaction).

The chi-square interaction statistic (χ^2_{INT}) has the general form

$$\chi^2_{INT} = \sum_{g=1}^{k} \frac{(\widehat{MA}_g - \widehat{aMA})^2}{\widehat{VAR}\,(\widehat{MA}_g)} \tag{11.1}$$

where $\widehat{MA}_g$ represents the measure of association on a logarithmic scale in stratum g (see Table 11.2 for formulas), $\widehat{VAR}\,(\widehat{MA}_g)$ represents the variance estimate for the measure of

TABLE 11.2. Measures of Association and Their Variance Estimates

Notation for Cumulative Incidence Ratio Data and Odds Ratio Data

	Exposure +	Exposure −	
Disease +	a	b	m_1
Disease −	c	d	m_0
	n_1	n_0	n

Notation for Incidence Ratio (Person-Time) Data

	Exposure +	Exposure −	
Disease +	a	b	m
Disease −	—	—	—
Person-Time	L_1	L_0	L

Measure of Association MA	Point Estimate, Stratum g $\widehat{MA}_g$	Variance Estimate, Stratum g $\widehat{VAR}(\widehat{MA}_g)$
ln (cumulative incidence ratio)	$\ln\left(\dfrac{a_g/n_{1g}}{b_g/n_{0g}}\right)$	$\dfrac{m_{0g}\,n_g}{m_{1g}\,n_{1g}\,n_{0g}}$
ln (incidence density ratio)	$\ln\left(\dfrac{a_g/L_{1g}}{b_g/L_{0g}}\right)$	$\dfrac{L_g^2}{m_{1g}\,L_{1g}\,L_{0g}}$
ln (odds ratio)	$\ln\left(\dfrac{a_g d_g}{b_g c_g}\right)$	$\dfrac{1}{a_g}+\dfrac{1}{b_g}+\dfrac{1}{c_g}+\dfrac{1}{d_g}$

association in stratum g (also see Table 11.2 for formulas), and $\widehat{aMA}$ represents the adjusted measure of association based on the following formula:

$$\widehat{aMA} = \frac{\Sigma w_g \widehat{MA}_g}{\Sigma w_g} \tag{11.2}$$

where MA_g represents the measure of association on a logarithmic scale in stratum g (see Table 11.2 for formulas) and $w_g = [\widehat{VAR}(\widehat{MA}_g)]^{-1}$. Note that this adjusted measure of association is a weighted average based on the inverse of intrastrata variance estimates.

The χ^2_{INT} statistic is translated to a p value using a chi-square table with k-1 of freedom. By convention, p values greater than .05 are considered insignificant, in which case the null hypothesis of no interaction is retained. p Values less than .05 are considered significant, in which case the null hypothesis of no interaction is rejected.

To simplify matters, let us focus on a case-control study of smoking and cervical cancer while considering the extraneous factor "the number of sexual partners a women has had." Data appear in Table 11.3. The null and alternative hypotheses for the test of interaction are

$$H_0: OR_1 = OR_2$$
$$H_1: OR_1 \neq OR_2$$

For case-control data, the chi-square statistic for interaction is

TABLE 11.3. Illustrative Data: E = Smoking, D = Cervical Cancer, F = Number of Sexual Partners

	Stratum 1 Zero or One Partner		Stratum 2 Two or More Partners		Pooled	
	E+	E−	E+	E−	E+	E−
D+	12	26	96	92	108	117
D−	21	118	142	150	163	268
	400	400	600	600	1,000	1,000

$$\widehat{OR_1} = 2.70 \qquad \widehat{OR_2} = 1.10 \qquad \widehat{cOR} = 1.52$$

$$\ln \widehat{OR_1} = .9922 \qquad \ln \widehat{OR_2} = .0974$$

$$\widehat{VAR}(\ln \widehat{OR_1}) = \frac{1}{12} + \frac{1}{25} + \frac{1}{21} + \frac{1}{11} \qquad \widehat{VAR}(\ln \widehat{OR_2}) = \frac{1}{96} + \frac{1}{92} + \frac{1}{142} + \frac{1}{150}$$

$$= .1794 \qquad\qquad\qquad = .0350$$

$$w_1 = (.1794)^{-1} = 5.5733 \qquad w_2 = (.0350)^{-1} = 28.5714$$

$$a(\ln \widehat{OR}) = \frac{\sum (w_g)(\ln \widehat{OR_g})}{\sum w_g} = \frac{(5.5733)(.9922) + (28.5714)(.0974)}{5.5933 + 28.5714} = 0.2435$$

$$\chi^2_{INT} = \sum_{g=1}^{k} \frac{[\ln \widehat{OR_g} - a(\ln \widehat{OR})]^2}{\widehat{VAR}(\ln \widehat{OR_g})} = \left[\frac{(.9922 - .2435)^2}{.1794} \frac{(.0974 - .2435)^2}{.0350} \right] = 3.73$$

Chi-square test for interaction: $.05 < p < .10$

$$a(\widehat{OR}) = \exp[a(\ln \widehat{OR})] = \exp[0.2436] = 1.28$$

Source: Nishan et al. (1988), as reported by Pagano & Gauvreau (1993), p. 359.

$$\chi^2_{INT} = \sum_{g=1}^{G} \frac{[\ln \widehat{OR_g} - a(\ln \widehat{OR})]^2}{\widehat{VAR}(\ln \widehat{OR_g})} \qquad (11.3)$$

where

$$\ln \widehat{OR_g} = \ln\left(\frac{a_g d_g}{b_g c_g}\right) \qquad (11.4)$$

$$\widehat{VAR}(\ln \widehat{OR_g}) = \frac{1}{a_g} + \frac{1}{b_g} + \frac{1}{c_g} + \frac{1}{d_g} \qquad (11.5)$$

$$a(\ln \widehat{OR}) = \frac{\Sigma(w_g)(\ln \widehat{OR_g})}{\Sigma w_g} \qquad (11.6)$$

$$w_g = [\widehat{VAR}(\ln \widehat{OR_g})]^{-1} = \left(\frac{1}{a_g} + \frac{1}{b_g} + \frac{1}{c_g} + \frac{1}{d_g}\right)^{-1} \qquad (11.7)$$

The χ^2_{INT} statistic for the illustration data set is 3.73 with 1 degree of freedom (see Table 11.3 for calculations). This translates to $.05 < p < .10$ ("marginal significance"). Using the standard .05 significance level, the null hypothesis of no interaction is retained. Therefore, although strata-specific odds ratio estimates vary $(\widehat{OR}_1 = 2.70; \widehat{OR}_2 = 1.10)$, this difference is assumed to be due to chance. (*Note:* This points out one of the limitations of the chi-square tests of interaction—it has limited power.)

Identifying and Adjusting for Confounding

After ruling out interaction, potential confounding is addressed. To aid in the evaluation of confounding, the adjusted measure of association is compared to the crude measure of association. If these values are similar, the potential for confounding is small. If the crude and adjusted measures of association are dissimilar, the potential for confounding is great. Thus, a working definition of confounding is $\widehat{cMA} \neq \widehat{aMA}$ Note, however, that formal hypothesis tests for confounding are ill advised. Confounding is a matter of systematic error that cannot be addressed by hypothesis testing. In practice, the axiom "a difference that makes no difference is no difference" applies. If the statistical adjustment for confounding alters the interpretation of the measure of association, the adjustment for confounding is warranted. If, on the other hand, the adjustment does not alter interpretation, the crude measure of association may be used.

A general formula for adjustment was introduced as formula 11.2. Note that this formula is a weighted average of strata-specific measures of association with weights based on the inverse of intrastrata-specific variance estimates. (It makes sense to give more weight to precise estimates.) Application of this general formula to the odds ratio appears as formula 11.6. Its use is illustrated in Table 11.3.

Application of the inverse variance adjustment formula to cumulative incidence ratios results in

$$a(\ln \widehat{CIR}) = \frac{\Sigma(w_g)(\ln \widehat{CIR}_g)}{\Sigma w_g}$$

where   (11.8)

$$w_g = [\widehat{VAR}(\ln \widehat{CIR}_g)]^{-1} = \left(\frac{m_{0g}n_g}{m_{1g}n_{1g}n_{0g}}\right)$$

Application of the inverse variance adjustment formula to incident density ratios is

$$a(\ln \widehat{IDR}) = \frac{\Sigma(w_g)(\ln \widehat{IDR}_g)}{\Sigma w_g}$$

where   (11.9)

$$w_g = [\widehat{VAR}(\ln \widehat{IDR}_g)]^{-1} = \left(\frac{L_g^2}{m_{1g}L_{1g}L_{0g}}\right)^{-1}$$

Because we have been dealing with logarithmic measures of association, we take their exponent to bring them back to nonlogarithmic form:

$$\widehat{aOR} = \exp[a(\ln \widehat{OR})] \tag{11.10}$$

$$\widehat{aCIR} = \exp[a(\ln \widehat{CIR})] \tag{11.11}$$

$$\widehat{aIDR} = \exp[a(\ln \widehat{IDR})] \tag{11.12}$$

For example, the adjusted log-odds ratio for the illustrative data set in Table 11.3 is 0.2435 and the adjusted odds ratio is 1.28.

Epidemiologists and statisticians have many different methods of confounding and interaction assessment and control at their disposal. Further consideration of these topics is beyond the scope of this text. For additional methods, please see the following:

Kleinbaum, D. G., Kupper, L. L., & Morgenstern, H. (1982). *Epidemiologic Research. Principles and Quantitative Methods.* New York: Van Nostrand Reinhold.

Selvin, S. (1991). *Statistical Analysis of Epidemiologic Data.* New York: Oxford University Press.

Rothman, K. J. (1986). *Modern Epidemiology.* Boston: Little, Brown.

Breslow, N. E., & Day, N. E. (1987). *Statistical Methods in Cancer Research. Volume II—The Design and Analysis of Cohort Studies.* Lyon: International Agency for Research on Cancer.

Breslow, N. E., & Day, N. E. (1980). *Statistical Methods in Cancer Research. Volume 1—The Analysis of Case-Control Studies.* Lyon: International Agency for Research on Cancer.

SUMMARY

1. Bias in analytic research refers to any element of study design, data collection, or data analysis that systematically distorts study accuracy. Three forms of analytic bias exist. These are selection bias, information bias and confounding bias.

2. Selection bias occurs when a sample is unrepresentative of the target population. This type of bias will occur when faulty sampling mechanisms are used to collect data. It may also result whenever a significant number of subjects refuse to participate in or withdraw from a study.

3. Information bias refers to errors in the measurement or classification of study factors. This type of bias may be caused by measurement device defects, inaccurate questionnaires and interviewing procedures, inaccurate diagnostic procedures, and incomplete or incorrect data sources. The probability of misclassification may be the same in all study groups (nondifferential misclassification) or may vary between groups (differential misclassification). Nondifferential misclassification will bias a measure of association toward the null. Differential misclassification can bias a measure of association toward or away from the null.

4. Confounding is a distortion of an association between an exposure and disease caused by one or more extraneous factors. This form of bias will occur if the extraneous factor and exposure are associated and the extraneous factor is an independent risk factor for the disease. If recognized, measures of association can be adjusted for the biasing effects of

confounders. Presented in this chapter is one such method that uses a weighted average of strata-specific measures of association to derive an adjusted measure of association.

5. Interaction refers to a difference in effect of one factor according to the level of another factor. Occurring whenever extraneous factors modify the exposure–disease association, interaction is the statistical analogue to the biologic notion of synergy, in which the combined effect of two factors is not fully predicted by the sum or product of their parts.

6. Presented in this chapter is a strategy for confounding and interaction assessment. The first step in the process is to check for interaction. A chi-square test for interaction can be used for this purpose. Interaction must be ruled out before methods of confounder adjustment can be used. Confounding assessment involves a comparison of an adjusted summary measure of association with the crude measure of association. Hypothesis tests for confounding are ill advised. (Confounding is a matter of systematic error that cannot be addressed by hypothesis testing.) However, if the statistical adjustment for confounding alters the interpretation of the measure of association, the adjustment for confounding is warranted. If, on the other hand, the adjustment does not alter interpretation, crude measures of association may be used.

NOTATION

$\widehat{MA}$	Measure of association, point estimate (either $\ln \widehat{OR}$, $\ln \widehat{CIR}$, or $\ln \widehat{IDR}$)
MA	Measure of association, parameter (either OR, CIR, or IDR)
χ^2_{INT}	Chi-square interaction statistic
$\widehat{aMA}$	Adjusted measure of association estimate
$\widehat{MA}_g$	Measure of association estimate, stratum g
$\widehat{VAR}(\widehat{MA}_g)$	Variance estimate for measure of association, stratum g
w_g	Weighting factor, stratum g
k	Number of strata

EXERCISES

1. For each survey described below, prognosticate whether selection or information bias would be present and, if so, predict whether this bias would tend to overestimate or underestimate prevalence:

   (A) a survey of prior venereal disease based on self-reporting

   (B) a survey of disability in the elderly based on a sample of senior citizens attending dance lessons

   (C) a survey of coronary artery disease based on the question "Has a doctor ever told you that you have coronary artery disease?"

   (D) a survey of smoking in teenagers

   (E) a survey of carpal tunnel syndrome based on self-reporting among employees who are not eligible for disability compensation

   (F) a telephone survey of senile dementia

2. In a 1958 study of psychiatric diagnoses and socioeconomic status (SES), Hollingshead and Redlich documented a strong positive association between low SES and psy-

TABLE 11.4. Prevalence of Hypertension by SES and Race, Hypothetical Data for Exercise 3

Race	SES		
	Low	Intermediate	High
White	17%	16%	16%
Black	29%	28%	27%

chosis, as well as a strong negative association between low SES and neurosis. How could information bias and selection produce these results?

3. When an association is found between two factors, E and D, there is always the possibility that the relationship is due to a third factor, F. By stratifying on F, it is possible to assess whether interaction or confounding is present. Let us assume that we have discovered an association between low socioeconomic status (SES) and hypertension so that the prevalence of hypertension in low, intermediate, and high SES 50- to 54-year-old men is 33%, 21%, and 17%, respectively. The hypertension literature reveals that African Americans have higher blood pressure, on average, than people of other races. We also know that race and SES are associated.

   (A) Is it likely that the association between SES and hypertension is confounded by race?

   (B) Table 11.4 shows hypertension rates by race and SES. What do you conclude?

4. A case-control study investigated asbestos exposure (E), lung cancer (D), and cigarette smoking (F) in men who worked in an asbestos plant. Data appear in Table 11.5.

   (A) Calculate the crude odds ratio.

   (B) Calculate the odds ratio for smokers.

   (C) Calculate the odds ratio for nonsmokers.

   (D) Calculate the chi-square statistic for interaction. Report a p value and state your conclusion.

5. The Nurses' Health Study is a large cohort study in which female nurses were mailed an initial questionnaire in 1976. Follow-up questionnaires are issued every other year. Data on breast cancer risk in current users and never users of postmenopausal hormones are displayed in Table 11.6 with data stratified by age. Based on these data:

   (A) Calculate the incidence density ratio in 39- to 54-year-olds.

   (B) Calculate the incidence density ratio in 55- to 64-year-olds.

TABLE 11.5. Case-Control Study of Lung Cancer and Asbestos, Stratified by Smoking Status

	Stratum 1 (Smokers)		Stratum 2 (Nonsmokers)		Pooled	
	Asbestos +	Asbestos −	Asbestos +	Asbestos −	Asbestos +	Asbestos −
Lung Cancer+	75	5	5	10	80	15
Lung Cancer−	20	80	18	72	38	152

TABLE 11.6. Current Use of Postmenopausal Hormones and Incidence Densities of Breast Cancer in Postmenopausal Participants in the Nurses' Health Study

	Age Stratum 1 39–54 years			Age Stratum 2 55–64 years			Pooled	
	E+	E−		E+	E−		E+	E−
D+	85	160	245	95	194	289	180	354
	—	—		—	—		—	—
Person-Years	49,191	97,280	146,471	26,452	89,186	115,638	74,643	186,466

Sources: Colditz et al. (1990), as reported by Rosner (1995), p. 594. Age groups have been merged.

(C) How might you explain the apparent discrepancies in the two incidence density ratios calculated in parts A and B?

6. Data on breast cancer risk in previous users and never users of postmenopausal hormones are displayed in Table 11.7. Data are stratified by age group. Based on these data, calculate the statistics requested in A–D and answer questions E and F.

(A) The incidence density ratio in 39- to 54-year-olds.

(B) The incidence density ratio in 55- to 64-year-olds.

(C) The chi-square statistic for interaction.

(D) The adjusted incidence density ratio.

(E) Is there evidence of interaction in the data?

(F) Is there evidence of confounding in the data?

ANSWERS TO EXERCISES

1. A Information bias would result in an underestimation of prevalence. (Persons with prior venereal disease may tend to deny it.)

 B Selection bias would result in an under-ascertainment of prevalence. (Seniors afflicted with disabilities would not be likely to attend dancing lessons.)

TABLE 11.7. Past Use of Postmenopausal Hormones and Incidence Densities of Breast Cancer in Postmenopausal Participants in the Nurses' Health Study

	Age Stratum 1 39–54 years			Age Stratum 2 55–64 years			Pooled	
	E+	E−		E+	E−		E+	E−
D+	62	160	222	111	194	305	173	354
	—	—	—	—	—	—	—	—
Person-Years	39,012	97,280	136,292	51,750	89,186	140,936	90,762	186,466

Sources: Colditz et al. (1990), as reported by Rosner (1995), p. 594. Age groups have been merged.

C   Information bias would tend to underestimate prevalence. (Many people will be unfamiliar with the term "coronary artery disease.")

D   Information bias would result in an underestimation of prevalence. (Teenagers are likely to deny their smoking, especially if confronted by an authority figure.)

E   Information bias would tend to underestimate prevalence if there is a disincentive to miss work.

F   Selection bias would result in an underestimate of prevalence. (People with severe dementia may no longer live at home.)

2. Mentally disturbed poor people may be labeled as psychotic, whereas wealthy people with similar signs could simply be called neurotic. There may also be an association between diagnostic tendencies and clinic type; that is, psychiatrists working for public agencies may be more likely to diagnose psychosis (perhaps to justify the need for continued care), while private psychiatrists may be more likely to diagnose neurosis (perhaps to avoid the stigma of psychosis).

3. A   Yes. The preconditions for confounding have been established.

   B   Black race is associated with hypertension, but there is no association between SES and hypertension. Apparently, race confounds the relationship between SES and hypertension.

4. A   21.3.

   B   60.0.

   C   2.0

   D $\chi^2_{INT} = 17.93$; p value $< .001$; reject the null hypothesis of no interaction; smoking modifies the effects of asbestos exposure. The following intermediate calculations are provided to help with calculations of the chi-square statistic for interaction:

   $$\ln (\widehat{OR_1}) = 4.0943$$

   $$\widehat{VAR} (\ln \widehat{OR_1}) = .2758$$

   $$w_1 = 3.625$$

   $$\ln (\widehat{OR_2}) = .6931$$

   $$\widehat{VAR} (\ln \widehat{OR_2}) = .3694$$

   $$w_2 = 2.707$$

   $$a(\ln \widehat{OR}) = 2.6403$$

5. A   1.05.

   B   1.65.

   C   One possible explanation is that older women are exposed for longer duration than younger menopausal women. (The average age of menopause is 51.)

6. A   0.97.

   B   0.99.

   C   0.00 ($p > .10$).

   D   0.98.

   E   No evidence of interaction.

   F   No evidence of confounding ($c\widehat{IDR} \approx a\widehat{IDR}$).

REFERENCES

Berkson, J. (1946). Limitations of the application of fourfold table analysis to hospital data. *Biometrics, 2,* 47–53.

Bross, I. D. J. (1954). Misclassification in 2 × 2 tables. *Biometrics, 10,* 478–486.

Colditz, G. A., Stampfer, M. J., Willett, W. C., Hennekens, D. H., Rosner, B., & Speizer, F. E. (1990). Prospective study of estrogen replacement therapy and risk of breast cancer in postmenopausal women. *JAMA, 264,* 2648–2653.

Freedman, D., Pisani, R., Purves, R., & Adhikari, A. (1991). *Statistics* (2nd ed.) New York: W. W. Norton.

Huff, D. (1954). *How to Lie with Statistics.* New York: W. W. Norton.

Jewell, N. (1984). Introduction to Risk and Intervention Research Methods. Unpublished manuscript, University of California, Berkeley.

Kleinbaum, D. G., Kupper, L. L., & Morgenstern, H. (1982). *Epidemiologic Research. Principles and Quantitative Methods.* New York: Van Nostrand Reinhold.

Kupper, L. L., & Hogan, M. D. (1978). Interaction in epidemiologic studies. *American Journal of Epidemiology, 108,* 447–453.

Miettinen, O. (1974). Confounding and effect modification. *American Journal of Epidemiology, 100,* 350–353.

Mosteller, F. (1949). *The Pre-election Polls of 1948.* New York: Social Science Research Council.

Hirayama, T. (1990). *Life-style and Mortality: A Large-Scale Census-Based Cohort Study in Japan.* Basel: S. Karger.

Horwitz, R. I., & Feinstein, A. R. (1978). Alternative analytic methods for case-control studies of estrogen and endometrial cancer. *New England Journal of Medicine, 299,* 1089–1094.

Mantel, N., & Haenszel, W. (1959). Statistical aspects of the analysis of data from retrospective studies of disease. *Journal of National Cancer Institute, 22,* 719–748.

Nishan, P., Ebeling, K., & Schindler, C. (1988). Smoking and invasive cervical cancer risk: results from a case-control study. *American Journal of Epidemiology, 128,* 74–77.

Pagano, M., & Gauvreau, K. (1993). *Principles of Biostatistics.* Belmont, CA: Duxbury Press.

Rosner, B. (1995). *Fundamentals of Biostatistics* (4th ed.). Belmont, CA: Duxbury Press.

12

From Association
To Causation

Causal inference allows us to determine cause and effect by reasoning from knowledge and factual evidence. This chapter reviews epidemiologic notions of cause and considers causal inferential criteria recommended by Austin Bradford Hill in the early 1960s. The addendum to this chapter is a CDC case study that integrates concepts and methods from Chapters 9 through 12.

12.1 BACKGROUND

Before delving into causal inference, it is worth reviewing epidemiologic notions of cause, first introduced in Section 2.3. Recall that the epidemiologic notion of cause is one in which a causal factor is any event, condition, or characteristic that increases the likelihood of disease, all other things being equal. Moreover, an association is thought to be causal if an alteration in the frequency of exposure E is followed by a measurable change in the frequency or severity of disease D. This contrasts with the classic microbiologic definition of cause initially proposed by Jacob Henle in 1840 and later modified by his student Robert Koch in 1882. The **Henle–Koch's postulates** explained disease etiology in terms of a near one-to-one ("deterministic") relationship between an agent and disease. The following criteria form the basis of Henle-Koch's postulates:

- The agent must be present in each and every case of the disease (i.e., the agent is **necessary**).
- The agent can occur in no other disease as a fortuitous or nonpathologic parasite (i.e., the agent is **specific**).
- The agent must be isolated from the body and be capable of causing disease anew in a susceptible host (i.e., the agent is **sufficient**).

Limitations of these criteria in explaining both infectious and nonfectious diseases are now widely recognized. Rarely can we explain disease occurrence in terms of a single

necessary, sufficient, and specific cause. To do so would require a near complete understanding of all the factors that contribute to the disease. Practically speaking, this degree
of knowledge is seldom available. Without complete knowledge of pathogenesis, adopting a fully deterministic view of disease etiology is limiting and impractical. This view is
eloquently stated in the following passages from Lilienfeld et al. (1967):

> In considering the question of causal associations it is well to digress a little and consider
> briefly the meaning of causality in biological phenomena. In medicine and public health, it is
> reasonable to adopt a pragmatic concept of causality. We therefore recognize that a causal re-
> lationship exists whenever there is evidence that possible etiological factors form part of the
> complex circumstances which increases the probability of developing a [disease], and that in
> its diminution or absence the frequency of the [disease] is diminished. After all, the reason
> for determining etiological factors in disease is to use this knowledge to prevent the develop-
> ment of the disease.
>
> This concept is not as logically rigorous as the more formalistic one held by some investiga-
> tors, one which requires evidence indicating that a factor is both a necessary and sufficient
> condition for a disease before it can qualify as a cause. In biological phenomena, these two
> requirements do not have to be met because of the existence of multiple causative factors. In
> tuberculosis the tubercle bacillus is a necessary, but not a sufficient condition for tuberculo-
> sis. Additional factors which are usually included under the term susceptibility are important.
> In diseases generally considered noninfectious, such as cancer, the concept of causation may
> have to be broadened further, since one particular etiologic factor may not even be a neces-
> sary one because of the probable existence of multiple causative agents.
>
> Actually, in both infectious and noninfectious diseases, the differences in these two concepts
> depends upon the frame of reference. To illustrate, the cause and effect relationships with
> multiple etiologic factors, labeled A_1, A_2, A_3, and so forth, each acting independently, are
> presented in Figure [12.1]. These factors produce a change in B at a cellular level and the
> changed cell B could then develop into C, the disease. Surely the cellular change in B can be
> considered the necessary and sufficient condition for the disease C. Therefore, to meet the
> more rigorous definition of causality, the biological mechanisms relating A to B and B to C
> must be determined. Pragmatically, however, the determination of each of the A factors is
> important, since attention must be focused on them to be able to apply preventive measures.

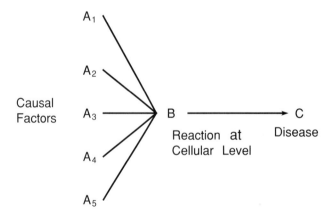

Figure 12.1. *Causal relationship with multiple, alternative causal factors.* (Source: *Lilienfeld, A. M.,
Pedersen, E., & Dowd, J. E.* Cancer Epidemiology: Methods of Study. *p. 88. © 1967. The Johns Hopkins University Press. Reproduced with permission.)*

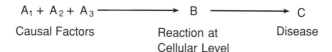

Figure 12.2. *Causal relationship with cumulative causal factors. (*Source: *Lilienfeld, A. M., Pedersen, E., & Dowd, J. E.* Cancer Epidemiology: Methods of Study. *p. 88. © 1967. The Johns Hopkins University Press. Reproduced with permission.)*

One can visualize different types of models with multiple etiological factors. In Figure [12.2] a model is shown in which each of the factors A_1, A_2, A_3 is necessary, but any individual one is not sufficient. Various types of additional combinations of causal factors can also be postulated.*

The goal, then, is to create a framework for taking action in the face of varying levels of certainty. In adopting a pragmatic inferential framework, epidemiologic thinking is divided into two distinct stages. Stage one searches for statistical associations between E and D. This stage usually involves planning studies, collecting and analyzing data, formulating tentative conclusions, and evaluating the roles of random and systematic error in explaining apparent associations. Satisfied with the knowledge that the statistical association is not artifactual, the epidemiologist moves to a second stage of reasoning that involves the derivation of biological meaning. This second stage is called **causal inference.**

Important debates over how best to infer causality from epidemiologic data intensified in the period following World War II. Many of these debates centered around the role of cigarettes in the development of lung cancer. In 1964, the Surgeon General of the United States convened a panel of scientists to advise him on this issue. This panel wrote a landmark report that established standards to address this and other issues related to the use of observational human data (U.S. Department of Health, Education, and Welfare, 1964). Acceptance of these standards and constructs has provided a framework for epidemiologic debates ever since. Some of the key constructs established by this report are:

- When coupled with [clinical, pathological, and experimental] data, results from the epidemiologic studies can provide the basis upon which judgments of causality may be made.
- In carrying out studies through the use of this epidemiologic method, many factors, variables, and results of investigations must be considered to determine first whether an association actually exists between an attribute or agent and disease.
- If it [is] shown that an association exists, then the question is asked: "Does the association have a causal significance?"
- Statistical methods cannot establish proof of a causal relationship in an association. The causal significance of an association is a matter of judgement which goes beyond any statement of statistical probability.
- To judge or evaluate causal significance . . . a number of criteria must be utilized, no one of which is an all-sufficient basis for judgment. These criteria include:
  (a) The consistency of the association
  (b) The strength of the association
  (c) The specificity of the association

*Lilienfeld, A. M., Pedersen, E., & Dowd, J. E. *Cancer Epidemiology: Methods of Study.* pp. 87–88. © 1967. The Johns Hopkins University Press. Reproduced with permission.

   (d) The temporal relationship of the association

   (e) The coherence of the association

(pp. 19–20)

Today, many of these points may seem rather tepid. At the time, however, they provided an important link in helping to change the way in which the world thought about nonexperimental epidemiologic data. Although the above causal criteria were not a *de novo* innovation of the committee, having been developed gradually over time by many different epidemiologists and scientists, the value of these criteria of judgment cannot be overlooked (Wynder, 1997). The criteria first propounded by the Surgeon General's Advisory Committee on Smoking and Health were later expanded and refined by British scientist A. Bradford Hill in a classic 1965 work (Hamill, 1997). These criteria are briefly discussed in the section that follows.

12.2 HILL'S CRITERIA

Criterion 1 (Strength) holds that strong association provide firmer evidence of causality than do weak ones and that the most direct measure of the strength of an association is found in the form of ratio measures of association such as the incidence density ratio, cumulative incidence ratio, odds ratio, and standardized mortality ratio. According to this criteria, the larger the risk ratio, the stronger the evidence for causality. Professor Hill (1965) explains it this way:

> To take a more modern and more general example upon which I have now reflected for over fifteen years, prospective inquiries into smoking have shown that the death rate from cancer of the lung in cigarette smokers is nine to ten times the rate in non-smokers and the rate in heavy cigarette smokers is twenty to thirty times as great. On the other hand the death rate from coronary thrombosis in smokers is not more than twice, possibly less, the death rate in non-smokers. Though there is good evidence to support causation it is surely much easier in this case to think of some features of life that may go hand-in-hand with smoking—features that might conceivably be the real underlying cause or, at the least, an important contributor, whether it be lack of experience, nature of diet or other factors. But to explain the pronounced excess in cancer of the lung in any other environmental terms requires some feature of life so intimately linked with cigarette smoking and with the amount of smoking that such feature should be easily detectable. If we cannot detect it or reasonably infer a specific one, then in such circumstances I think we are reasonably entitled to reject the vague contention of the armchair critic 'you can't provide it, there *may* be such a feature.' (pp. 295–296)*

Note that the basis of this criterion is the difficulty in "explaining away" a strong association as compared to a weak one. To explain a strong association as noncausal, an undiscovered risk factor (confounder) with an association at least as strong as the proposed risk factor would have to exist. Although conceivable, overlooking such a risk factor would be unlikely when dealing with a large risk ratio, especially if the disease is well understood. In contrast, explaining a modest association in terms of confounding factors is more conceivable.

*Reproduced with permission of the Journal of the Royal Society of Medicine.

Hill (1965) is quick to point out that the converse argument—that weak associations provide evidence that the association is noncausal—is untrue. As he puts it:

> We must not be too ready to dismiss a cause-and-effect hypothesis merely on the grounds that the observed association appears slight. There are many occasions in medicine when this is in truth so. (p. 296)*

Criterion 2 (Consistency) suggests that it is important to show similar findings in studies using diverse methods of study in different populations under a variety of circumstances. The greater the number of consistent studies, the stronger the causal evidence. Note, however, that consistency alone does not prove causation if, in fact, multiple studies suffer from similar biases.

Criterion 3 (Specificity) holds that the causal factor should lead to only one disease and that the disease should result from only this single cause. The importance of this criterion, however, should not be overemphasized, noting that specificity is difficult to establish without knowledge of reactions at the cellular level. For example, smoking's propensity to contribute to cardiovascular disease, cancer, chronic lung disease, musculoskeletal disease, and perhaps even neurologic disease cannot be used as an argument against its contribution to each. Thus, we cannot rule out causality based on the inability to confirm specificity. However, when specificity is evident, it can be a powerful argument in support of causality.

Criterion 4 (Temporarily) requires that exposure to the causal factor precede the onset of disease (Fig. 12.3). The importance of this may seem self-evident, but its demonstration is not always clear-cut. The problem in sorting out the proper temporal sequence of events is especially troublesome when studying conditions with long latency and insidious clinical onset. Consider the association between *Toxocara canis* infection in children and impaired neuropsychological development (Shofer et al., 1985; Worley et al., 1984). Visceral larval migrans is a clinical syndrome caused by the internal migration of the canine roundworm, *T. canis*, in human tissues. The parasite is a soil-transmitted nematode that, when ingested by humans, remains immature and fails to complete its life cycle. During the migration of the immature worm, the larva may encyst in various locations in the body, causing associated pathologies. For example, if the larval worm encysts in the central nervous system, impaired neuropsychological development may ensue. Indeed, case-control studies have found just such an association (Glickman and Shofer, 1987). However, even though *T. canis* is a common environmental contaminant, is neurotropic, and is capable of producing neurologic disease in humans, this association is not necessarily causal—it is equally plausible that children with behavioral problems and pica (a depraved or perverted appetite manifested by a hunger for substances not fit for consumption) are more likely to become infected with *T. canis*. Pica is also associated with lower socioeconomic status and deficient caregiving, and this, too, can explain the association.

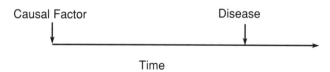

Figure 12.3. *Temporal relationship for causality.*

---

*Reproduced with permission of the Journal of the Royal Society of Medicine.

Thus, the uncertain and insidious onset of symptoms and the complex interrelationship among environmental contamination with *T. canis,* pica, socioeconomic status, and behavioral disorders in children make it difficult to sort out the correct temporal relationships among these factors (Fig. 12.4).

Criterion 5 (Biologic Gradient) holds that an increase in the level, intensity, duration, or total level of exposure to an agent leads to progressive increases in risk. This is in keeping with the general toxicologic principle of quantal **dose–response relationships** in populations. In a quantal dose–response relationship, the percentage of the population affected increases as the dose is raised. In an epidemiologic dose–response relationship, the incidence of disease increases as the level of the risk factor is raised. Examples of well-established and important epidemiologic dose–response relationships are the dose–response relationship between smoking and lung cancer (Fig. 12.5, Table 12.1); serum cholesterol levels, systolic blood pressure, and coronary heart disease (Fig. 12.6); and oral contraceptive estrogen dose and thrombotic disease (Fig. 12.7).

Epidemiologic dose–response relationships come in different forms and shapes (e.g., linear, log-normal, "U" shaped, and inverted "U" shaped), depending on the underlying pathophysiologic mechanism causing the elevation in risk. The type of dose–response relationship can have public health and regulatory implications. For in-

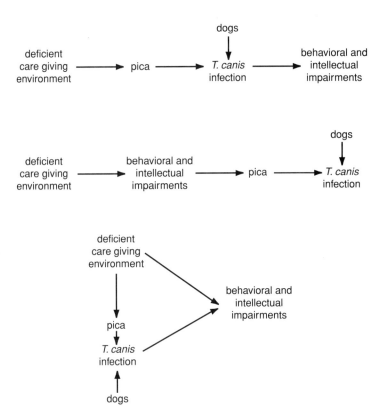

Figure 12.4. *Postulated temporal sequences that could explain the association between* Toxocara canis *infection and impaired psychological development in children. (*Source: Glickman & Shofer, 1987, p. 50, reproduced with permission of W. B. Saunders.)

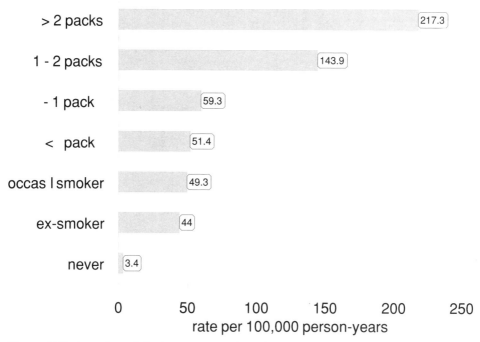

Figure 12.5. *Age-adjusted death rates due to bronchogenic carcinoma exclusive of adenocarcinoma by current amount of cigarette smoking (Based on data from Hammond & Horn, 1958, p. 1301.)*

stance, if there is a threshold response below which no further harm is done, further reduction in exposure is unwarranted; however, if risks are linearly related to cumulative dose throughout all potential levels of exposure, cumulative exposures must be minimized.

Criterion 6 (Plausibility) holds that the association should be plausible with known biologic facts about the pathophysiology of the disease. Statistical solutions are often unjustified without an understanding of the reasoning behind observations. Consider the fact that most people die in bed. This undeniable statistical association has little meaning given common sense and known biologic fact. However, we must not be too ready to dismiss other associations as noncausal just simply because a plausible explanation is as yet unavailable. Biological plausibility is contingent on the state of knowledge of the day, and the current state of knowledge can be inadequate in explaining associations that are in fact causal.

Criterion 7 (Coherence) holds that available evidence concerning the natural history, biology, and epidemiology of the disease should "stick together" (cohere) to form a cohesive whole. That is, the proposed causal relationship should not conflict or contradict information from experimental (human and animal), laboratory (*in vivo* and *in vitro*), clinical, pathological, and epidemiologic (both descriptive and analytic) sources of knowledge. For example, in considering smoking and lung cancer, the rise of smoking in Western countries during the early and mid-20th century was accompanied by a corresponding increase in lung cancer mortality, as one would expect given our current knowledge. This effect was more pronounced in men than in women, paralleling gender differences in the propensity to smoke.

TABLE 12.1. Cohort Studies of Smoking and Lung Cancer Mortality

Authors	Doll and Hill (1956)	Hammond and Horn (1958)	Dorn (1958, 1959)	Dunn et al. (1960)	Dunn et al. (1964)	Best et al. (1961)	Hammond (1964)
Study subject	British doctors	White men in nine states	U.S. veterans	California occupational groups	California American Legion members	Canadian pensioners (veterans and dependents)	Men in 25 states
Number of subjects	34,000	188,000	248,000	67,000	60,000	78,000+	448,000
Age range	35–75+	50–59	30–75+	35–69	35–75+	35–75+	35–89
Months followed	120	44	78	About 48	About 24	72	About 22
Lung cancer deaths in study	129	448	535	139	98	221	414
Lung cancer deaths, nonsmokers	3	25	56	3	12	8	16
Current cigarettes Smoked per Day	Standardized Mortality Ratios (Lung Cancer)						
None	Reference	Reference	Reference	Reference	Reference	Reference	Reference
<10	4.4	5.8	5.2	(5)[a] 8.3	(≤ 20)[a] 4.2	8.4	(current smoker)[a]
10–20	10.8	7.3	9.4	(10)[a] 9.0	13.5	13.5	9.6
21–39	(21+)[a] 43.7	15.9	18.1	(20)[a] 19.4 (30)[a] 25.1	(20+)[a] 7.4	15.1	
40+		24.7	23.3	(40)[a] 28.7			

Source: U.S. Department of Health, Education, and Welfare (1964), pp. 83, 164.

[a]indicates daily number of cigarettes smoked in which classes have been split or combined.

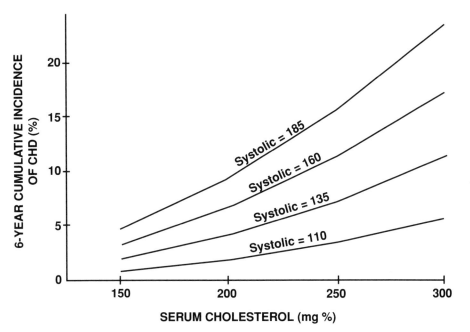

Figure 12.6. Six-year cumulative incidence of coronary heart disease (CHD) according to serum cholesterol levels at specified systolic blood pressures, men 45 to 62 years old. (Source: Kannel et al., 1961, p. 43.; reproduced with permission of the Annals of Internal Medicine.)

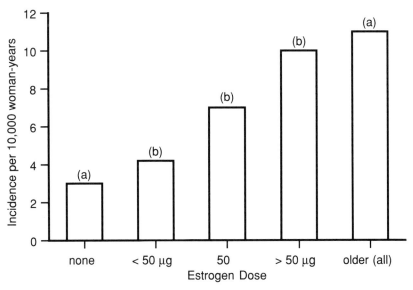

Figure 12.7. Oral contraceptive dose and risk of idiopathic deep venous thromboembolic disease. (Data sources: (a) Stadel, 1981, p. 614; (b) Gerstman et al., 1991, p. 34.)

More recently, declines in the age-adjusted death rates for lung cancer in men parallel recent declines in the prevalence of smoking (National Center for Health Statistics, 1992, p. 3). Moreover, animal experiments support the presence of carcinogenic factors in cigarette smoke, and histopathology evidence demonstrates the cytotoxic effect of smoking on the bronchial epithelium of smokers. These and other observations from a coherent whole in supporting the smoking and lung cancer causal hypothesis.

Criterion 8 (Experimentation) requires experimental epidemiologic studies, natural experiments, *in vitro* laboratory experiments, and animal models in support of a causal hypothesis. The strength of **experimental epidemiologic studies** (i.e., clinical trials and community trials) lies in the investigator's ability to control the allocation of the experimental intervention directly, thus negating the influence of extraneous factors in their potential to confound results. Experimental epidemiologic data, therefore, can provide strong evidence in support of a causal hypothesis. However, as discussed in Chapter 9, epidemiologic experimentation is often impractical or unethical, thus precluding its use.

When true experiments are unavailable, **natural experiments** can be considered. This term, first used by John Snow during his 19th century investigations of cholera, implies that the study factor is distributed in a way that resembles what would occur if randomization were permissible. Although not a true experiment, natural experiments provide the next best thing.

Testing of causal theories in the lab is also an important part of many causal arguments. This may occur in the form of *in vitro* experiments or *in vivo* experiments in animal models. *In vitro* **experimentation** (literally meaning "within a glass" experimentation) involves study within an artificial environment. Such experimentation is necessary to establish specific agents and their etiologic role in the pathogenesis of disease. It is also important in determining specific physiologic and environmental contributions to disease at the cellular and subcellular level.

Animal models provide the opportunity to study pathological phenomena and conditions in animals for the purpose of understanding human disease. This approach, sometimes called comparative medical research, may involve inducing a disease in laboratory species or studying a spontaneous disease of animals in nature.

When available, experimental evidence of all types provide strong evidence in support of causal theories. However, as with most of these criteria, its absence does not necessarily weaken the causal argument, especially if pragmatic and ethical concerns preclude their use.

Criterion 9 (Analogy) implies a similarity between things that are otherwise different. Analogy is one of the weaker forms of evidence, but it can be useful in providing insights into the cause of a disease, especially during early phases of investigation. An example of analogic thinking in epidemiology is that if one pharmaceutical drug (such as thalidomide) causes severe birth defects, so might others. Another example of analogic thinking is discussed by Fraser (1987):

When testing of serum specimens from the patients in Sierra Leone confirmed the diagnosis of Lassa fever, an investigation was organized to determine how the disease was spreading and—if it was not from one person to another—what the ultimate source might be. Because Lassa virus under the electron microscope resembles lymphocytic choriomeningitis virus and other arenaviruses (which also cause chronic infections in particular rodents), the investigators reasoned, by analogy with the spread of lymphocytic choriomeningitis virus, that some

West African rodent may be susceptible of Lassa virus infection and may infect humans through contaminated urine. (p. 311)

Thus, similar structures of otherwise dissimilar viruses led to clues about the source and transmission of the Lassa fever agent. As with all the criteria, this type of reasoning is incapable of providing hard-and-fast proof of cause and effect. In fact, no single criterion can be required as a necessary condition or indispensable need. Instead, a compilation of fact, judgment, experimental support, and perhaps even good fortune is required. In time, the truth will become known. However, for the sake of saving lives, there is often the need to take action in the face of incomplete scientific knowledge. Hill reminds us of this responsibility with these parting word from his 1965 article:

> All scientific work is incomplete—whether it be observational or experimental. All scientific work is liable to be upset or modified by advancing knowledge. This does not confer upon us a freedom to ignore the knowledge we already have, or to postpone action that it appears to demand at a given time. . . . Who knows, asked Robert Browning, but the world may end tonight? True, but on available evidence most of us make ready to commute on the 8.30 next day. (p. 12)*

SUMMARY

1. The epidemiologic notion of cause suggests that a causal factor is any event, condition, or characteristic that increases the likelihood of disease, all other things being equal. A statistical association is supported as causal when an alteration in the frequency of the exposure is followed by a change in the frequency or severity of disease. Note that this connotes a probabilistic (nondeterministic) etiologic model. In creating a framework for taking action in the face of varying degrees of certainty, epidemiologic reasoning is divided into two distinct stages. Stage one (statistical inference) searches for a statistical association between the exposure and disease. Stage two (causal inference) involves the derivation of biological meaning.

2. Important debates concerning the use of causal inference in modern epidemiologic research began in the period following World War II. Central to these debates was the Surgeon General's Report on Smoking and Health in 1964. This report validated the use of nonexperimental data for scientific decisions about health while establishing that statistical methods alone cannot provide proof of causality, especially for diseases in which the coexistence of many factors may be necessary to result in cause. The Surgeon General's Report used the following criteria to judge or evaluate causal significance: (a) the consistency of the association, (b) the strength of the association, (c) the specificity of the association, (d) the temporal relationship of the association, and (e) the coherence of the association.

3. Many of the causal criteria accepted by the Surgeon General's Report were based on the theoretical work of A. Bradford Hill. Hill's criteria are: (a) strength, (b) consistency, (c) specificity, (d) temporality, (e) biological gradient, (f) plausibility, (g) coherence, (h) experimentation, and (i) analogy. Although no single criterion is *sine quo non,* the criteria as a whole may be used as a framework for considering cause and effect.

---

*Reproduced with permission of the Journal of the Royal Society of Medicine.

EXERCISES

Matching Exercises

Exercises 1 and 2 are matching exercises in which you select the causal criterion that best fits the description below. The short titles for the causal criteria are:

Strength
Consistency
Specificity
Temporality
Biological gradient
Plausibility
Coherence
Experimentation
Analogy

1. Match the definition with the causal criterion it describes.
   (A) This criterion holds that all available clinical, experimental, and observational evidence should form a cohesive whole in the argument for causation.
   (B) This criterion holds that an increase in the level, intensity, duration, or total level of exposure leads to progressive increases in the magnitude of risk.
   (C) This criterion holds that it is helpful for an association to be explainable in terms of known biological fact.
   (D) This criterion requires that exposure to the causal factor precede the onset of disease.
   (E) This criterion is based on supporting evidence from community and clinical trials, *in vitro* laboratory experiments, and animal models.
   (F) This criterion is based on similarities from otherwise dissimilar sources.
   (G) This criterion holds that the cause should lead to only one disease and that the disease should result from only this single cause.
   (H) The criterion holds that diverse methods of study carried out in different populations under a variety of circumstances by different investigators provide similar measures of association.
   (I) This criterion holds that strong associations provide firmer evidence of causality than do weak ones.

2. The association between oral contraceptives and cardiovascular disease has been the subject of considerable debate. Indicate which of Hill's causal criteria is addressed by each of the statements below.
   (A) The risk of cardiovascular disease increases with increasing the estrogen dose of the oral contraceptive formulation.
   (B) Studies have shown that oral contraceptives cause endothelial proliferation, decrease the rate of venous blood flow, and increase the coagulability of blood by altering platelet function, coagulation factors, and fibrinolytic activity.

(C) The relative risk of oral contraceptive use and mortality from all circulatory disease in the 1970s was approximately 4.

(D) Most studies completed to date have demonstrated a positive association between oral contraceptive use and cardiovascular disease risk.

(E) Other steroidal sex hormones, such as testosterone, have known effect on cardiovascular disease risk.

(F) Altered parameters of hemostasis are measurable soon after oral contraceptives are begun. These alterations return to baseline within a month of discontinuing oral contraceptives.

Multiple Choice Exercises

3. The first stage of epidemiologic inference involves determining a statistical association between an exposure and disease. The next stage usually involves:

(A) formulating preventive strategies

(B) determining cost effectiveness

(C) communicating findings

(D) inference regarding cause and effect

4. Hill's criterion for "consistency" holds that the exposure will always lead to the disease.

(A) True

(B) False

5. A survey finds that patients who suffer from chronic back pain are more likely to be depressed than a series of age- and sex-matched controls. Can it be concluded that stress causes back pain. (After selecting your response, justify your answer.)

(A) Yes

(B) No

ANSWERS TO EXERCISES

1. A   Coherence.
   B   Biologic gradient.
   C   Plausibility.
   D   Temporality.
   E   Experimentation.
   F   Analogy.
   G   Specificity.
   H   Consistency.
    I   Strength.

2. A   Biologic gradient.
   B   Plausibility.
   C   Strength.
   D   Consistency.
   E   Analogy.
   F   Temporality.

3. D   Statistical inference is followed by causal inference.

4. B   (False) Consistency implies that studies are consistent in the estimation of association. If an exposure consistently causes disease in a given person, it is said to be sufficient. Sufficiency is not one of Hill's criteria for causality.

5. B   (No) The proper temporal sequence has not been established. It is just as likely that chronic back pain causes depression.

REFERENCES

Best, E. W. R., Josie, G. H., & Walker, C. B. A. (1961). Canadian study of mortality in relation to smoking habits, a preliminary report. *Canadian Journal of Public Health,* 52, 99–106.

Doll, R., & Hill, A. B. (1956). Lung cancer and other causes of death in relation to smoking. *British Medical Journal,* 2, 1071–1081.

Dorn, H. F. (1958). The mortality of smokers and non-smokers. *Proc. Soc. Stat. Sect. Am. Statist. Assoc.,* 34–71. [As cited in U.S. Department of Health, Education, and Welfare, 1964.]

Dorn, H. F. (1959). Tobacco consumption and mortality from cancer and other diseases. *Public Health Reports,* 74, 581–593.

Dunn, J. E. Jr., Linden, G., & Breslow, L. (1960). Lung cancer mortality experience of men in certain occupations in California. *American Journal of Public Health,* 50, 1475–1487.

Dunn, J. E. Jr., Linden, G., & Breslow, L. (1964). California State Department of Public Health. *Special Report to the Surgeon General's Advisory Committee on Smoking and Health.* [Data published in U.S. Department of Health, Education and Welfare, 1964.]

Fraser, D. W. (1987). Epidemiology as a liberal art. *New England Journal of Medicine,* 316, 309–314.

Gerstman, B. B., Piper, J. M., Tomita, D. K., Ferguson, W. J., Stadel, B. V., & Lundin, F. E. (1991). Oral contraceptive estrogen dose and the risk of deep venous thromboembolic disease. *American Journal of Epidemiology,* 133, 32–37.

Glickman, L. T., & Shofer, F. S. (1987). Zoonotic visceral and ocular larva migrans. *Veterinary Clinics of North America: Small Animal Practice,* 17(1), 39–53.

Hamill, P. V. V. (1997). Re: "Invited commentary: response to *Science* article, 'Epidemiology faces its limits.'" *American Journal of Epidemiology,* 146, 527.

Hammond, E. C. (1964). Prospective study of 1,085,000 men and women in 25 of the United States aged 35–89. *Special Report to the Surgeon General's Advisory Committee on Smoking and Health.* [Data published in U.S. Department of Health, Education and Welfare, 1964.]

Hammond, E. C., & Horn, D. (1958). Smoking and death rates—report of forty-four months of follow-up of 187,783 men. Part I. Total mortality. Part II. Death rates by cause. *JAMA,* 166, 1159–1172, 1294–1308.

Hill, A. B. (1965). The environmental and disease: association or causation? *Proceedings of the Royal Society of Medicine,* 58, 295–300.

Kannel, W. B., Dawber, T. R., Kagan, A., Revotskie, N., & Stokes, J. (1961). Factors of risk in the development of coronary heart disease—six year follow-up experience. *Annals of Internal Medicine,* 55, 33–50.

Lilienfeld, A. M., Pedersen, E., & Dowd, J. E. (1967). *Cancer Epidemiology: Methods of Study.* Baltimore, MD: The Johns Hopkins University Press.

National Center for Health Statistics (1995). *Health, United States, 1994.* Hyattsville, MD: Public Health Service.

Shofer, F. S., Glickman, L. T., Marmor, M., et al. (1985). Zoonotic dog roundworm (*Toxocara canis*) infection of children: epidemiologic and neuropsychologic findings. *American Journal of Epidemiology,* 122, 515 (abstract).

Stadel, B. V. (1981). Oral contraceptives and cardiovascular disease. *New England Journal of Medicine,* 305, 612–618, 672–677.

U.S. Department of Health, Education, and Welfare. (1964). *Smoking and Health. Report of the Advisory Committee to the Surgeon General of the Public Health Service.* USPHS Publication No. 1103. Washington: U.S. Government Printing Office. [Also published by D. Van Nostrand Company, Princeton, New Jersey.]

Worley, G., Green, J. A., Frothingham, T. E., Sturner, R. A., Walls, K. W., Vytautas, A. P., & Ellis, G. S. Jr. (1984). *Toxocara canis* infection: clinical and epidemiological associations with seropositivity in kindergarten children. *The Journal of Infectious Diseases,* 149, 591–597.

Wynder, E. L. (1997). The author replies. *American Journal of Epidemiology,* 146, 527–528.

CHAPTER ADDENDUM (CASE STUDY): CIGARETTE SMOKING AND LUNG CANCER

Source   Centers for Disease Control. *Cigarette Smoking and Lung Cancer. 1992 EIS Course.*

Terminology and notation have been altered to be consistent with this text.

Objectives

This exercise uses the classic studies by Doll and Hill, which demonstrated a relationship between smoking and lung cancer. After completing this case study, the student should be able to:

1. Discuss the elements of case-control and cohort study designs and identify their respective advantages and disadvantages.
2. Discuss some of the biases that might have affected these studies.
3. Calculate and interpret the following measures of association and potential impact: exposure odds ratio, incidence density ratio, incidence density difference, and attributable fraction.
4. Appreciate how the above measures of association and potential impact do or do not reflect the strength of association and public health importance of the association.
5. Review the criteria for causation.

Part I

A causal relationship between cigarette smoking and lung cancer was first suspected in the 1920s on the basis of clinical observations. To test this apparent association, numerous epidemiologic studies were undertaken between 1930 and 1960. Two studies were conducted by Doll and Hill in Great Britain. The first was a case-control study begun in 1947 comparing the smoking habits of lung cancer patients with the smoking habits of other patients. The second was a cohort study begun in 1951 recording causes of death among British physicians in relation to smoking habits. This exercise deals first with the case-control study, then with the cohort study.

Data for the case-control study were obtained from hospitalized patients in London and vicinity over a 4-year-period (April 1948 to February 1952). Initially, 20 hospitals, and later more, were asked to notify the investigators of all patients admitted with a new diagnosis of lung cancer. These patients were then interviewed concerning smoking habits, as were controls selected from patients with other disorders (primarily nonmalignant) hospitalized in the same hospitals at the same time.

Data for the cohort study were obtained from the population of all physicians listed in the *British Medical Register* who resided in England and Wales as of October 1951. Information about present and past smoking habits was obtained by questionnaire. Information about lung cancer came from death certificates and other mortality data recorded during ensuing years.

Question 1a   What makes the first study a case-control study?

Question 1b   What makes the second study a cohort study?

The remainder of Part I deals with the case-control study.

Question 2   Why were hospitals chosen as the setting for this study? What other sources of cases and controls might have been used?

Question 3   What are the advantages of selecting controls from the same hospitals as cases?

Question 4a   How representative of all persons with lung cancer are hospitalized patients with lung cancer?

Question 4b   How representative of all persons without lung cancer are hospitalized patients without lung cancer?

Question 4c   How may these representativeness issues affect interpretation of the study's results?

Over 1700 cases of lung cancer, all under age 75, were eligible for the case-control study. About 15% were not interviewed because of death, discharge, severity of illness, or inability to speak English. An additional group of patients were interviewed but later excluded when initial lung cancer diagnosis proved mistaken. The final study group included 1465 cases (1357 males and 108 females).

Table 12.2 shows the relationship between cigarette smoking and lung cancer among male cases and controls.

Question 5a   From this table, calculate the exposure proportion in cases $(\widehat{EP}_1)$ and controls $(\widehat{EP}_0)$.

Question 5b   What do you infer from these proportions?

Question 6   Calculate the odds of smoking for cases and controls $(\widehat{EO}_1$ and $\widehat{EO}_0$, respectively). Calculate the exposure odds ratio $(\widehat{EOR})$ and a 95% confidence interval for the exposure odds ratio. Interpret these results.

TABLE 12.2. Cigarette Smoking and Lung Cancer, Case-Control Study: Data for Case Study Questions 5 and 6

	E_1 Cigarette Smokers	E_0 Nonsmoker	
Cases	1350	7	1357
Controls	1296	61	1357
	2646	67	2714

Exposure proportion, cases $(\widehat{EP}_1)$ = _____

Exposure proportion, controls $(\widehat{EP}_0)$ = _____

Exposure odds, cases $(\widehat{EO}_1)$ = _____

Exposure odds, controls $(\widehat{EO}_0)$ = _____

Exposure odds ratio $(\widehat{EOR})$ = _____

95% Confidence interval for the EOR = (_____ , _____)

Table 12.3 shows the frequency distribution of male cases and controls by average number of cigarettes smoked per day.

Question 7 Compute the odds ratio by category of daily consumption, comparing each smoking category to nonsmokers. Interpret these results.

While the study appears to demonstrate a clear association between smoking and lung cancer, cause-and-effect is not the only explanation.

Question 8 What are the other possible explanations for the apparent association?

Part II

Part II of this exercise deals with the cohort study.

As you may recall, data for the cohort study were obtained from the population of all physicians listed in the *British Medical Register* who resided in England and Wales as of

TABLE 12.3. Daily Consumption of Cigarettes in Cases and Controls: Data for Case Study Question 7

	Exposure Category (Cigarettes per day)				
	E_3 25+	E_2 15–24	E_1 1–14	E_0 0	
Cases	340	445	565	7	1357
Controls	182	408	706	61	1357
	522	853	1271	68	2714

October 1951. Questionnaires were mailed in October 1951, to 59,600 physicians. The questionnaire asked the physician to classify himself into one of three categories: (1) current smoker, (2) ex-smoker, or (3) nonsmoker. Smokers and ex-smokers were asked the amount they smoked, their methods of smoking, the age they started to smoke, and, if they had stopped smoking, how long it had been since they last smoked. Nonsmokers were defined as persons who had never consistently smoked as much as one cigarette a day for as long as one year.

Usable responses to the questionnaire were received from 68% or 40,637 physicians, of whom 34,445 were males and 6192 were females.

Question 9   How might the response rate of 68% affect the study's results?

The remainder of this exercise is concerned exclusively with male physician respondents, 35 years of age or older.

The occurrence of lung cancer in physicians responding to the questionnaire was documented over the period of 10 years (November 1951 through October 1961) from death certificates filed with the Registrar General of the United Kingdom and from lists of physician deaths provided by the British Medical Association. All certificates indicating that the decedent was a physician were abstracted. For each lung cancer case, medical records were reviewed to confirm the diagnosis.

Diagnoses of lung cancer were based on the best evidence available; about 70% were from biopsy, autopsy, or sputum cytology (combined with bronchoscopy or X-ray evidence); 29% from cytology, bronchoscopy, or X-ray alone; and only 1% from just case history, physical examination, or death certificate.

Of 4597 deaths in the cohort over the 10-year period, 157 were reported to have been due to lung cancer; in 4 of the 157 cases this diagnosis could not be documented, leaving a net total of 153 cases of lung cancer.

Table 12.4 shows numbers of lung cancer deaths by daily number of cigarettes smoked at the time of the 1951 questionnaire (for male physician nonsmokers and current smokers only). Age-standardized person-years at risk are given for each smoking category. The number of cigarettes smoked was available for 136 of the lung cancer cases.

TABLE 12.4. Lung Cancer Deaths by Daily Number of Cigarettes Smoked

	Exposure Category (Cigarettes per day)			
	E_3 25+	E_2 15–24	E_1 1–14	E_0 0
Deaths	57	54	22	3
Person-Years at Risk	25,100	38,900	38,600	42,800
Incidence Density (per 1000 person-years)				0.07
Incidence Density Ratio (no units)				1.0
Incidence Density Difference (per 1000 person-years)				0.00

TABLE 12.5. Lung Cancer Deaths in Smokers and Nonsmokers

	E_1 Cigarette Smokers	E_0 Nonsmokers	Totals
Deaths	133	3	136
Person Years at Risk	102,600	42,800	145,400

Question 10a Compute lung cancer incidence densities, incidence density ratios, and incidence density differences for each smoking category in the table. What do each of these measures mean?

Question 10b Table 12.5 shows numbers of lung cancer deaths in smokers and non-smokers. Calculate the incidence density of cancer death in smokers, the incidence density in nonsmokers, and the incidence density for the entire population. If no one had smoked, what proportion of cases of lung cancer would have been averted? What is this proportion called?

Question 10c What proportion of lung cancer cases in smokers is attributed to smoking? What is this proportion called?

Table 12.6 shows the relationship between smoking and lung cancer mortality in terms of the effects of stopping smoking.

Question 11 What do these data imply for the practice of public health and preventive medicine?

The cohort study also provided mortality rates for cardiovascular disease among smokers and nonsmokers. Table 12.7 presents data for comparing lung cancer with cardiovascular disease.

Question 12a Which disease has a stronger association with smoking? Why?

Question 12b If the excess number of deaths due to smoking is used as an index of public health importance, for which disease is smoking of greater public health importance?

TABLE 12.6. Lung Cancer Mortality in Current, Former, and Nonsmokers

Cigarette Smoking Status	Number of Cases	Incidence Density (per 1000 person-years)	Incidence Density Ratio
Current smokers	133	1.30	18.5
Former smokers, years since quitting:			
<5 years	5	0.67	9.6
5–9 years	7	0.49	7.0
10–19 years	3	0.18	2.6
20+ years	2	0.19	2.7
Nonsmokers	3	0.07	1.0 (ref)

TABLE 12.7. Lung Cancer and Cardiovascular Disease Rates in the Population, and in Smokers and Nonsmokers

	Incidence Density (per 1000 person-years) (All)	Incidence Density (per 1000 person-years) (Nonsmokers)	Incidence Density (per 1000 person-years) (Smokers)	Incidence Density Ratio	Incidence Density Difference (per 1000 person-years)	Attributable Fraction (Population)
Lung cancer	0.94	0.07	1.30	18.5	1.23	95%
Cardiovascular disease	8.87	7.32	9.51	1.3	2.19	23%

As noted at the beginning of this problem, Doll and Hill began their case-control study in 1947. They began their cohort study in 1951. The odds ratios and incidence density ratios from the two studies by numbers of cigarettes smoked are given in Table 12.8.

Question 13 Compare the results of the two studies. Comment on the similarities and differences in the computed measures of association.

Question 14a What are the advantages and disadvantages of case-control versus cohort studies? (Fill in Table 12.9.)

Question 14b Which type of study (cohort or case-control) would you have done first? Why? Why do a second study? Why do the other type of study?

Question 15 Which of the following criteria for causality are met by the evidence presented from these two studies?

Strength of the association (Y/N)
Consistency with other studies (Y/N)
Temporality (exposure precedes disease) (Y/N)
Biologic gradient (dose–response effect) (Y/N)
Specificity of effect (Y/N)
Biologic plausibility (Y/N)

TABLE 12.8. Incidence Density Ratios and Odds Ratios from the Doll and Hill Cohort and Case-Control Studies

Daily Number of Cigarettes Smoked	Incidence Density Ratio from Cohort Study	Odds Ratio from Case-Control Study
0	1.0 (reference)	1.0 (reference)
1–14	8.1	7.0
15–24	19.8	9.5
25+	32.4	16.3
All smokers combined	18.5	9.1

TABLE 12.9. Comparison of Cohort and Case-Control Studies (Fill in)

	Case-Control	Cohort
Sample size		
Costs		
Study time		
Rare disease		
Rare exposure		
Multiple exposures		
Multiple outcomes		
Natural history		
Disease rates		
Selection bias		
Recall bias		
Loss to follow-up		

ANSWERS TO CASE STUDY: CIGARETTE SMOKING AND LUNG CANCER

Part I

Answer 1a   In the case-control study, people diagnosed as having a disease (in this case lung cancer) are compared with others who do not have the disease (controls). The purpose is to detect if the two groups differ in the proportion of persons who had been exposed to a specific factor (in this instance, cigarette smoking).

Answer 1b   A cohort study involves a well-defined group of people, some exposed to the risk factor under investigation, and some unexposed. In a cohort study the people are followed forward in time to detect disease occurrence.

Answer 2   Hospitals provide for a high likelihood of finding cases, ease of finding cases, accurate diagnosis, and a captive audience for study. Other sources are the following: cases—cancer registries, death certificates, insurance files, doctors' offices, and occupational records; controls—neighbors, acquaintances, and population-based.

Answer 3   Advantages are convenience, temporal match, control for socioeconomic status, place of residence, access to care, and diagnostic practices.

Answer 4a   Representative, because most cases are hospitalized. However, they may be sicker or in advanced stages of disease, may have more complications or other diseases, or, conversely, be less sick (survivors).

Answer 4b Usually, hospitalized patients are not very representative of the general population.

Answer 4c The purpose of a control group in a case-control study is to provide the prevalence of exposure in the population from which the cases are drawn. Hospitalized controls may be in the hospital for other smoking-related diagnoses; the prevalence of smoking in a hospitalized population is greater than that found in the general population. The net effect of a higher prevalence of smokers among the controls is that the true risk of lung cancer associated with smoking will be underestimated. The resulting bias can be classified as a form of selection bias.

Answer 5a

Exposure proportion, cases $(\widehat{EP}_1)$ = .995

Exposure proportion, controls $(\widehat{EP}_0)$ = .955

Exposure odds, cases $(\widehat{EO}_1)$ = 192.1

Exposure odds, controls $(\widehat{EO}_0)$ = 21.2

Exposure odds ratio $(\widehat{EOR})$ = 9.1

95% Confidence interval for the EOR = (4.0, 21.8)

Answer 5b Although cases have a slightly higher proportion of smokers than controls, the proportions are remarkably close. Note the overall prevalence of smoking (more than 95%)!

Answer 6 Strictly speaking, the interpretation is that the odds of being a smoker are 9.1 times higher in lung cancer cases than among noncases. In this instance, lung cancer is a rare disease and the odds ratio is a good estimator of the relative risk. Assuming that the study is not biased, one can infer that the risk of lung cancer is 9 times higher in cigarette smokers than in nonsmokers.

Answer 7

$\widehat{EOR}_1$ = 7.0 (odds ratio comparing people smoking 1–14 cigarettes per day and non-smokers)

$\widehat{EOR}_2$ = 9.5 (odds ratio comparing people smoking 15–24 cigarettes per day and non-smokers)

$\widehat{EOR}_3$ = 16.3 (odds ratio comparing people smoking 25+ cigarettes per day and non-smokers)

Values of the odds ratio rise steadily, consistent with a dose–response relationship between the daily number of cigarettes smoked and the strength of the association.

Answer 8 Selection bias, information bias, confounding, and chance (although the statistical tests suggest that chance is an unlikely explanation) are possible explanations.

An example of a likely selection bias in this study is that the controls were chosen from among hospitalized patients, who are more likely to be smokers than the general population. (The effect of the bias, however, would be to underestimate, rather than overestimate, the risks associated with smoking.)

Information bias could have occurred if lung cancer cases were more likely to recall their smoking history accurately than the controls. This type of bias is not highly likely in this instance, since the hypothesis regarding an association between smoking and lung cancer was not widely known and also because controls were other hospitalized patients who were probably as likely as the cases to be introspective about previous exposures or events.

Age might be a potential confounder in this study. To be a confounder, a factor must be associated with, but not a consequence of, an exposure and must be an independent risk factor for the outcome. If lung cancer is more likely to occur among older people and being older is associated with an increased likelihood of being a smoker, then the observed association between smoking and lung cancer might simply reflect the confounding by age.

Part II

Answer 9 As a general rule of thumb, we like to see response rates of 80% or better in epidemiologic studies. Realistically, a 68% response rate is good for a small study. If participation in a prospective cohort study is not related to both exposure and disease status, then a suboptimal response rate will only decrease the power of the study and will not bias the measure of association. If participation in a cohort study is related to both exposure and disease status, then selection bias may be a problem. Therefore, if possible, you should characterize the nonrespondents as best you can and determine whether the respondents differ on important factors.

Answer 10a See Table 12.10

Answer 10b

$$\widehat{ID}_1 = 133/102600 = 0.001296$$
$$\widehat{ID}_0 = 3/42800 = 0.00007009$$
$$\widehat{cID} = 136/145400 = 0.0009354$$
$$\widehat{IDR} = 0.001296/0.000070009 = 18.5$$
$$\widehat{AF}_p = (0.0009354 - 0.00007009)/.0009354 = .925 \text{ (formula 8.13)}$$

This proportion is called the attributable fraction in the population.

TABLE 12.10. Answer to Case Study Question 10a

	Exposure Category (Cigarettes per day)			
	E_3 25+	E_2 15–24	E_1 1–14	E_0 0
Deaths	57	54	22	3
Person-Years at Risk	25,100	38,900	38,600	42,800
Incidence Density (per 1000 person-years)	2.27	1.39	0.57	0.07
Incidence Density Ratio	32.4	19.8	8.1	1.0
Incidence Density Difference (per 1000 person-years)	2.20	1.32	0.50	0.00

Answer 10c
$$\widehat{AF}_e = (18.5 - 1)/18.5 = .950$$

Overall 95% of cases among smokers are attributable to smoking. Therefore, if none of the smokers had smoked, 95% of 133 cases, or 126 cases, would have been averted.

Answer 11   The lowest risk is seen among those who never smoked. However, the risk of lung cancer mortality decreases with time since last cigarette smoked, although even after 20 years of abstinence the risk is nearly three times greater than for never smokers. Hence, smoking cessation efforts are worthwhile from a public health point of view, but smoking prevention efforts would be most valuable.

Answer 12a   The incidence density ratio is the primary measure of an association's strength. Thus, there is a much stronger association betweeen smoking and lung cancer mortality than between smoking and cardiovascular mortality as indicated by a 14-fold greater incidence density ratio for smokers (18.5 vs. 1.3).

Answer 12b   The incidence density difference per 1000 person-years is greater for cardiovascular disease than for lung cancer even though the incidence density ratio is considerably lower. Thus, if no one smoked, more cardiovascular deaths would be prevented than lung cancer deaths.

Answer 13   The odds ratio in the case-control study consistently underestimates the incidence density ratios, probably because of the use of hospital patients as controls (hospitalized controls with other diseases were very likely to be smokers). However, overall, the

TABLE 12.11. Comparison of Cohort and Case-Control Studies (Filled in)

	Case-Control	Cohort
Sample size	Small	Large
Costs	Less	More
Study time	Short	Long
Rare disease	Advantage	Disadvantage
Rare exposure	Disadvantage	Advantage
Multiple exposures	Advantage	Disadvantage
Multiple outcomes	Disadvantage	Advantage
Natural history	Disadvantage	Advantage
Disease rates	Cannot measure	Advantage
Recall bias	Potential problem	Less problem
Loss to follow-up	Advantage	Potential problem
Selection bias	Potential problem	Less problem

two studies provide very consistent results, including evidence of a dose–response effect in both.

Answer 14a   See Table 12.11.

Answer 14b   Generally, a case-control study is quicker and easier than a cohort study. If the case-control study provides results that warrant further investigation, then it is appropriate to do a second study to confirm the findings. The cohort study, which is more difficult and expensive to mount and is slower to yield results, provides confirmation, gives better assessment of natural progression from exposure to disease, allows calculation of disease rates, and, depending on choice of study subjects, may be more generalizable.

Answer 15   Data from these studies fulfill the strength, consistency, exposure precedes disease, and biologic gradient criteria. However, the specificity of effect and biologic plausibility criteria are not directly addressed.

BIBLIOGRAPHY

Berkson, J. (1960). Smoking and cancer of the lung. *Proceedings of the Staff Meetings of the Mayo Clinic,* 35, 367–385.

Burch, P. R. J. (1978). Smoking and lung cancer: the problem of inferring cause. *Journal of the Royal Statistics Society A (General),* 141, 437–477.

Burch, P. R. J. (1980). Smoking and lung cancer: tests of a causal hypothesis. *Journal of Chronic Disease,* 33, 221–238.

Burch, P. R. J. (1981). Smoking and mortality in England and Wales, 1950 to 1976. *Journal of Chronic Disease,* 34, 87–103.

Doll, R., & Hill, A. B. (1950). Smoking and carcinoma of the lung. *British Medical Journal,* 2, 739–748.

Doll, R., & Hill, A. B. (1952). A study of the aetiology of carcinoma of the lung. *British Medical Journal,* 2, 1271–1286.

Doll, R., & Hill, A. B. (1954). The mortality of doctors in relation to their smoking habits. *British Medical Journal,* 1, 1451–1455.

Doll, R., & Hill, A. B. (1956). Lung cancer and other causes of death in relation to smoking. *British Medical Journal,* 2, 1071–1081.

Doll, R., & Hill, A. B. (1964). Mortality in relation to smoking: 10 years' observation of British doctors. *British Medical Journal,* 1, 1399–1410, 1460–1467.

Fisher, R. A. (1957). Dangers of cigarette smoking. *British Medical Journal,* 2, 43, 297.

13

Clusters

13.1 BACKGROUND

Outbreaks, Epidemics, and Clusters

An **epidemic** is a clear and often profound excess in the occurrence of a disease or disease-related condition in a community or region. The term **outbreak** is usually reserved to refer to a localized epidemic, although it may also be applied to an epidemic of broad geographic distribution if a common exposure source is suspected or involved. The term **cluster** refers to a close grouping of disease or disease-related events in space, time, or both space and time and is usually reserved to describe the aggregation of rare diseases such as specific forms of cancer. Thus, all three terms refer to a nonuniform distribution of cases over a study area, but each has a different connotation.

Cancer Clusters and Perceived Cancer Clusters

There is considerable public concern that environmental hazards cause cancer in some communities. In 1989, state health departments in the United States received approximately 1500 requests to investigate cancer clusters (Greenberg & Wartenberg, 1991). Although cancer cluster investigations are often mounted in response to this type of concern, most fail to find a true excess of cases in the region, and those that do are usually unable to identify a specific environmental cause. People are often unaware of how common cancer is in the United States and that cancer is not just one disease but is in fact many different diseases caused by a wide variety of environmental and nonenvironmental factors. Consequently, most anecdotal reports of clusters are simply normal occurrences or are artifacts of inflated reporting. Therefore, the term cluster is sometimes construed to imply that the observed aggregation of cases is believed or perceived to be greater than expected but is not necessarily so. Effort must then be expended to determine whether a perceived cluster represents a true increase in occurrence.

Difficulties in Studying Cancer Clusters

In 1989, the Centers for Disease Control and Prevention convened a national conference to discuss concerns about the study of cancer clusters. This conference was able to clarify some of the following difficulties surrounding cluster investigations (Rothman, 1990):

- Perceived clusters often include different types of cancers, thus reducing the likelihood that they resulted from a common exposure.
- Many reported clusters include too few cases to reach reliable statistical conclusions.
- Regional boundaries of clusters are rarely demarcated, making it difficult to determine the size of the population at risk that gave rise to the cases in question.
- Regional boundaries of clusters may be altered to make the cluster seem more substantial or inclusive.
- Conclusions about perceived clusters may not be reliable because of differences in the sensitivity of statistical and mapping techniques used for their detection.
- Causal exposures are often unspecified and, when specified, are often insufficiently intense to explain the perceived cluster.
- Chance can never really be ruled out as a *post hoc* explanation for a cluster—even when the statistical likelihood of an observation is small, rare events are inevitable if enough possibilities are considered.

Why Bother Investigating Clusters?

Despite difficulties encountered when studying clusters, most public health agencies consider it good public health practice, and good public relations, to respond to community concerns about every possible cluster. If a true cluster does exist, citizens' can take appropriate action. If a true cluster does not exist, citizens' concerns can be alleviated.

From a political, economic, and psychological point of view, the perception of a risk may be almost as important as an actual risk. Instances in which property values have fallen following publicity about a cluster have been documented. Once the cluster was disproved, property values returned to normal (Guidotti and Jacobs, 1993). Moreover, cluster investigations provide the opportunity for public health agencies to be "responsibly responsive" to public concerns and educate the public (Bender et al., 1990). Accordingly, several states have adopted standardized protocols for investigating clusters reported by citizens. Typically, the investigation of a cluster will include:

- Talking with the person reporting the cluster
- Verifying diagnoses of reported cases
- Reviewing potentially important exposure information
- Obtaining population data to determine if the observed number of cases is significantly greater than expected (see Section 13.2)

At each step of the investigation, the need for more extensive and costly research is evaluated while findings are simultaneously reported to the public.

Some cluster investigations are conducted because the law requires an agency to do so. For example, the National Institute of Occupational Safety and Health is required to evaluate the risks of health and safety in a workplace if requested to do so by three or more workers (CDC, 1992, p. 351).

Informative Cancer Cluster Investigations

Cluster investigations occasionally result in important scientific findings. For example, the Centers for Disease Control (1981a,b) discovered AIDS by investigating clusters of Kaposi's sarcoma and pneumocystis pneumonia in young men, Herbst et al. (1971) found that a cluster of adenocarcinomas of the vagina in young women was caused by *in utero* exposure to diethylstilbestrol, Baris et al. (1987) found a high rate of mesothelioma associated with lifelong inhalation of fine silica fibers from the erionite rock used for house construction in a village in Turkey, and Austin and Roe (1979) traced elevated rates of uterine cancer in the San Francisco Bay Area to the increased use of estrogens. Thus, cluster investigations can occasionally be informative, especially when chemical exposures are documented, routes of human exposure are traced, subpopulations at highest risk are identified, reliable denominator data are available, the diagnosis of the outcome has been consistent over time, and specific health outcomes are studied.

13.2   THE POISSON DISTRIBUTION

Random Fluctuations in Occurrence

Before more extensive research can be ordered in follow-up to a cluster investigation, we must evaluate whether the observed number of cases is greater than expected and, if so, whether this excess could be due to chance. Random fluctuations in the number of observed events are inevitable. For example, if a computer randomly assigns 50 dots to a grid with 50 equally sized squares, some squares will have no dots, some squares will have one dot, some will have two dots, and so (Fig. 13.1). Similarly, a community may experience a wide range in the number of cases in a given year with no change in the underlying risk of disease. The question: "At what point do we declare the observed increase to be above normal?" is now relevant. We can answer this question only after understanding the way in which random events distribute themselves in time and space.

Definition of Random Occurrence

A random distribution of cases in time and space is one in which (a) each population has the same probability of containing a case as any other population and (b) the occurrence of a case is not influenced by the occurrence of any other case.

   An example of a random distribution of cases in time might be the number of fatal motor vehicle accidents per year along a given stretch of highway (assuming no change in conditions or traffic). An example of a random distribution of cases in space might be the number of new diabetes cases in adjacent communities (assuming the communities have comparable age distribution). Nonrandom distributions are seen with contagion and other epidemic-related phenomena.

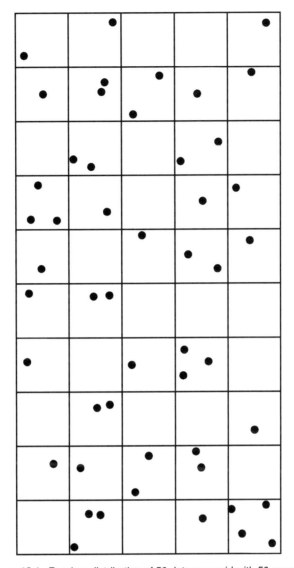

Figure 13.1. *Random distribution of 50 dots on a grid with 50 squares.*

The Poisson Distribution

Definition and Formula   The Poisson distribution is a probability distribution that describes the random occurrence of uncommon, discrete events. The formula for calculating Poisson probabilities is

$$Pr(X = x) = \frac{e^{-\mu}\mu^x}{x!} \tag{13.1}$$

where X represents the variable number of cases in a population, $Pr(X = x)$ represents the probability of observing x cases, e is the universal constant that forms the base of the natural logarithm ($\approx$2.718281), μ represents the expected number of cases, and $x!$ is the mathematical operation "x factorial" $= (x)(x-1)(x-2)\cdots(1)$. For example, $4! = (4)(3)(2)(1) = 24$. By definition, $0! = 1$.

Use of the Formula   To illustrate the Poisson formula, let us consider the probability of observing no case ($x = 0$) assuming one case is expected ($\mu = 1$). Accordingly,

$$Pr(X = 0) = \frac{e^{-1}1^0}{0!} = .3679$$

The probability of observing one case ($x = 1$) when one case is expected ($\mu = 1$) is

$$Pr(X = 1) = \frac{e^{-1}1^1}{1!} = .3679$$

The probability of observing two cases when one is expected is

$$Pr(X = 2) = \frac{e^{-1}1^2}{2!} = .1839$$

The probability of observing three cases when one is expected is

$$Pr(X = 3) = \frac{e^{-1}1^3}{3!} = .0613$$

The probability of observing four cases when one is expected is

$$Pr(X = 4) = \frac{e^{-1}1^4}{4!} = .0153$$

and so on. Figure 13.2 shows the Poisson distribution for $\mu = 1$ graphically.

Computational Formula for a Series of Calculations   In calculating a series of Poisson probabilities, the following computational formula may be used:

$$Pr(X = x) = \frac{Pr(X = [x-1])\mu}{x} \tag{13.2}$$

For example, based on the knowledge that $Pr(X = 0) = .3679$ when $\mu = 1$, the probability of observing one case is

$$Pr(X = 1) = \frac{Pr(X = 0)(1)}{1} = \frac{(.3679)(1)}{1} = .3679$$

The probability of seeing two cases is

$$Pr(X = 2) = \frac{Pr(X = 1)(1)}{2} = \frac{(.3679)(1)}{2} = .1839$$

and so on.

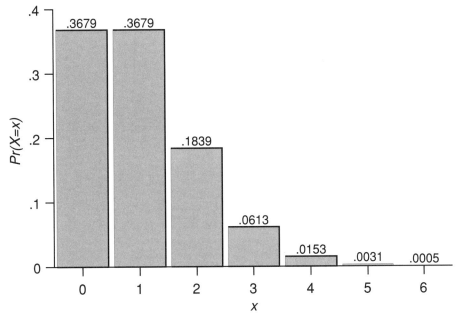

Figure 13.2. Poisson distribution, $\mu = 1$.

Calculating the Expected Number of Cases

Use of the Poisson formula requires knowledge of the expected number of cases in the population. This value can often be calculated as the product of the population size (n) and an expected rate (R_0):

$$\mu = (n)(R_0) \tag{13.3}$$

The size of the study population is based on census information or other enumeration data. The expected rate can be based on the age-adjusted rate in the country as a whole or in a comparable region. For example, if the study population size is 100,000 and the expected rate of disease is 1 per million person-years, the expected number of cases is

$$(100,000 \text{ persons})\left(\frac{1}{1,000,000 \text{ person-years}}\right) = 0.1 \text{ year}^{-1}$$

Illustrative Example 1: "Rare Cancer"

Let us assume a rare cancer normally occurs at the rate of 1 case per 1,000,000 person-years. We wish to calculate the probability of observing a given number of cases of this cancer in a community of 100,000. The expected number of cases (μ) is 0.1 (see above). Poisson probabilities for various numbers of occurrences are shown in Table 13.1. Figure 13.3 displays this distribution graphically. With this information in hand, we can say that the community will show either zero or one case in most years.

TABLE 13.1. Poisson Distribution, $\mu = 1$, Illustrative Example 1

x	$Pr(X = x)$
0	.9048[a]
1	.0905[b]
2	.0045[c]
3	.0002[d]
4	.0000[e]

$$^{a}Pr(X = 0) = \frac{e^{-0.1}\mu^0}{0!} = \frac{(.9048)(1)}{1} = .9048$$

$$^{b}Pr(X = 1) = \frac{(.9048)(.1)}{1!} = .0905$$

$$^{c}Pr(X = 2) = \frac{(.9048)(.01)}{2!} = .0045$$

$$^{d}Pr(X = 3) = \frac{(.9048)(.001)}{3!} = .0002$$

$$^{e}Pr(X = 4) = \frac{(.9048)(.0001)}{4!} = .0000$$

Quantifying Chance

Working Definition of "Not Likely to Be Due to Chance" When Events Are Defined Retrospectively Let X represent the variable number of cases in a population. By making certain assumptions, we can use the Poisson distribution to calculate whether an observed number of cases (x) is likely to be due to chance. If the probability of observing x or more cases is "sufficiently small," we might conclude that the observed fluctuation is nonrandom. Although no standard definition of "sufficiently small" exists in

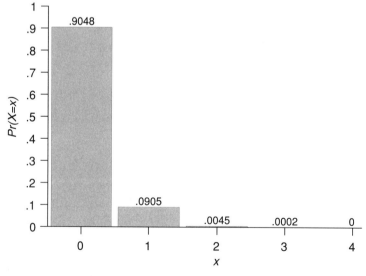

Figure 13.3. Poisson distribution, $\mu = 0.1$.

this context, let us use a cutoff point of 1 in 200 (.005).[*] That is, we will conclude that the observed number of cases is not likely to be due to chance if $Pr(X \geq x) < .005$.

Law of Complements   To calculate $Pr(X \geq x)$, two laws of probability must be introduced. The first law is the Law of Complements. In set theory, the complement of event A is "not A" (i.e., everything other than A). For example, if a set is made up of the numbers 1 to 5, and subset A represents 1, 2, and 3, the complement of A is the subset 4 and 5. The symbol $\overline{A}$ is used to represent the complement of A. The law of complements states

$$Pr(\overline{A}) = 1 - Pr(A) \qquad (13.4)$$

For example, if the probability of A is .1, then the probability of "not A" is $1 - .1 = .9$.

Law of Addition for Mutually Exclusive Events   To calculate the probability of observing x or fewer cases, we use the fact

$$Pr(X \leq x) = Pr(X = 0) + Pr(X = 1) + \cdots + Pr(X = x) \qquad (13.5)$$

For example, the probability of seeing two or fewer cases in illustrative example 1 is $Pr(X \leq 2) = Pr(X = 0) + Pr(X = 1) + Pr(X = 2) = .9048 + .0905 + .0045 = .9998$

Probability of Observing at Least x Cases   By combining the Law of Complements and Law of Addition for Mutually Exclusive Events, we have

$$Pr(X \geq x) = 1 - Pr(X \leq x - 1) \qquad (13.6)$$

For example, the probability of observing at least three cases in illustrative example 1 is $Pr(X \geq 3) = 1 - Pr(X \leq 2) = 1 - .9998 = .0002$. This suggests the likelihood of observing three or more cases under the assumption of randomness is very small, thus representing a true cluster.

Post Hoc Definitions of Chance Are Inherently Troublesome

Clustering, however, can never definitively be identified after the fact. The *post hoc* discovery of a cluster comes with at least two conceptual problems. First, drawing artificial boundaries in time and space can create the illusion of a cluster when none exists. This has been compared with randomly shooting a bullet at the broad side of a barn and then drawing the bull's-eye around the bullet hole after the fact. Second, even when the statistical likelihood of an observation is small, rare events will and do occur if enough possibilities are considered. In fact, the random occurrence of three or more cases in the illustrative example is possible although unlikely—it will occur once per 5000 observations.

---

[*]Note that this nonstandard definition of "significance" is different from the commonly accepted standard of .05 or .01 used in most hypothesis-testing situations. This difference stems from a fundamental distinction between *a priori* and *post hoc* evaluations of chance. More explicitly, *post hoc* evaluations of chance should be more stringent than those used to test new data. Perhaps even more importantly, *post hoc* evaluations of chance are inherently troublesome.

These fundamental conceptual problems suggest that there is often little scientific or public health purpose in investigating individual disease clusters (see Rothman, 1990). Perhaps, clustering can only be addressed on a larger scale.

13.3   GOODNESS OF FIT OF THE POISSON DISTRIBUTION

Comparing an Observed Distribution to a Theoretical Distribution

The best way to decide if events are clustered is to use a **goodness of fit test.** Goodness of fit tests compare the observed distribution of cases to a theoretical distribution predicted by the Poisson model. If events are truly random, the Poisson distribution will be an effective model. If the Poisson distribution does not fit the data, evidence of clustering is established. The first step in testing a Poisson model's goodness of fit is to collect data from multiple, comparably aged and sized "risk units" of observation.

Illustrative Example 2: "Fatal Horse Kicks"

Table 13.2 contains data from an early application of the Poisson model. Data represent the frequency of fatal horse kicks in Prussian army corps in the years between 1875 and 1894. Since 10 army corps units are observed for 20 years, the study includes 200 risk units of observation.

Estimating Poisson Parameter μ

If Poisson parameter μ is unavailable, it is estimated by the **sample mean** $(\bar{x})$ using the formula

$$\bar{x} = \frac{\Sigma f_i x_i}{n} \tag{13.7}$$

TABLE 13.2. Fatal Horse Kicks in the Prussian Army, 1875–1894, Illustrative Example 2

Number of Fatalities x_i	Frequency f_i
0	109
1	65
2	22
3	3
4	1
5+	0
	$\Sigma f_i = 200$

$n = \Sigma f_i = 200$

$\Sigma f_i x_i = (109)(0) + (65)(1) + (22)(2) + (3)(3) + (1)(4) + (0)(5) = 122$

$\bar{x} = \dfrac{\Sigma f_i x_i}{n} = \dfrac{122}{200} = .610$

Source: Bortkiewicz (1898), as cited in Sokal & Rohlf (1995), p. 93.

TABLE 13.3. Poisson Distribution, $\mu = 0.610$, Fatal Horse Kick Data, Illustrative Example 2

Number of Fatalities x_i	Poisson Probability $Pr(X = x_i)$	Expected Frequency $\hat{f}_i = [Pr(X = x_i)][n]$
0	.543351[a]	108.68
1	$(.543351)(.61)/1 = .331444$[b]	66.28
2	$(.331444)(.61)/2 = .101090$[b]	20.22
3	$(.101090)(.61)/3 = .020556$[b]	4.12
4	$(.020556)(.61)/4 = .003135$[b]	0.62
5+	$(.003135)(.61)/5 = .000382$[b]	0.08
	1.000	200.00

[a]$Pr(X = 0) = \dfrac{e^{-0.61}\mu^0}{0!} = .543351$.

[b]See formula 13.2.

where Σ is interpreted to mean "summation of all values," x_i represents the observed number of events, f_i represents the frequency with which x_i occurs, and n represents the number of risk units in the sample. (*Note:* $n = \Sigma f_i$.)

Based on formula 13.7, the average number of fatal horse kicks per army corp unit is 0.610 (see Table 13.2 for calculations). Poisson probabilities using $\bar{x}$ as the estimated value for μ are shown in Table 13.3.

Expected Frequencies

Our next task is to calculate the expected number of events for each category of x_i under the Poisson model. The *expected number of events* ($\hat{f}_i$) is

$$\hat{f}_i = [Pr(X = x_i)][n] \tag{13.8}$$

where $Pr(X = x_i)$ represents the probability of observing x_i cases and n represents the number of risk units in the sample. Expected frequencies for illustrative example 2 are displayed in Table 13.3.

Testing the Poisson Model

Observed and expected frequencies (f_i and $\hat{f}_i$, respectively) are compared to determine whether the Poisson model fits the data (Table 13.4; Fig. 13.4). Based on Figure 13.4, it appears that the Poisson model fits the data well. To test this model, we set up the hypotheses

H_0: events are distributed randomly (the Poisson model fits data well)

H_1: events are not distributed randomly (the Poisson model does not fit data well)

Falsity of the null hypotheses of randomness can be due to one of two situations. Either cases are uniformly distributed or cases are clustered. Figure 13.5 shows these possibilities diagrammatically.

By convention, an alpha level of .05 is used to test this hypothesis. (See Section 10.3 for a discussion of alpha levels.)

TABLE 13.4. Observed Frequencies, Expected Frequencies, and the Log-Likelihood Ratio Statistic G, Illustrative Example 2

Number of Fatalities x_i	Observed Frequency f_i	Expected Frequency $\hat{f}_i = [Pr(X = x_i)][n]$	$f_i \ln \dfrac{f_i}{\hat{f}_i}$
0	109	108.68	0.320471
1	65	66.28	−1.267560
2	22	20.22	1.856145
3+	4	4.82	−0.745918
			$\Sigma f_i \ln \dfrac{f_i}{\hat{f}_i} = 0.163138$

[a]Categories with fewer than one case are pooled in preparation for the goodness of fit test.

$G = 2\Sigma f_i \ln \dfrac{f_i}{\hat{f}_i} = (2)(0.163138) = .326276$

$df = k-2 = 4 - 2 = 2$
$p > .05$

In preparation for the goodness of fit statistic, categories with fewer than one expected observation are pooled. This is necessary to ensure proper functioning of the goodness of fit statistic (Cochran, 1954).

Log-Likelihood Goodness of Fit Statistic G

The hypothesis-testing statistic of choice is **log-likelihood ratio goodness of fit statistic G:**

$$G = 2\sum_{i=1}^{k} f_i \ln \frac{f_i}{\hat{f}_i} \qquad (13.9)$$

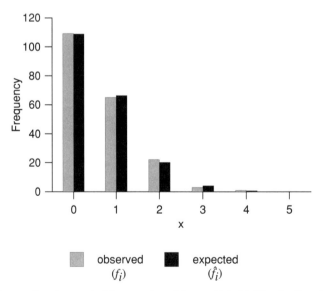

Figure 13.4 Observed and expected frequencies of horse kick fatalities in Prussian army corps, 1875–1894.

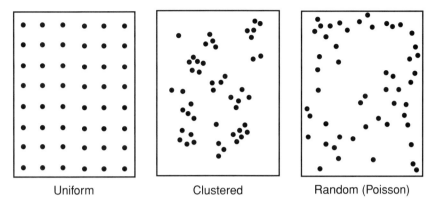

Figure 13.5. *Distribution of dots in two-dimensional space.*

where there are k categories of X, f_i represents the observed frequency of value x_i, and $\hat{f}_i$ represents the expected frequency of value x_i. Although other goodness of fit statistics are available (e.g., the chi-square goodness of fit statistic), the log-likelihood ratio goodness of fit statistic shows superior performance (Rao & Chakravarti, 1956). Large values of G will suggest poor model fit; small values will suggest good fit. Here, "large" and "small" have standard definitions. Under the null hypothesis, the G statistic is distributed as a chi-square random variable with $k - 2$ degrees of freedom. (*Note:* When μ is known and *not* estimated by $\bar{x}$, the goodness of fit statistic has $k - 1$ degrees of freedom.) An abbreviated chi-square table is provided as Table 13.5. This table is used to transform the G statistics to a p value. For example, a G statistic of 5.99 with 2 degrees of freedom is transformed into a p value of .05; a G statistic of 9.21 with 2 degrees of freedom is transformed to a p value of .01; a G statistic greater than 9.21 with 2 degrees of freedom is transformed to a p value of less than .01; and so on. If the calculated p value is less than .05, the null hypothesis of randomness is rejected.

Table 13.4 calculates a G statistic of .326 with 2 degrees of freedom for the fatal horse kick illustrative data. Therefore, $p > .05$ and the null hypothesis of randomness is retained.

TABLE 13.5. Critical Values of the Chi-Square Distribution

Degrees of Freedom	Alpha					
	.10	.05	.025	.01	.005	.001
1	2.706	3.841	5.024	6.635	7.879	10.828
2	4.605	5.991	7.378	9.210	10.597	13.816
3	6.251	7.815	9.348	11.345	12.838	16.266
4	7.779	9.488	11.143	13.277	14.860	18.467
5	9.236	11.070	12.832	15.086	16.750	20.515
6	10.645	12.592	14.449	16.812	18.548	22.458
7	12.017	14.067	16.013	18.475	20.278	24.322
8	13.362	15.507	17.535	20.090	21.955	26.124
9	14.684	16.919	19.023	21.666	23.589	27.877
10	15.987	18.307	20.483	23.209	25.188	29.588

Illustrative Example 3: "Frequency of War"

A second example of a goodness of fit test evaluates the frequency of war in the 432 years between 1500 and 1931. War, for this analysis, was defined as a military action that either was legally declared, involved more than 50,000 troops, or resulted in a significant border realignment. To achieve greater uniformity in the analysis, major confrontations were split into smaller subwars. For example, World War I was treated as five separate wars. According to this definition of war, war occurred 299 times during these 432 years of observation. Table 13.6 shows the distribution of the number of wars initiated in a given year (Richardson, 1944, as cited in Larson and Marx, 1981, pp. 148–149, 367). Calculations are shown in the table. The hypotheses to be tested are H_0: wars are distributed randomly versus H_1: wars are not distributed randomly. The average number of wars per year is 0.69. The G statistic is 2.48 with 3 degrees of freedom. The G statistic translates to $p > .05$, resulting in retention of the null hypothesis of a random time distribution of wars. One interpretation of this test is that human hostility levels as measured by the initiation of war is constant over time—a rather grim view of human nature.

TABLE 13.6. Yearly Frequency of War Between 1500 and 1931, Illustrative Example 3

Number of Wars X	Observed Frequency f_i
0	233
1	142
2	48
3	15
4+	4
	$\Sigma f_i = 442$

$n = \Sigma f_i = 442$

$\Sigma f_i x_i = (233)(0) + (142)(1) + (48)(2) + (15)(3) + (4)(4) = 299$

$\bar{x} = \dfrac{\Sigma f_i x_i}{n} = \dfrac{299}{443} \approx .69$

Poisson probabilities, expected frequencies, and intermediate calculations for the log-likelihood goodness of fit statistic are shown below.

Number of Wars X	Observed Frequency f_i	Poisson Probability $Pr(X = x_i)$	Expected Frequency $\hat{f}_i = [Pr(X = x_i)][n]$	Intermediate Calculation for G $f_i \ln \dfrac{f_i}{\hat{f}_i}$
0	233	.5016[a]	221.71	6.41
1	142	.3461	152.98	−7.32
2	48	.1194	52.77	−3.45
3	15	.0275	12.16	3.52
4+	4	.0055	2.39	2.08
Sums	$\Sigma f_i = 442$	1.000	442	$\Sigma f_i \ln \dfrac{f_i}{\hat{f}_i} = 1.24$

[a]$Pr(X = 0) = \dfrac{e^{-0.69}\mu^0}{0!} = .5016$

$G = 2 \Sigma f_i \ln \dfrac{f_i}{\hat{f}_i} = (2)(1.24) = 2.48;\ \mathrm{df} = k - 2 = 3;\ p > .05.$

Source: Richardson (1944) as cited in Larson and Marx (1981), p. 367.

SUMMARY

1. A cluster is a close grouping of disease or disease-related events in time or space. Many perceived clusters are, in fact, not really clusters at all, representing random fluctuations in occurrence. Despite the many difficulties encountered when investigating a cluster, most clusters are investigated for policy and legal reasons.

2. The Poisson distribution is a probability distribution that describes the random occurrence of uncommon, discrete events. This distribution can be used to quantify chance explanations for clusters. Examples of Poisson calculations are presented throughout this chapter.

3. The best way to learn whether a distribution of cases is random or clustered is to use a goodness of fit test. Goodness of fit statistics compare the observed distribution of cases to a theoretical distribution predicted by the Poisson model. If the Poisson model fits the data, we conclude events are random. If the Poisson model does not fit the data, we conclude events are clustered.

NOTATION AND FORMULA REFERENCE

X	Variable number of cases in a population
x	Observed number of cases in a population
μ	Expected number of cases (formula 13.3)
n	Sample size
R_0	Expected rate
e	Universal constant of the natural logarithm
$Pr(X = x)$	Probability of observing x cases (formulas 13.1 and 13.2)
$x!$	x Factorial
A	Event A
$\overline{A}$	Complement of A (formula 13.4)
$Pr(X \leq x)$	Probability of observing x or fewer cases (formula 13.5)
$Pr(X \geq x)$	Probability of observing at least x cases (formula 13.6)
$\bar{x}$	Sample mean/estimator of μ (formula 13.7)
$\hat{f}_i$	Expected frequency (formula 13.8)
f_i	Observed frequency
G	Log-likelihood ratio goodness of fit statistic (formula 13.9)

EXERCISES

1. Several classes of drugs are used to treat gastric and duodenal ulcers by reducing the volume and acidity of gastric secretions. Although millions of people have been treated with these drugs and the incidence of adverse drug reactions is low, an issue of ongoing concern is that they may increase the risk of gastric cancers by causing a profoundly hypochlorhydric stomach. Suppose we find 3 cases of gastric cancer in a cohort of people taking gastric acid reducers. Further suppose that, based on the size and age distribution of the cohort, 1.2 cases were expected ($\mu = 1.2$).

   (A) Calculate the probability of observing no cases in the cohort.

   (B) Calculate the probability of observing one case in cohort.

(C) Calculate the probability of observing two cases in the cohort.

(D) Calculate the probability of observing *at least* three cases in the cohort.

(E) Was the observation of three cases *significantly* more than expected?

2. Assuming the expected number of cases in a population is 2, what is the likelihood of observing:

(A) no cases

(B) exactly 1 case

(C) exactly 2 cases

(D) exactly 3 cases

(E) at least 4 cases

3. One of the best studied leukemia clusters to date occurred in Niles, Illinois, from 1956 to 1960 (Heath & Hasterlik, 1963). In the 5.3-year period from 1956 to the first four months of 1961, eight cases of childhood leukemia were reported among the 7076 white children less than 15 years of age in Niles. These cases were concentrated in the St. John Brebeuf Parish (Fig. 13.6). During the same period, 286 cases of childhood leukemia occurred among the 1,152,695 children in Cook County, Illinois, exclusive of Niles.

(A) Based on the occurrence rate in Cook County, how many cases were expected in Niles?

(B) Assuming randomness, how likely were the eight cases in Niles?

(C) Would you say that the eight cases in Niles represent a true cluster?

4. Although currently lacking in support, an ongoing theory suggests that the electro-magnetic fields from cellular phones may cause brain tumors. Suppose the expected

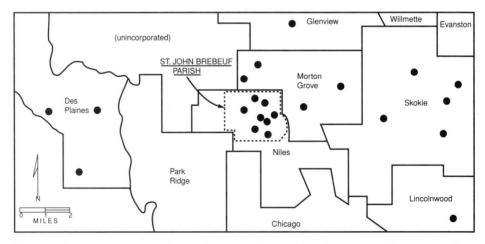

Figure 13.6. *Leukemia among children in Niles, Illinois, and vicinity, 1956–1960. Each dot indicates a single case. (Source: Reprinted by permission of the publisher from Health, C. W. Jr., & Hasterlik, R. J. Leukemia among children in a suburban community, American Journal of Medicine, 34, p. 797. Copyright © 1963 by Excerpta Medica, Inc., P.O. Box 882 Madison Square Station, New York, NY 10159-0882.)*

number of brain tumors in a cohort of cellular telephone users is 1.8 and 4 cases are observed. Would this be considered excessive? Justify the response with a probability statement.

5. Suppose the expected number of motor vehicle fatalities on a given highway is 0.75 per year.

(**A**) What is the probability of observing exactly 0 fatalities?

(**B**) What is the probability of observing exactly 1 fatality?

(**C**) What is the probability of observing exactly 2 fatalities?

(**D**) What is the probability of observing exactly 3 fatalities?

(**E**) What is the probability of observing at least 4 motor vehicle fatalities?

ANSWERS TO EXERCISES

1. A $Pr(X = 0) = \dfrac{e^{-1.2}1^0}{0!} = .301194$ (by formula 13.1).

B $Pr(X = 1) = (.301194)(1.2)/1 = .361433$ (by formula 13.2).

C $Pr(X = 2) = (.361433)(1.2)/2 = .216860$ (by formula 13.2).

D $Pr(X \geq 3) = 1 - Pr(X \leq 2) = 1 - (3012 + .3614 + .2169) = .1205$ (by   formula 13.6).

E   No.

2. A   .1353.

B   .2706.

C   .2706.

D   .1804.

E   .1431.

3. A $\mu = (n)(R_0) = (7076)(286/1,152,695) = 1.76.$

B   .00049.

C   Yes. This probability is small enough to reject the notion that the eight cases occurred randomly. However, there is still a small chance that the observation is an unusual chance occurrence. This is one of the difficulties in interpreting *post hoc* clusters—rarities do occasionally occur.

4. No, this would not be considered excessive since $Pr(X \geq 4) = .1087.$

5. A   .4724.

B   .3543.

C   .1329.

D   .0332.

E $Pr(X \geq 4) = 1 - (.4724 + .3543 + .1329 + .0332) = .0072.$

REFERENCES

Austin, D. F., & Roe, K. M. (1979). Increase in cancer of the corpus uteri in the San Francisco–Oakland Standard Metropolitan Statistical Area. *Journal of the National Cancer Institute, 62,* 13–16.

Baris, Y., Simonato, L., Artvinli, M., Pooley, F., Saracci, R., Skidmore, J., & Wagner, C. (1987). Epidemiological and environmental evidence of the health effects of exposure to erionite fibers: a four year study in the Cappadocian region of Turkey. *International Journal of Cancer,* 29, 10–17.

Bender, A. P., Williams, A. N., Johnson, R. A., & Jagger, H. G. (1990). Appropriate public health responses to clusters: the art of being responsibly responsive. *American Journal of Epidemiology,* 132, S48–S52.

Bortkiewicz, L von. (1898). *Das Gesetz Der Kleinen Zahlen.* Leipzig: Tuebner.

Centers for Disease Control [CDC]. (1981a). Pneumocystis pneumonia—Los Angeles. *MMWR,* 30, 250–252.

Centers for Disease Control [CDC]. (1981b). Kaposi's sarcoma and pneumocystis pneumonia among homosexual men—New York City and California. *MMWR,* 30, 305–308.

Centers for Disease Control and Prevention [CDC]. (1992). *Principles of Epidemiology. Self-Study Course 3030-G* (2nd ed.). Atlanta, GA: U.S. Department of Health and Human Services.

Cochran, W. G. (1954). Some methods for strengthening the common χ^2 test. *Biometrics,* 10, 417–451.

Greenberg, M., & Wartenberg, D. (1991). Communicating to an alarmed community about cancer clusters: a fifty state survey. *Journal of Community Health,* 16, 71–82.

Guidotti, T. L., & Jacobs, P. (1993). The implications of an epidemiologic mistake: a community's response to a perceived excess cancer risk. *American Journal of Public Health,* 83, 233–239.

Heath, C. W. Jr., & Hasterlik, R. J. (1963). Leukemia among children in a suburban community. *American Journal of Medicine,* 34, 796–812.

Herbst, A. L., Ulfelder, H., & Poskanzer, D. C. (1971). Adenocarcinoma of the vagina: association of maternal stibestrol therapy with tumor appearance in young women. *New England Journal of Medicine,* 284, 878–881.

Larson, R. J., & Marx, M. L. (1981). *An Introduction of Mathematical Statistics and Its Applications.* Englewood Cliffs, NJ: Prentice Hall.

Rao, C. R., & Chakravarti, I. M. (1956). Some small sample tests of significance for a Poisson distribution. *Biometrics,* 12, 264–282.

Richardson, L. F. (1944). The distribution of wars in time. *Journal of the Royal Statistical Society,* 179, 242–250.

Rohlf, F. J., & Sokal R. R. (1995). *Statistical Tables* (3rd. ed.) New York: W. H. Freeman.

Rothman, K. J. (1990). A sobering start for the cluster buster's conference. *American Journal of Epidemiology,* 132(Suppl. 1), S6–S13.

Sokal, R. R., & Rohlf, F. J. (1995). *Biometry. The Principles and Practice of Statistics in Biologic Research* (3rd ed.). New York: W. H. Freeman.

14

Outbreak Investigation

This chapter considers the investigation of outbreaks and epidemics. The following ten investigatory steps, as prescribed in CDC training materials, are considered: (1) preparation for field work, (2) establishing the existence of an outbreak, (3) verifying diagnoses of cases, (4) establishing a case definition and searching for additional cases, (5) conducting descriptive epidemiologic studies, (6) developing hypotheses, (7) evaluating hypotheses, (8) refining hypotheses and performing additional studies, (9) implementing control and prevention measures, and (10) communicating findings.

14.1 BACKGROUND

Initial Detection of Epidemics And Outbreaks

Outbreaks come to the attention of public health agencies in two primary ways. Either (a) epidemiologic surveillance systems warn of an emerging health problem or (b) individuals directly or indirectly affected by the outbreak (e.g., caregivers, cases, relations) notify the authorities directly.

Epidemiologic surveillance systems are organizations and structures set in place for the express purpose of collecting, analyzing, and interpreting outcome-specific health data for planning, carrying out, and evaluating public health practices (Thacker & Berkelman, 1988). Surveillance methods are distinguished by their practicability, uniformity, and rapidity. It is important to note that surveillance systems are often limited in scope and accuracy. For example, they commonly exhibit an incomplete enumeration of cases, time lags between the reporting of cases and actual occurrences, insensitivities to subtle change in occurrence, lack of information on important contributors to disease, and other deficiencies in information. Therefore, changes in the incidence of a disease may be missed and, when evident, may indicate an artifact of the system. Consequently, the more common way to become aware of an outbreak is by direct notification from a affected individual. The initial detection of acquired immunodeficiency syndrome (AIDS) provides an interesting illustration.

One of the first clues that led to the discovery of AIDS came from an astute pharmacist responsible for filling prescriptions for the drug used to treat *Pneumocystis* pneumonia (Centers for Disease Control, 1981a,b). Normally, *Pneumocystis* pneumonia occurs only in immune-compromised individuals, such as those undergoing chemotherapy for cancer. When physicians treating cancer-free young men started requesting the drug in increasing numbers, the astute pharmacist suspected something was amiss. This led to an investigation and eventual discovery of the new form of immunodeficiency now called AIDS.

When Are Outbreaks Investigated?

The decision whether to mount a large-scale investigation of an apparent outbreak is based on some of the following factors:

· The ability to confirm that the observed number of cases is significantly greater than expected (see Chapter 13)
· The scale and severity of the outbreak
· Whether the outbreak disproportionally affects an identifiable subgroup
· The potential for spread
· Political and public relations considerations
· Availability of resources

Goals of Outbreak Investigations

The goals of outbreak investigations are:

· To assess the range and extent of the outbreak
· To reduce the number of cases associated with the outbreak
· To prevent future occurrences by identifying and eliminating the source of the problem
· To identify new disease syndromes
· To identify new causes of known disease syndromes
· To assess the efficacy of currently employed prevention strategies
· To address liability concerns
· To train epidemiologists
· To provide for good public relations and educate the public

Components of Outbreak Investigations

Outbreak investigations have **diagnostic** (research) and **directed action** components. These components are not mutually exclusive. The epidemiologist researching the outbreak must clearly define the problem, describe the epidemiology of the epidemic, formulate hypotheses as to cause and transmission, test causal and prevention hypotheses, and draft conclusions and specific recommendations (Table 14.1).

Who Investigates Outbreaks?

The responsibility of investigating outbreaks usually falls on the shoulders of the local health department. However, if the investigation requires further resources, attracts sub-

TABLE 14.1. Components of Outbreak Investigations

1. *Define the Problem*

   Confirm diagnoses

   Show that an epidemic exists (observed number of cases is significantly greater than expected)

2. *Describe the Epidemiology of the Outbreak*

   Time: determine dates and times of onset; draw epidemic curve; determine attack rates over time

   Place: draw spot map of cases; consider environments of home, work, recreational, and special meeting places

   Person: calculate attack rates by age, sex, occupation, ethnic group, and other personal factors; consider rates of infection, disease and death; note possible means of transmission; address both common denominators and notable exceptions

3. *Formulate Hypotheses*

   Source of infection

   Method of contamination and spread

   Possible control mechanisms

4. *Test Hypotheses*

   Conduct special epidemiologic, laboratory, and environmental investigations

5. *Draw Conclusions and Devise Practical Applications*

   Long-term surveillance

   Prevention

Source: Evans (1982), p. 7 (some modification), reproduced with permission of Plenum Publishing.

stantial public concern, or is associated with a high attack rate or serious complications (hospitalization or death), state and federal agencies are called in. Outbreaks of regional or national importance are investigated by the Centers for Disease Control and Prevention (CDC). In fulfillment of this responsibility, the CDC has prepared excellent outbreak investigation training materials. Much of the discussion in this chapter is based on these materials.

14.2 INVESTIGATORY STEPS

Ten Investigatory Steps

Although no single way to investigate an outbreak works in all situations, some common steps prevail. For the sake of efficiency and completeness, the CDC (1992a) recommends the following 10-step approach:

1. Prepare for field work.
2. Establish the existence of an outbreak.
3. Verify diagnoses of cases.
4. Establish a case definition and search for additional cases.
5. Conduct descriptive epidemiologic studies.
6. Develop hypotheses.

7. Evaluate hypotheses.

8. As necessary, reconsider or refine hypotheses and conduct additional studies.

9. Implement control and prevention measures.

10. Communicate findings.

Step 1: Prepare for Field Work

Preparation for an investigation includes completing the administrative and personal measures required to begin the inquiry. Travel preparations must be made, supplies and equipment readied, knowledge updated, and administrative and scientific contacts established. Investigators must have a clear understanding of their role in the field and must know the chain of authority involved in the process.

Step 2: Establish the Existence of an Outbreak

One of the first tasks in outbreak investigation is to confirm that the reported cases represent a true outbreak with a common cause. Often, purported outbreaks represent sporadic occurrences of unrelated disease. The investigator must therefore identify and confirm all prospective cases and submit each case to standard diagnostic criteria. After confirming all cases, the observed rate of occurrence must be compared to an expected rate. Expected rates of occurrence can be gleaned from public health surveillance databases, national morbidity and mortality statistics, special registries (e.g., cancer or birth defect registries), data from neighboring states, or special surveys. Comparisons must account for both chance and systematic sources of variation. Quantifying the role of chance involves comparing the observed number of cases to the expected number under the Poisson model (see Sections 13.2 and 13.3). Systematic fluctuations in the number of cases can be due to any of the biases discussed in Chapter 11. Some of the important biases to consider when evaluating potential outbreaks are:

General Information Bias: Has there been a change in the reporting procedure or case definition, thus resulting in an artifactual increase in the number of cases? Does the increase represent a miscellaneous fad or false alarm?

Change in Population Size: Can a sudden increase in population size, such as might occur in a resort area, college town, or farming area with migrant labor, reflect an increase in the population at risk rather than a change in the rate of disease?

Diagnostic Suspicion Bias: Can diagnostic suspicion bias, such as might occur with improved diagnostic procedures, screening campaigns, or a new physician or infection control nurse in town, explain the apparent increase?

Publicity Bias: Can publicity bias, such as might occur when media attention stimulates the reporting of cases that would have previously gone unnoticed, explain the apparent increase?

The task of verifying an outbreak is made simple if a common cause is identified (as might be expected with foodborne illnesses). When this is the case, mechanisms of transmission and means of control will be well known, allowing for routine and rapid completion of the investigation.

Steps 3 and 4: Verify Diagnoses of Cases and Search for Additional Cases

If the initial signal of an outbreak is verified, the next task is to establish a reliable case definition. Briefly, the case definition is the set of standardized criteria used to decide whether an individual should be classified as having the disease in question (see Chapter 5). Once a reliable case definition is established, the epidemiologist submits each prospective case to these standard criteria for inclusion or exclusion in the study.

The investigation team also searches for previously unidentified cases. In searching for additional cases, the investigator checks local hospitals, clinics, and clinical laboratories that are likely to participate in the diagnosis or treatment of cases. It often proves useful to question directly those individuals who might treat or encounter the disease. For example, in studying a disease of the blood, the investigator might query hematologists and laboratory personnel who might treat or study the disease; in studying neoplastic diseases, the investigator questions oncologists, cancer registry personnel, cancer support groups, and other people likely to encounter prospective cases. Because direct inquiry may require a fair amount of walking about, it has traditionally been called **"shoe-leather" epidemiology.**

Previously unreported cases may also be discovered by issuing a plea for reports through a media appeal or by direct mailing of requests to physicians. Note, however, that blanket requests such as these may elicit duplicate reports, false-positive cases, reports of old cases irrelevant to the current outbreak, and other dubious information.

Step 5: Conduct Descriptive Epidemiologic Studies

Objectives and Approach   Descriptive epidemiology is used to explore and describe the general pattern of disease in the population at risk. This type of analysis is done early in the investigation, when little is known about the outbreak. To begin descriptive epidemiology, we collect the following information:

- Case identification information (name, address, telephone number, and other information that will allow investigators to contact the subjects for notification or follow-up purposes)
- Demographic information (age, sex, race, occupation, and other "person" factors that allow for the description of rates)
- Clinical information (time of disease onset, time of exposure to the etiologic agent, signs, symptoms, and test results as are relevant to the case definition)
- Risk factor information (relevant exposures and extraneous factors that might influence the probability of disease; specific items must be tailored to the disease in question)
- Reporter information (to allow for further questioning, if needed, and reporting back of the results of the investigation)
- Denominator data (census and *ad hoc* information that might provide reasonable estimates for denominators of prevalence and incidence calculations)

Once data are collected, the investigator describes the outbreak according to the **epidemiologic variables** of time, place, and person (see Section 2.4). Descriptive epidemiology has the following objectives:

- To assess data quality for completeness and accuracy
- To learn about the range and extent of the outbreak

- To assess the possible source of exposure, mode of transmission, incubation period, environmental contributors, host risk factors, and agent characteristics
- To generate hypotheses about the outbreak

Although principles concerning the description of disease according to person, place, and time have already been considered in Section 2.4, a brief review relevant to outbreak investigation is in order.

Time   Epidemiologic analyses of outbreaks by **time** are routinely presented in the form of an **epidemic curve.** Epidemic curves provide pictorial insights into:

- The past and future course of the epidemic
- The incubation period of the disease
- Whether the epidemic pattern is common exposure or propagating

The y axis of an epidemic curve represents the number (or percentage) of incident cases at a given time. The x axis represents a unit of time. In selecting a time scale for the x axis, we use units (e.g., hours, hour groupings, days, day groupings, weeks, months, years) appropriate to the incubation period of the disease. The CDC suggests, as a rule of thumb, using a time unit that is one-eighth to one-third the average incubation period (CDC, 1992a, pp. 363–364). For example, if the typical incubation period is one week, the x axis might be displayed in single day units. However, since time signals are extremely sensitive to the choice of intervals and inappropriate aggregations may mask relevant detail, it is best to draw several epidemic curves using different time scales and then select the one that best represents the data. When drawing the curve, the x axis should begin before the epidemic period (to show the endemic level of disease prior to the outbreak's onset) and extend to the period after the epidemic is over (to demonstrate whether disease levels have returned to normal).

Epidemic curves are useful for predicting the past and future temporal course of an epidemic. For example, Figure 14.1 shows an epidemic curve for the 1854 cholera epidemic investigated by John Snow (see Section 1.3). Ironically, this graph suggests that removal of the handle from the Broad Street pump had little to do with ending this notorious outbreak, thus contradicting the folklore surrounding this decisive (and largely symbolic) act. Sir A. Bradford Hill (1955) eloquently describes the course of events:

> Though conceivably there might have been a second peak in the curve, and though almost certainly some more deaths would have occurred if the pump handle had remained *in situ*, it is clear that the end of the epidemic was not dramatically determined by its removal. (p. 1010)

John Snow (1855), himself, recognized that the epidemic might have burned itself out before his removal of the pump handle, leaving few susceptibles on which the disease could prey:

> . . . but the attacks had so far diminished before the use of the water was stopped, that it is impossible to decide whether the well still contained the cholera poison in an active state, or whether, from some cause, the water had become free from it. (pp. 51–52)

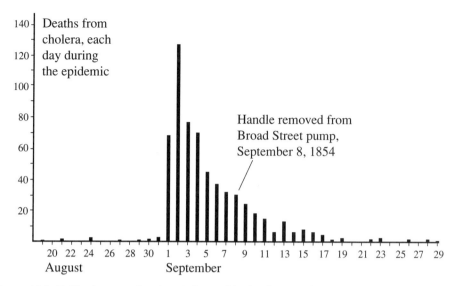

Figure 14.1. *Epidemic curve, London cholera epidemic of 1854. (*Source: *Tufte, 1997, p. 33;* Data originally from: *Snow, 1855, p. 49; reproduced with permission of Graphics Press.)*

Analysis of the typical **incubation period** associated with the disease is another important element of descriptive epidemiology. Recall that (a) the incubation period of a disease is the time interval between invasion of the agent into the host's body and appearance of first signs or symptoms of disease and (b) the incubation period of an agent varies considerably according to the pathogenicity of the agent, level of exposure, and susceptibility of the host. If the probable time of exposure to the agent is known, the incubation period can be summarized by its minimum, maximum, and average (Fig. 14.2). The average incubation period can be expressed as an arithmetic average, geometric average, or median. Knowledge of these values is helpful in identifying the etiologic pathogen.

The shape of the epidemic curve is useful in determining the epidemic pattern of the disease. **Point-source epidemics** are caused by exposure to the agent from a single source over a brief time. When this is the case, the epidemic exhibits a sudden rise followed by a rapid falloff (Fig. 2.9C, 14.1, and 14.2). **Propagating epidemics** depend on serial propagation from person to person or continuing exposure from a single source. Propagating epidemics exhibit a plateau or continual rise in the number of cases (Fig. 2.9D).

Place Describing the occurrence of cases by **place** can provide powerful evidence about the cause and transmission of the agent. Epidemic maps may take the form of simple dot maps or more complex maps of area-specific rates.

Dot maps may serve to document the geographic extent of the problem and provide evidence of clustering. Snow's celebrated dot map of clustering of cholera deaths around the Broad Street pump (Fig. 1.2) provides an important historical example. By combining this picture with other sources of information, John Snow was able to support his idea that the etiologic agent was waterborne.

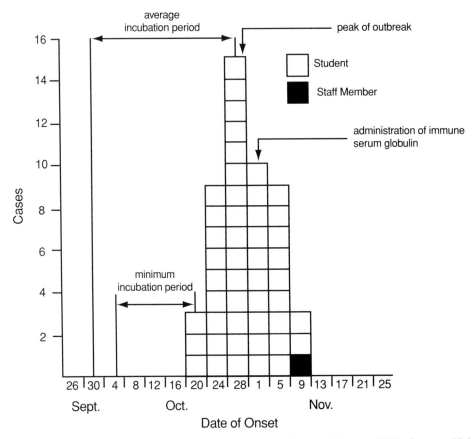

Figure 14.2 *Epidemic curve, hepatitis A outbreak, Colbert County, Alabama, 1972. (Source: CDC, 1992a, p. 367.)*

The problem with dot maps, however, is that they fail to account for the number of people at risk in a given area. If populations in areas being compared are unequal in size, dot maps can be misleading. Tufte (1997) puts it this way:

> If the population of central London had been distributed just as the deaths were, then the cholera map would have merely repeated the unimportant fact that more people lived near the Broad Street pump than elsewhere. (p. 35)

To compensate for this inherent weakness of dot maps, the epidemiologist might choose to map area-specific rates. One such map of an Ebola virus outbreak is shown in Figure 14.3. This figure displays Ebola disease attack rates (per 100 inhabitants) in the epidemic zone. The attack rates are epicentered around Yambuku, the town where the mission hospital was located. The decreasing attack rates with increasing distance from the hospital suggest iatrogenic spread of the agent (i.e., acquired by a patient during the course of treatment).

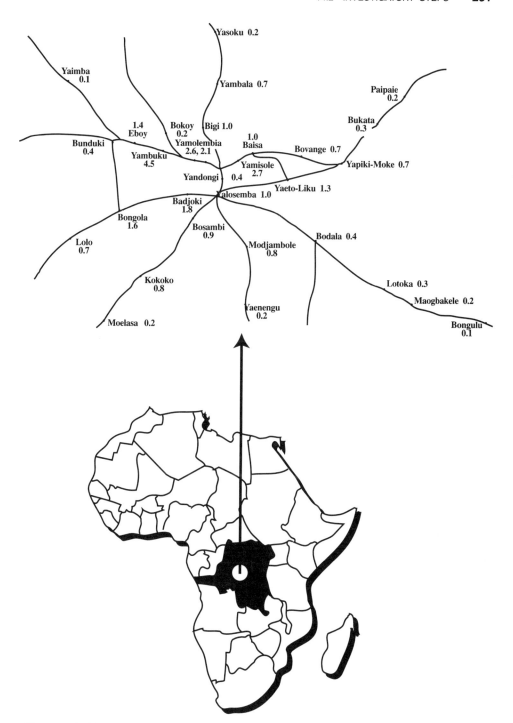

Figure 14.3. *Ebola virus epidemic zone, Zaire, 1976. (Source: Adapted from CDC, 1992b, p. 10.)*

Person   Description of disease rates by **person variables** is useful in identifying high-risk groups. Risk, in turn, is presumptively related to the opportunity for exposure or susceptibility to disease. Examples of person factors relevant to outbreak investigation include demographic characteristics (age, sex, ethnicity), personal activities and practices (occupation, customs, leisure activities, religious activities, knowledge, attitudes, and beliefs), genetic predispositions, physiologic states (pregnancy, parity, distress, nutritional status), concurrent diseases, immune status, and marital status.

Description of disease frequency by personal characteristics may be limited by the availability of numerator (number of cases) or denominator (size of the population at risk) information. At minimum, the frequency of disease is described by age and sex, since these are important determinants of disease. Occupation is also often important in determining the risks of exposure. Other analyses cater to the type of disease being investigated. For example, when investigating AIDS, the epidemiologist is interested in describing disease rates according to sexual practices and contacts, intravenous drug use, and potential iatrogenic exposures.

Step 6: Develop Hypotheses

A hypothesis is a tentative explanation that accounts for a set of facts and can be tested by further investigation. In the investigation of outbreaks, hypotheses should address the most likely source of exposure to the etiologic agent, the means of transmission, the next steps in the investigation, and future control measures.

Keep in mind, however, that hypothesis generation and development is more art than science. It begins when the first clues that an epidemic might exist come to light and continues until the investigation is complete. Hypothesis development requires an understanding of the disease process and population at risk. It is supported by discussions with patients, health-care providers, local public health officials, community activists, and other interested parties and should include the review of all relevant clinical, epidemiologic, and laboratory information. In generating and developing hypotheses one should consider:

- What is generally known about the disease itself
- All relevant clinical and laboratory findings
- What patients say about the disease
- Descriptive epidemiologic findings
- Other intuitive insights

Table 14.2 is a checklist of items that may be useful when generating and developing hypotheses. When generating hypotheses, we search for common denominators and notable exceptions. When searching for common denominators, the objective is to search for the specific exposure having the highest (or lowest) relative risk of disease. Important clues, however, may also come from investigating why certain people exposed to the putative agent did not become ill and why apparently unexposed people developed the illness. Exceptions to the observed pattern, or **outliers** as they are occasionally called, can provide important clues about the source of infection and mode of transmission. John Snow, in his classic 19th century cholera investigations, used this technique on repeated

TABLE 14.2. Hypothesis-Generating Checklist

1. Review what is known about the disease itself:
     Agent
     Usual reservoir
     Mechanisms of transmission (portal of entry, portal of exit, life cycle of agent in nature, etc.)
     Natural history of disease
     Clinical spectrum of disease
     Pathogenic mechanisms
     Known risk factors
2. Study clinical and laboratory findings:
     Review clinical and laboratory records
     Check to see if lab tests are confirmed and the lab is accurate
     Determine if specialized lab work (e.g., DNA "fingerprinting") is necessary
     Describe frequency of symptoms, signs, and test results among cases
3. Consider what patients and caregivers say:
     Determine potentially relevant exposure sources
     Hear what they think about cause
     Gain additional insights into clinical features
     See if they are aware of other cases
     Infer commonalities and differences in cases
4. Review descriptive epidemiology results:
     Epidemic curve and pattern (point source, propagating, combination)
     Geographic distribution
     Incubation statistics (minimum, maximum, mean, median)
     Events occurring around the most likely period of exposure of each case
     Significant "person" risk factors
5. Ruminate critical facts:
     Deduction
     Intuition
     Analogy
     Coherence
     Credibility of sources
     Quality of information
     Missing keys and explanations
     Exceptions and outliers

occasions. For example, he pointed out the relative absence of fatal cholera cases in brewery workers living near the epidemic's center (see Fig. 1.2) and attributed this deficiency to a daily allowance of malt liquor. (The proprietor of the brewery believed his workers did not drink water at all and most certainly did not obtain water from the pump on the street.) Snow also noted a fatal case in a 59-year-old widow living outside the epidemic area and traced this to water transported from the pump. These notable exceptions provided strong clues in support for the waterborne theory.

Steps 7 and 8: Evaluate Hypotheses; As Necessary, Reconsider or Refine Hypotheses and Conduct Additional Studies

Hypotheses developed in step 6 are continually reexamined, refined, and tested throughout the investigation. The scientific method is iterative, cyclic, and self-correcting by nature, thus requiring a continual process of hypothesis generation, hypothesis testing, and hypothesis refinement. Since the usefulness of an analytic study is dictated by the clarity and quality of the hypothesis, time devoted to hypothesis refinement is well spent. It is an axiom of epidemiology that if you cannot generate insightful hypotheses, then continuing to analytic epidemiology is likely to be a waste of time (CDC, 1992a, p. 384).

Working hypotheses can be tested using informal methods, analytic epidemiology, laboratory studies, and environmental evaluations. Informal methods can be adequate when a clear-cut or nearly deterministic ("one-to-one") relationship exists between the etiologic exposure and disease. The *CDC Self-Study Course* (1992) describes one such example as follows:

> In an outbreak of hypervitaminosis D that occurred in Massachusetts in 1991, it was found that all the case-patients drank milk delivered to their homes by a local dairy. Therefore, investigators hypothesized that the dairy was the source and the milk was the vehicle. When they visited the dairy, they quickly recognized that the dairy was inadvertently adding far more than the recommended dose of vitamin D to the milk. No analytic epidemiology was really necessary to evaluate the basic hypotheses in this setting. (p. 375)

Nevertheless, in most outbreaks, analytic epidemiologic studies are necessary to draw inferences about the etiology of the outbreak and source of exposure. Analytic studies may take the form of a cohort study, case-control study, cross-sectional study, clinical-trial study, or community trial study. The choice of a study design depends on many factors, including the timing of the investigation (i.e., whether the outbreak is ongoing or has resolved), the availability of resources, past experience of the investigator, the size of the population at risk, the prevalence of the exposure, and the incidence of the disease. In general, small, well-circumscribed outbreaks in which the incidence of disease is large are well suited for a cohort study design. In contrast, outbreaks in large, poorly circumscribed populations in which the disease is rare may be better suited for case-control methods. (Readers may wish to consult the more thorough presentation of study design options that is undertaken in Chapter 9.)

Laboratory and environmental studies are used to support causal hypotheses by isolating the etiologic agent from cases or the environment. The laboratory investigation should determine the presence of the pathogenic organism and whether it is present in large enough numbers to be considered significant. Environmental and sanitary conditions should be studied to help explain why the outbreak occurred in the first place and what might prevent it from happening again. Special laboratory tests (e.g., DNA, chemical, or immunologic fingerprinting) can occasionally be used to link the agent isolated from patients to various environmental sites. When available, laboratory evidence can "clinch the findings" established by the epidemiologic investigation. Note, however, that since many outbreaks are investigated after the fact, appropriate specimens and isolates are often lacking or incomplete.

TABLE 14.3. Elements of Epidemic Control

Action	Example
1. Control the source of the pathogen	Remove the source of contamination
	Remove persons from exposure
	Inactivate or neutralize the pathogen at its source
	Isolate and treat the infected person
2. Interrupt the transmission (environmental control)	Sterilize or interrupt animate (vertebrate host) and inanimate (water, food, soil, air) environmental transmission
	Control insect vectors
	Improve sanitation
3. Control or modify the host response to exposure	Immunize susceptibles
	Use prophylactic chemotherapy

Source: Methods in Observational Epidemiology, Second Edition by Jennifer L. Kelsey et al. Copyright © 1996 by Oxford University Press, Inc. Used by permission of Oxford University Press, Inc.

Step 9: Implement Control and Prevention Measures

Two of the main objectives of outbreak investigation are to bring the current epidemic to a halt and prevent future occurrences. Elements of control should be directed at the weakest link in the chain of infection. This can involve efforts directed toward any of the agent, host, or environmental factors that constitute the ecology of the disease. Elements of infection control are summarized in Table 14.3.

Demonstration of the efficacy of control measures also provides support of associated causal hypotheses. Termination of the outbreak, however, does not offer direct proof. The population may simply have run out of susceptibles or the cessation of cases may be coincidental with other events.

Step 10: Communicate Findings

The investigation is not complete until the results are disseminated to the appropriate parties. Study findings should be reported to initial informants, those involved in the investigation, local, state, and federal public health agencies, and the community of people affected by the outbreak. This is done in the form of oral briefings and written reports. The "what, why, when, how, where, and who" of reporting are summarized in Table 14.4.

REFERENCES

Centers for Disease Control [CDC]. (1981a). Pneumocystis pneumonia—Los Angeles. *MMWR*, 30, 250–252.

Centers for Disease Control [CDC]. (1981b). Kaposi's sarcoma and pneumocystis pneumonia among homosexual men—New York City and California. *MMWR*, 30, 305–308.

Centers for Disease Control and Prevention [CDC]. (1992a). *Principles of Epidemiology: Self-Study Course 3030-G* (2nd ed.). Atlanta, GA: U.S. Department of Health and Human Services.

Centers for Disease Control and Prevention [CDC]. (1992b). *An Outbreak of Hemorrhagic Fever in Africa. 1992 EIS Course.* Washington, DC: Association of Teachers of Preventive Medicine.

Evans, A. S. (1982). Epidemiological concepts and methods. In A. S. Evans (Ed.). *Viral Infections of Humans. Epidemiology and Control* (pp. 3–42). New York: Plenum Medical Book Company.

TABLE 14.4. The "What, Why, When, How, Where, and Who" of Outbreak Reporting

What: oral briefings

Why: to disseminate information and defend conclusions and recommendations, to promote good public relations, and to allow for constructive criticism

When: at the beginning and end of the investigation and whenever information for prevention and control comes to light

How: use scientifically objective language (avoid emotional terms), consider the audience (many people may not be epidemiologists), and explain epidemiologic principles and methods (avoid jargon)

Where: the appropriate venue is dictated by the audience; presentations should be given in the locality affected by the outbreak and at the sponsoring agency; findings can also be presented at regional and national professional conferences

Who: audience may vary but should include local, state, and federal authorities and people responsible for control and prevention measures

What: written reports

Why: to document the investigation, to disseminate information and defend conclusions and recommendations, to promote good professional relations, to increase credibility of the work, to allow for constructive criticism, to prevent future occurrences, and to add to the public health information base

When: at the conclusion of the investigation

How: use standard scientific reporting format with introduction, methods, results, discussion, ($\pm$ recommendations); sponsoring agency may have additional reporting requirements

Where: internal documents should be filed with the local health department and all supporting agencies; if appropriate, a manuscript should be submitted to a general or discipline-specific peer-reviewed journal for publication

Who: audience may vary but might include epidemiologists in training, field epidemiologists, and researchers in the discipline

Hill, A. B. (1955). Snow—an appreciation. *Proceedings of the Royal Society of Medicine, 48,* 1008–1012.

Kelsey, J. L., Thompson, W. D., & Evans, A. S. (1986). *Methods in Observational Epidemiology.* New York: Oxford University Press.

Snow, J. (1936). *Snow on Cholera.* New York: The Commonwealth Fund. (Originally published as *On the Mode of Communication of Cholera* in 1855)

Thacker, S. B., & Berkelman, R. L. (1988). Public health surveillance in the United States. *Epidemiologic Reviews,* 10, 164–190.

Tufte E. R. (1997). *Visual Explanations.* Cheshire, CT: Graphic Press.

CHAPTER ADDENDUM 1 (CASE STUDY): A DRUG–DISEASE OUTBREAK

Author: Joyce Murat Piper

Acronyms

CJD	Creutzfeldt–Jakob disease
FDA	(U.S.) Food and Drug Administration
hGH	Human growth hormone

Background

As your first assignment working for the U.S. Food and Drug Administration (FDA), you are to act as an epidemiologic consultant to the division that reviews and approves the use of endocrinologic and metabolic drugs. One day in late February (1985), a medical officer from the reviewing division comes to you with an unusual problem and asks for your help. The medical officer has just received a report of the death of a 20-year-old man with Creutzfeldt–Jakob disease (CJD). It is noted that this case received human growth hormone (hGH) for 13 years as a child, between the ages of 3 and 16 (from 1966 to 1980). You note that hGH is used to prevent pituitary dwarfism when given during the growth years.

Question 1   What is your first step in investigating this case? What is your reaction to this single case of CJD?

Question 2   What additional information do you need to evaluate the relevance of this case?

Question 3   What immediate action, if any, do you think the FDA should take?

Preparatory Research

You find an excellent review article on the epidemiology of CJD (Brown, 1980). Through this and other sources (e.g., Benenson, 1995) you learn:

- CJD is a subacute degeneration of the central nervous system that occurs most often in people of late middle age. Death usually results within six months of onset.
- CJD affects men and women equally.
- Few cases have been reported in patients in their twenties and early thirties, although the youngest reported patient died at the age of 17. It is not until the age of 40 that CJD begins to occur with any consistency. Most cases occur in 50- to 75-year-old people. The average age of death is approximately 60 years of age.
- In 1968, Gibbs and co-workers proved the CJD agent to be a membrane-associated unconventional virus of very small size and unusual resistance to physical and chemical means of inactivation. The pathogen is similar to the unconventional agent that causes kuru in people and scrapie in sheep. (These agents are currently called "prions.")
- The virus can be found in cerebrospinal fluid and the central nervous system of patients. Transmission of the disease to primates is accomplished by inoculation through intracerebral and peripheral routes. The incubation period is up to 6 years when primates are inoculated through the intracerebral route.
- Incubations as long as 20 to 30 years are found in naturally occurring kuru.
- Approximately 10,000 children had received hGH from the National Hormone and Pituitary Program. (The program started in 1963.) There is no commercial distribution of hGH in the United States.
- A U.S. Vital Statistics report suggests there was a total of two deaths from CJD in persons less than 40 years of age in the United States in 1979. The age-specific mortality rate of the disease in persons less than 40 is therefore approximately 1 per 10 million.

Question 4   Knowing these new facts, would you have answered question 1 any differently? If so, how?

How hGH Is Prepared

Every good epidemiologist can think of a reason why just about any association is biologically plausible (or, so it has been said). You learn that the hGH used during the interval when the case was exposed was extracted from human pituitaries obtained at autopsies. You also learn that: (a) it takes approximately 16,000 human pituitaries to make a single lot of hGH, (b) the average child undergoing treatment receives hGH injections 2–3 times a week for 4 years, and (c) a patient usually receives hGH from three different lots during each year of treatment.

Questions 5   To how many pituitaries is the average hGH-treated child exposed?

Source of the Agent

Although CJD is a rare disease among young people it is not as rare as you might suspect when deaths from all age groups are considered. For example, in 1979 there were 148 CJD cases among the 1,913,841 deaths in the United States.

Question 6   What proportion of deaths in the United States is CJD-related?

Question 7   If there were no screening criterion of pituitary donors, to how many infected pituitaries would the average treated child have been exposed?

Question 8   Even with careful screening of pituitaries, is it biologically plausible to suspect pituitaries as the vehicle of transmission? Why or why not?

More Cases

Meanwhile, your medical officer friend has been on the phone to pediatric endocrinologists who have used hGH supplied by the National Hormone and Pituitary Program. She finds an additional two cases of CJD-like death occurring in the 10,000 hGH-exposed children. The first death is a 22-year-old man treated with hGH from 1969 to 1977. The second death is a 34-year-old man treated from 1963 to 1969. These two additional cases await pathological confirmation.

Question 9   How many cases of CJD were expected in the study population of 10,000 hGH-exposed children, assuming an expected rate of 1 in 10 million? (*Hint:* Use formula 13.3.) What is the *SMR* in this pituitary-exposed cohort? (*Hint:* Use formula 7.3.)

Question 10   Assuming a random (Poisson) distribution of cases, and using the expected number of cases calculated in question 9, calculate the Poisson probabilities of observing 0 cases in this cohort. What is the probability of observing exactly 1 case? What is the probability of observing exactly 2 cases? What is the probability of seeing 3 or more cases? Does this analysis confirm the existence of an epidemic (*Hint:* Use formulas 13.1, 13.5, and 13.6.)

Question 11   What additional information would you like to know about the exposure of each individual case?

Question 12   What action, if any, do you think the FDA should take as a regulatory agency?

Question 13   The Assistant Secretary of Health establishes an Interagency Task Force to review the problem and make recommendations. You are assigned to the Task Force subgroup charged with directing future epidemiologic studies. Your subgroup recommends a case-control study to learn which lots of hGH were contaminated and a cohort study to learn the incidence of CJD overall and among subgroups. Each study will also explore host risk factors that determine the likelihood of disease. Discuss the advantages and disadvantages of each study design.

ANSWERS TO CASE STUDY: A DRUG–DISEASE OUTBREAK

Answer 1   The first step in the investigation is to verify the case's diagnosis. Assuming this case checks out, further investigation might be necessary.

Answer 2   Information concerning the "who, what, when, where, why, and how" of CJD and hGH should be studied. For example, the descriptive epidemiology of CJD must be researched (e.g., age and sex distribution of cases, age-specific rates, risk factors). In addition, we need to learn about how hGH is made and how it is used to treat dwarfism.

Answer 3   Although beginning immediate regulatory action is premature, active follow-up of people in the hGH-exposed cohort might be warranted.

Answer 4   Yes. Rarity of CJD in this age group, its transmissibility, and the inoculation of possible infected pituitary glands into susceptible individuals have heightened our level of suspicion that the association might be causal and that additional cases may be forthcoming.

Answer 5   Based on the stated assumptions, the average hGH-treated child would be exposed to 16,000 pituitaries/lot $\times$ 3 lots/year $\times$ 4 year = 192,000 pituitaries.

Answer 6   The proportion of deaths from CJD = 148 /1,913,841 = .000077.

Answer 7   Number of infected pituitary per hGH-treated child = 192,000 pituitaries $\times$ .000077 = 14.8 infected pituitaries.

Answer 8   Yes. People dying of other causes may be incubating CJD.

Answer 9   Formula 13.3 states $\mu = (n)(R_0)$, where μ represents the expected number of cases, n represents the size of the study population, and R_0 represents the expected rate. Therefore, $\mu = (10,000)(1/10,000,000) = 0.001$.

Formula 7.3 states $SMR = x/\mu$, where x represents the observed number of cases and μ represents the expected number of cases. Therefore, the SMR is equal to 3/0.001 = 3000.

Answer 10 We calculate the following Poisson probabilities by using formula 13.1:

$$Pr(X = 0) = \frac{(e^{-0.001})(0.001^0)}{0!} = .99900$$

$$Pr(X = 1) = \frac{(e^{-0.001})(0.001^1)}{1!} = .00100$$

$$Pr(X = 2) = \frac{(e^{-0.001})(0.001^2)}{2!} = .00000$$

By using formulas 13.5 and 13.6, $Pr(X \geq 3) = 1 - Pr(X \leq 2) = 1 - (.999000 + .00010 + .00000) = .00000$. Therefore, the epidemic is confirmed.

Answer 11 Knowing if a common "hot" lot was involved would be useful.

Answer 12 Recommendations for immediate actions are to cease use of hGH, notify all exposed individuals, and inform the public.

Answer 13 See Table 9.5 for a summary listing of advantages and disadvantages of case-control and cohort studies. For these particular studies, we might expect difficulties in tracking exposures and identifying all cases regardless of the study design. A problem of particular concern when considering the cohort design is the lengthy incubation period associated with the disease.

REFERENCES

Benenson, A. S. (Ed.). (1995). *Control of Communicable Diseases in Man* (16th ed.) Washington, DC: American Public Health Association.

Brown, P. (1980). An epidemiologic critique of Creutzfeldt–Jakob disease. *Epidemiologic Reviews, 2*, 113–135.

Gibbs, C. J., Jr., Gajdusek, D. C., Asher, D. M., Alpers, M. P., Beck, E. , Daniel, P. M., & Matthews W. B. (1968). Creutzfeldt–Jakob disease (spongiform encephalopathy); transmission to the chimpanzee. *Science, 161*, 388–389.

CHAPTER ADDENDUM 2 (CASE STUDY): FOODBORNE DISEASE OUTBREAK

Source: Adapted from DHEW/CDC training materials as presented in the University of California, Berkeley Infectious Disease Epidemiology course, Spring 1984.

Comment

Foodborne disease outbreak investigations generally involve both a laboratory and an epidemiologic component. The **epidemiologic investigation** determines the number of cases, types and frequency of symptoms, location, date, and time of the suspect meal, onset time of symptoms in cases, history of food preparation and handling (including storage conditions), food and biologic samples (when possible), 24-hour food histories for all persons attending the suspect meal, and attack rates by food items eaten and not eaten. By piecing together these bits of information, the epidemiologists can usually determine the agent in question and its ultimate source.

The **laboratory investigation** is necessary to detect the presence of the agent in cases and the environment. The laboratory investigation is also useful in identifying other organisms in the environment that might be present in large enough numbers to suggest inadequacy of general sanitary conditions of food preparation. Laboratory procedures should include aerobic and anaerobic plate counts of samples collected during the epidemiologic investigation, with samples (e.g., stool, saliva, vomit) coming from both cases and foods, as appropriate, depending on the suspected etiologic agent. Culture and other diagnostic procedures aimed at the suspected agent should be pursued.

Background

The local medical center in a rural California county notifies the county health department of a hospitalized case of gastroenteritis. From interviewing this patient, you discover that the case had attended a church supper in Rhynedale, California, seven days earlier. You find out that approximately 50 other individuals had attended this church supper and that several participants had become ill with symptoms similar to those seen in the sentinel case. Your assignment is to investigate this case and determine whether it was the result of food poisoning.

The Locale

Rhynedale is a small, unincorporated town of 581 residents in northern California, not far from Sacramento.

Question 1 Discuss how you might prepare for the field work.

The Church Supper

Between the hours of 6:00 p.m. and 9:30 p.m. on Saturday, July 23, a Rhynedale community church held a pot luck supper in a wooded area near their church. The attending families each brought food from home, which was laid out on tables for all to share. Though many brought similar foods, none of these foods were mixed, and all food remained in its original container. No caterers or other persons were involved in handling the food. The bulk of the food was eaten between 6:30 and 7:30 p.m. All cases that were contacted denied having a diarrheal illness before or during the supper and denied knowledge of the same for others attending the supper.

The Involved Group

Fifty-one people from 16 family groups attended this affair. Thirteen of the families were from the Rhynedale area. One family was from a nearby town. Two families were from out-of-state.

Materials and Methods

You place phone calls to all families who had attended the supper. Family rosters are recorded and, for anyone reporting symptoms, the course and duration of their illness are described by onset, duration, symptoms, and the need for physician care or hospitalization. Food histories are obtained on all supper attendees—whether ill or not—for each item served at the supper. Inquiries are made of pet and other animal contacts, and of prior contacts with persons known to have had diarrheal illnesses.

You request each family to furnish a list of foods they brought to the supper. You also inquire where they purchased these foods, how they were prepared, what foods they took home from the supper, and whether food items were still available for laboratory testing. Visits are made to two families who did not have telephones. (This is a fairly old case study.) Out-of-state parties are not reached, although multiple telephone calls are attempted.

Data

Each study subject is uniquely identified with a record (REC) number. Information on case status and demographic factors appear in Table 14.5. Information on signs, symp-

TABLE 14.5. Case Status and Demographic Data: Foodborne Disease Outbreak Case Study

Variable Names and Descriptions

REC	Record (identification) number
CASE	Case of gastroenteritis (Y/N)
SEX	Gender (M/F)
AGE	Age (in years)

Data

REC	CASE	SEX	AGE	REC	CASE	SEX	AGE
1	Y	M	17	27	N	F	2
2	Y	F	8	28	N	F	15
3	Y	M	37	29	N	M	44
4	Y	F	7	30	N	F	42
5	Y	F	8	31	N	F	17
6	Y	M	26	32	N	F	19
7	Y	F	25	33	N	M	16
8	Y	F	5	34	N	M	3
9	Y	M	14	35	N	F	66
10	Y	M	48	36	N	F	18
11	Y	F	12	37	N	M	39
12	Y	M	10	38	N	F	17
13	Y	M	14	39	N	F	14
14	Y	M	13	40	N	M	46
15	Y	M	28	41	N	F	45
16	Y	F	9	42	N	F	16
17	Y	M	45	43	N	F	11
18	Y	F	35	44	N	M	26
19	Y	F	39	45	N	F	57
20	Y	M	10	46	N	M	60
21	Y	M	11	47	N	F	34
22	Y	M	7	48	N	F	16
23	Y	M	33	49	N	M	18
24	Y	F	41	50	N	F	4
25	Y	M	13	51	N	M	62
26	N	F	52				

TABLE 14.6. Signs, Symptoms, Duration of Illness, and Incubation Periods: Foodborne Disease Outbreak Case Study

Variable Names and Descriptions

CRMP	Cramps (Y/N/ · = missing)
DIAR	Diarrhea (Y/N/ · = missing)
BDIAR	Bloody diarrhea (Y/N/ · = missing)
NAUS	Nausea (Y/N/ · = missing)
VOMIT	Vomiting (Y/N/ · = missing)
FEV	Fever (Y/N/ · = missing)
CHIL	Chills (Y/N/ · = missing)
HEAD	Headache (Y/N/ · = missing)
MYAL	Myalgia (Y/N/ · = missing)
DUR	Duration of symptoms (in days)
INC	Incubation (hours between the beginning of supper and first symptoms)

Data

REC	CRAMPS	DIAR	BDIAR	NAUS	VOMIT	FEV	CHIL	HEAD	MYAL	DUR	INC
1	Y	Y	N	Y	Y	Y	N	Y	Y	9	9
2	Y	Y	N	Y	Y	Y	Y	Y	Y	7	15
3	Y	Y	N	N	N	Y	Y	Y	N	3	17
4	Y	Y	·	Y	Y	N	Y	Y	·	7	19
5	Y	Y	N	N	N	Y	N	Y	Y	5	20
6	Y	Y	N	Y	Y	Y	Y	Y	Y	7	23
7	Y	Y	N	Y	N	N	N	Y	·	3	25
8	Y	Y	·	Y	Y	Y	Y	Y	·	7	25
9	Y	Y	N	Y	Y	Y	Y	Y	Y	8	26
10	Y	Y	N	N	N	Y	Y	Y	Y	2	18
11	Y	Y	N	Y	Y	Y	N	Y	Y	7	19
12	Y	Y	·	Y	N	Y	Y	Y	Y	8	32
13	Y	Y	N	N	N	Y	N	Y	Y	6	32
14	Y	Y	N	Y	Y	Y	Y	Y	Y	7	36
15	Y	Y	N	N	N	Y	Y	Y	Y	3	43
16	Y	Y	N	Y	N	Y	Y	Y	Y	6	47
17	Y	Y	N	Y	Y	Y	Y	Y	Y	7	53
18	Y	Y	N	Y	Y	Y	Y	Y	Y	7	62
19	Y	Y	Y	Y	N	Y	Y	N	N	5	76
20	Y	Y	N	N	N	Y	N	Y	Y	4	77
21	Y	Y	N	Y	Y	Y	N	N	Y	7	89
22	Y	Y	·	N	N	Y	N	Y	·	7	97
23	Y	Y	N	Y	Y	Y	N	Y	Y	4	98
24	Y	Y	N	N	N	Y	Y	Y	Y	7	100
25	Y	Y	N	Y	N	Y	Y	Y	Y	8	111

toms, duration of illness, and time of onset relative to the beginning of the church supper appears in Table 14.6. Note that a dot indicates missing data. Information about food items consumed by people attending the church supper appears in Table 14.7.

Question 2 Draw an epidemic curve. Determine the minimum, maximum, and median incubation times.

The median is the data point that is greater than or equal to half the values in the sample. Before calculating the median, data are sorted in ascending order and ranked from 1 to n, where n represents the number of cases. The median value is the value halfway down the rank-ordered list. If n is odd, this corresponds to the value of the observation with rank $(n + 1)/2$. If n is even, this corresponds to the average of values associated with ranks $n/2$ and $(n/2) + 1$.

TABLE 14.7. Food Histories: Foodborne Disease Outbreak Case Study

Variable Names and Descriptions

SHRIMP	Shrimp salad (Y/N/ · = missing)
OLIVE	Olives (Y/N/ · = missing)
FRCHICK	Fried chicken (Y/N/ · = missing)
BBQCHICK	Barbecued chicken (Y/N/ · = missing)
BEANS	Beans (Y/N/ · = missing)
POTSAL	Potato salad (Y/N/ · = missing)
GJEL	Green Jell-O (Y/N/ · = missing)
RJEL	Red Jell-O (Y/N/ · = missing)
MAC	Macaroni salad (Y/N/ · = missing)
RBEER	Root beer (Y/N/ · = missing)
ROLL	Rolls (Y/N/ · = missing)
BUTTER	Butter (Y/N/ · = missing)
DEVEGG	Deviled eggs (Y/N/ · = missing)
POTCHIP	Potato Chips (Y/N/ · = missing)
PICK	Pickle (Y/N/ · = missing)
SCP	Strawberry cream pie (Y/N/ · = missing)
NCP	Neapolitan cream pie (Y/N/ · = missing)
CAKE	Cake (Y/N/ · = missing)
TOM	Tomato (Y/N/ · = missing)

Data, Part I (Shrimp Salad, Olives, Fried Chicken, Barbeque Chicken, Beans, Potato Salad, Green Jell-O, Red Jell-O, Macaroni Salad)

REC	CASE	SHRIMP	OLIVE	FRCHICK	BBQCHICK	BEANS	POTSAL	GJEL	RJEL	MAC
1	Y	N	Y	Y	Y	N	Y	Y	Y	N
2	Y	N	N	Y	·	N	N	Y	N	Y
3	Y	N	N	Y	Y	N	Y	·	N	N
4	Y	·	Y	Y	Y	N	Y	Y	Y	N
5	Y	N	Y	Y	·	Y	N	·	Y	Y
6	Y	Y	Y	Y	Y	Y	Y	N	Y	Y
7	Y	·	Y	·	Y	·	Y	Y	N	N
8	Y	N	Y	Y	Y	Y	Y	N	Y	N
9	Y	N	Y	Y	Y	Y	Y	N	Y	N
10	Y	Y	Y	Y	N	N	Y	·	N	·
11	Y	Y	Y	Y	N	Y	Y	Y	N	N
12	Y	Y	Y	Y	N	Y	Y	N	Y	Y
13	Y	N	N	N	Y	N	N	N	N	N
14	Y	N	Y	Y	Y	N	Y	N	·	N
15	Y	Y	Y	Y	Y	Y	N	·	·	·
16	Y	N	N	Y	Y	N	N	·	N	Y
17	Y	N	Y	·	Y	Y	Y	·	N	Y
18	Y	Y	Y	Y	·	N	N	N	Y	N
19	Y	Y	N	Y	N	Y	Y	N	Y	N
20	Y	N	Y	Y	N	N	Y	N	·	Y
21	Y	N	·	·	Y	Y	N	Y	Y	N
22	Y	N	Y	·	Y	N	Y	N	Y	N
23	Y	Y	Y	Y	Y	Y	N	Y	·	Y
24	Y	N	Y	·	Y	Y	Y	Y	N	Y
25	Y	N	Y	Y	N	N	Y	N	Y	N
26	N	Y	N	N	N	Y	Y	·	N	Y
27	N	N	N	Y	N	N	Y	N	Y	·
28	N	N	Y	Y	N	·	Y	Y	·	Y
29	N	N	N	Y	N	Y	Y	Y	N	N
30	N	N	Y	Y	N	N	N	Y	N	Y

TABLE 14.7. *(Continued)*

Data, Part I (Shrimp Salad, Olives, Fried Chicken, Barbeque Chicken, Beans, Potato Salad, Green Jell-O, Red Jell-O, Macaroni Salad)

REC	CASE	SHRIMP	OLIVE	FRCHICK	BBQCHICK	BEANS	POTSAL	GJEL	RJEL	MAC
31	N	N	N	Y	N	Y	Y	·	N	Y
32	N	Y	Y	Y	N	N	Y	N	Y	N
33	N	N	N	Y	N	N	Y	N	Y	Y
34	N	·	N	N	N	Y	Y	N	Y	Y
35	N	·	N	N	N	Y	Y	N	Y	Y
36	N	N	Y	Y	N	N	Y	·	·	Y
37	N	N	N	Y	N	N	Y	N	Y	N
38	N	N	N	Y	N	N	Y	·	·	N
39	N	N	N	Y	N	Y	Y	N	Y	N
40	N	N	N	Y	N	Y	Y	·	·	Y
41	N	N	N	Y	N	Y	N	N	Y	Y
42	N	N	Y	Y	N	Y	Y	Y	N	N
43	N	N	Y	Y	·	N	Y	Y	·	N
44	N	N	Y	Y	N	Y	Y	Y	N	Y
45	N	N	Y	Y	N	N	N	Y	·	N
46	N	N	N	Y	N	Y	Y	·	N	Y
47	N	N	Y	Y	N	Y	N	·	·	N
48	N	N	Y	Y	N	Y	N	Y	·	N
49	N	Y	Y	Y	N	·	Y	N	Y	Y
50	N	N	Y	Y	N	Y	Y	·	·	Y
51	N	Y	Y	Y	·	N	N	Y	·	Y

Data, Part II (Root Beer, Rolls, Butter, Deviled Eggs, Potato Chips, Pickles, Strawberry Cream Pie, Neapolitan Cream Pie Cake, Tomato)

REC	CASE	RBEER	ROLL	BUTTER	DEVEGG	POTCHIP	PICK	SCP	NCP	CAKE	TOM
1	Y	Y	N	N	·	Y	N	N	N	N	N
2	Y	Y	·	N	N	N	N	Y	N	N	N
3	Y	Y	N	N	Y	Y	Y	N	·	N	Y
4	Y	Y	N	N	Y	Y	N	N	·	N	N
5	Y	Y	N	N	Y	Y	N	N	Y	N	Y
6	Y	Y	N	N	N	Y	Y	Y	N	Y	Y
7	Y	Y	N	N	Y	Y	·	·	·	·	·
8	Y	Y	N	N	Y	Y	N	N	N	N	N
9	Y	Y	N	N	Y	Y	N	N	N	N	N
10	Y	Y	·	·	·	Y	Y	N	N	·	N
11	Y	Y	N	N	Y	Y	N	Y	N	N	N
12	Y	Y	N	N	Y	N	Y	N	N	·	N
13	Y	N	N	N	N	N	N	N	N	N	N
14	Y	Y	N	N	N	Y	Y	N	N	N	N
15	Y	Y	N	N	Y	Y	Y	Y	N	N	·
16	Y	Y	Y	Y	N	N	Y	Y	N	N	N
17	Y	Y	Y	Y	N	N	Y	Y	N	N	N
18	Y	Y	N	N	Y	Y	Y	Y	N	N	N
19	Y	Y	N	N	N	Y	N	N	N	N	N
20	Y	Y	N	N	Y	Y	N	N	N	N	N
21	Y	N	·	·	N	Y	Y	Y	N	·	Y
22	Y	Y	N	N	N	Y	Y	Y	N	N	N
23	Y	Y	Y	Y	Y	Y	Y	Y	N	N	N
24	Y	Y	Y	Y	N	Y	N	N	N	·	N
25	Y	Y	N	N	N	Y	N	N	N	N	Y

(continued)

TABLE 14.7. (Continued)

Data, Part II (Root Beer, Rolls, Butter, Deviled Eggs, Potato Chips, Pickles, Strawberry Cream Pie, Neapolitan Cream Pie Cake, Tomato)

REC	CASE	RBEER	ROLL	BUTTER	DEVEGG	POTCHIP	PICK	SCP	NCP	CAKE	TOM
26	N	Y	N	N	N	.	N	N	N	N	Y
27	N	Y	N	N	N	Y	N	N	N	N	Y
28	N	Y	Y	Y	Y	Y	N	N	N	Y	Y
29	N	Y	N	N	.	Y	Y	N	N	N	N
30	N	Y	Y	Y	N	Y	Y	N	N	N	Y
31	N	Y	N	N	N	Y	Y	N	N	Y	Y
32	N	Y	Y	Y	N	Y	N	Y	N	N	N
33	N	Y	N	N	N	Y	N	N	N	N	N
34	N	Y	N	N	N	Y	N	N	N	N	Y
35	N	Y	N	N	N	Y	N	N	N	N	Y
36	N	.	Y	.	N	Y	N	.	.	N	Y
37	N	Y	N	N	N	Y	N	N	N	.	Y
38	N	Y	N	N	Y	Y	N	N	N	.	N
39	N	N	Y	Y	N	N	N	.	N	N	Y
40	N	Y	Y	Y	N	N	N	N	Y	N	Y
41	N	Y	Y	Y	N	N	Y	N	N	N	N
42	N	Y	N	N	N	N	N	N	N	N	N
43	N	Y	Y	Y	.	Y	N	N	N	N	N
44	N	Y	N	N	Y	N	Y	N	N	Y	N
45	N	Y	Y	Y	Y	N	N	N	Y	N	Y
46	N	Y	Y	Y	Y	N	Y	N	.	N	Y
47	N	Y	N	N	Y	N	Y	Y	N	N	N
48	N	Y	N	N	N	N	N	N	N	N	Y
49	N	Y	Y	.	N	N	N	Y	N	N	Y
50	N	Y	N	.	N	Y	Y	.	.	Y	N
51	N	N	Y	Y	Y	Y	Y	N	N	.	Y

Question 3 Determine the frequency of symptoms by filling in Table 14.8. Exclude people with missing values from numerators and denominators of the frequency calculation in question.

Question 4 Calculate the food-specific attack rates (cumulative incidences) and relative risks (cumulative incidence ratios) associated with each food item. Attack rates are calculated as follows:

$$\text{Attack rate}_{exposed} = \frac{\text{no. of people who ate food and became ill}}{\text{total no. of people who ate food}} \quad (14.1)$$

$$\text{Attack rate}_{unexposed} = \frac{\text{no. of people who did not eat food and became ill}}{\text{total no. of people who did not eat food}} \quad (14.2)$$

The relative risk (*RR*) is

$$RR = \frac{\text{Attack rate}_{exposed}}{\text{Attack rate}_{unexposed}} \quad (14.3)$$

Write your answers in Table 14.9. Based on your calculations, what is the most likely source of exposure to the pathogen?

TABLE 14.8. Frequency of Symptoms: Foodborne Disease Outbreak Case Study

Symptom	Number Reporting Symptom	Number of Cases Responding to Question	Percentage
Cramps			
Diarrhea			
Bloody diarrhea			
Nausea			
Vomiting			
Fever			
Chills			
Headache			
Myalgia			

Question 5 Use the Abbreviated Compendium of Acute Foodborne Gastrointestinal Diseases that appears as Table 14.10 to create a list of the most likely agent. Base this list on the typical signs, incubation period, and most likely food source of the pathogen.

TABLE 14.9. Attack Rates and Relative Risks: Foodborne Disease Outbreak Case Study

Food Exposure	Attack Rate in Consumers	Attack Rate in Nonconsumers	Relative Risk
Shrimp salad	8/12 (66.7%)	15/35 (42.9%)	1.56
Olives			
Fried chicken			
Barbecued chicken			
Beans			
Potato salad			
Green Jell-O			
Red Jell-O			
Macaroni salad			
Root beer			
Rolls			
Butter			
Deviled eggs			
Potato chips			
Pickle			
Strawberry cream pie			
Neopolitan cream pie			
Cake			
Tomato			

TABLE 14.10. An Abbreviated Compendium of Acute Foodborne Gastrointestinal Diseases

I. Diseases Typified by Vomiting After a Short Incubation Period with Little or No Fever

Agent	Incubation Period Usual (and Range)	Symptoms[a] (Partial List)	Pathophysiology	Characteristic Foods	Specimens
A. Staphylococcus aureus	2–4 hours (1–6 hours)	N, C, V; D, F may be present	Preformed enterotoxin	Sliced/chopped ham and meats, custards, cream fillings	Food: enterotoxin assay (FDA), culture for quantitation and phage typing of staph, gram stain Handlers: culture nares, skin, skin lesions, and phage type staph Cases: culture stool and vomitus, phage type staph
B. Bacillus cereus	2–4 hours (1–6 hours)	N, V, D	? Preformed enterotoxin	Fried rice	Food: culture for quantitation Cases: stool culture
C. Heavy metals 1. Cadmium 2. Copper 3. Tin 4. Zinc	5–15 minutes (1–60 minutes)	N, V, C, D		Foods and beverages prepared/stored/cooked in containers coated/lined/contaminated with offending metal	Toxicologic analysis of food container, vomitus, stomach contents, urine, blood, feces

II. Diseases Typified by Diarrhea After a Moderate to Long Incubation Period, Often with Fever

Agent	Incubation Period Usual (and Range)	Symptoms[a] (Partial List)	Pathophysiology	Characteristic Foods	Specimens
A. Clostridium perfringens	12 hours (8–16 hours)	C, D (V, F rare)	Enterotoxin formed in vivo	Meat, poultry	Food: enterotoxin assay done as research procedure by FDA, culture for quantitation and serotyping Cases: culture feces for quantitation and serotyping of C. perfringens; test for enterotoxin in stool Cases: culture feces for quantitation and serotyping of C. perfringens

Organism	Incubation period	Symptoms	Mechanism	Food vehicle	Diagnosis
B. *Salmonella* (nontyphoid)	12–36 hours (6–72 hours)	D, C, F, V, H septicemia or enteric fever	Tissue invasion	Poultry, eggs, meat, raw milk (cross-contamination important)	*Food:* culture with serotyping; *Cases:* stool culture with serotyping; *Handlers:* stool culture with serotyping as a secondary consideration
C. *Vibrio parahaemolyticus*	12 hours (2–48 hours)	C, D; N, V, F, H, B	Tissue invasion, ?enterotoxin	Seafood	*Food:* culture on TCBS, serotype, Kanagawa test; *Cases:* stool cultures on TCBS, serotype, Kanagawa test
D. *Escherichia coli* enterotoxigenic	16–48 hours	D, C	enterotoxin	Uncooked vegetables, salads, water, cheese	*Food:* culture and serotype; *Cases:* stool cultures; serotype and enterotoxin production, invasiveness assay
Escherichia coli enteroinvasive	16–48 hours	C, D, F, H	Tissue invasion	Same	*Cases:* stool cultures; serotype and enterotoxin production. Look for common serotype in food and cases not found in controls; DNA probes
Escherichia coli enterohemorrhagic (*E. coli* O157.H7 and others)	48–96 hours	B, C, D, H; F infrequent	Cytotoxin	Beef, raw milk, water	Stool cultures on MacConkey's sorbitol; serotype
E. *Bacillus cereus*	8–16 hours	C, D	? Enterotoxin	Custards, cereals, puddings, sauces, meat loaf	*Food:* culture; *Cases:* stool cultures
F. *Shigella*	24–48 hours	C, F, D, B, H, N, V	Tissue invasion	Foods contaminated by infected foodhandler; usually not foodborne	*Food:* culture and serotype; *Cases:* stool culture and serotype; *Handlers:* stool culture and serotype

(continued)

TABLE 14.10. *(Continued).*

Agent	Incubation Period Usual (and Range)	Symptoms[a] (Partial List)	Pathophysiology	Characteristic Foods	Specimens
G. *Yersinia enterocolitica*	3–5 days (usual) range unclear	F, D, C, V, H	Tissue invasion, ? enterotoxin	Pork products and foods contaminated by infected human or animal	*Food:* culture *Cases:* stool, blood cultures, serology *Handlers:* stool cultures
H. *Vibrio cholerae* O-1	24–72 hours	D, V	Enterotoxin formed *in vivo*	Shellfish, water or foods contaminated by infected person or obtained from contaminated environmental source	*Food:* culture on TCBS, serotype *Cases:* stool cultures on TCBS, serotype Send all isolates to CDC for confirmation and toxin assay
I. *Vibrio cholerae* non O-1	16–72 hours	D, V	Enterotoxin formed *in vivo* ? Tissue invasion	Shellfish	*Food:* culture on TCBS, serotype *Cases:* stool cultures on TCBS, serotype
J. *Campylobacter jejuni*	3–5 days	C, D, B, F	Unknown	Raw milk, poultry, water	*Food:* culture on selective media (5%O$_2$, 42°C) *Cases:* culture on selective media (5%O$_2$, 42°C), serology
K. Parvovirus-like agents (Norwalk, Hawaii, Colorado, cockle agents)	16–48 hours	N, V, C, D	Unknown	Shellfish, water	Stool for immune electron microscopy and serology by special arrangement
L. Rotavirus	16–48 hours	N, V, C, D	Unknown	Foodborne transmission not well documented	*Cases:* stool examination by EM or ELISA; serology

270

III. Botulism

Organism	Incubation	Symptoms	Toxin	Food source	Diagnostic tests
Clostridium botulinum	12–72 hours	V, D, descending paralysis	Preformed toxin	Improperly canned or similarly preserved foods	*Food:* toxin assay *Cases:* serum and feces for toxin assay by CDC or State Lab; stool culture for *C. botulinum*

IV. Diseases Most Readily Diagnosed from the History of Eating a Particular Type of Food

Disease	Incubation	Symptoms	Toxin	Food source	Diagnostic tests
A. Poisonous mushrooms	Variable	Variable		Wild mushrooms	*Food:* speciation by mycetologist.
B. Other poisonous plants	Variable	Variable		Wild plant	*Cases:* vomitus, blood, urine *Food:* speciation by botanist; feces may sometimes be helpful in confirmation
C. Scombroid fish poisoning		N, C, D, H, flushing, urticaria	Histamine	Mishandled fish (i.e., tuna)	*Food:* Histamine levels
Ciguatera poisoning		D, N, V, paresthesias, reversal of temperature sensation	Ciguatoxin	Large ocean fish (i.e., barracuda, snapper)	*Food:* Stick test for ciguatoxin (not widely available)
D. Other poisonous food sources	Variable	Variable	Variable		

Source: Centers for Disease Control, Epidemic Intelligence Service, Summer 1992.

[a]*Abbreviations:* B = bloody stools, C = cramps, D = diarrhea, F = fever, H = headache, N = nausea, V = vomiting.

Question 6   What are the mechanisms by which such vehicles usually become contaminated with the pathogen you suspect caused this outbreak?

Question 7   What measures are possible to prevent such contamination?

Question 8   What can be done to prevent illness if foods do become contaminated?

ANSWERS TO CASE STUDY: FOODBORNE DISEASE OUTBREAK

Answer 1   The following text comes from the CDC *Principles of Epidemiology: Self-Study Course*: (1992a)

> Anyone about to embark on an outbreak investigation should be well prepared before leaving for the field. Preparations can be grouped into three categories: investigation, administration, and consultation. Good preparation in all three categories will facilitate a smooth field experience.
>
> *Investigation*   First, as a field investigator, you must have the appropriate scientific knowledge, supplies, and equipment to carry out the investigation. You should discuss the situation with someone knowledgeable about the disease and about field investigations, and review the applicable literature. You should assemble useful references such as journal articles and sample questionnaires. Before leaving for a field investigation, consult laboratory staff to ensure that you take the proper laboratory material and know the proper collection, storage, and transportation techniques. Arrange for a portable computer, dictaphone, camera, and other supplies.
>
> *Administration*   Second, as an investigator, you must pay attention to administrative procedures. In a health agency, you must make travel and other arrangements and get them approved. You may also need to take care of personal matters before you leave, especially if the investigation is likely to be lengthy.
>
> *Consultation*   Third, as an investigator, you must know your expected role in the field. Before departure, all parties should agree on your role, particularly if you are coming from "outside" the local area. For example, are you expected to lead the investigation, provide consultation to the local staff who will conduct the investigation, or simply lend a hand to the local staff? In addition, you should know who your local contacts will be. Before leaving, you should know when and where you are to meet with local officials and contacts when you arrive in the field. (pp. 353–354)

Answer 2   The epidemic curve appears as Figure 14.4. This curve is unimodal with a long right tail, reflecting the point source nature of this epidemic. The median incubation time is 32 hours. The minimum incubation time is 9 hours, and the maximum is 111 hours.

Answer 3   The frequency of symptoms is seen in Table 14.11. This table suggests that the disease is characterized by cramping, diarrhea, nausea, vomiting, fever, chills, headache, and myalgia. Bloody diarrhea is generally absent.

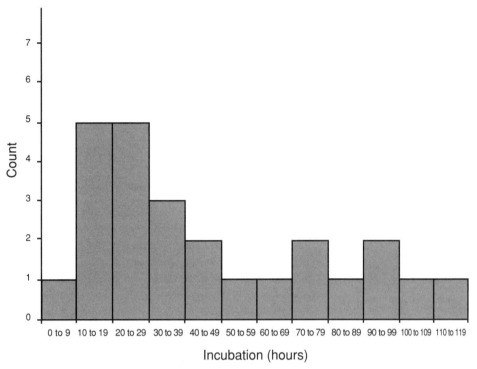

Figure 14.4. *Epidemic curve, foodborne disease outbreak case study.*

Answer 4 Attack rates and relative risks associated with each food appear in Table 14.12. Based on these data, the most likely source of the pathogen is the barbecued chicken (*RR* = 5.0).

Answer 5 The most likely agent is *Salmonella. Salmonella* is the only agent typified by diarrhea, a moderate to long incubation period, cramps, fever, and vomiting. It is

TABLE 14.11. Frequency of Symptoms: Foodborne Disease Outbreak Case Study Answer Key

Symptom	Number Reporting Symptom	Number Responding to Question	Percentage
Cramps	25	25	100%
Diarrhea	25	25	100%
Bloody diarrhea	1	21	5%
Nausea	17	25	68%
Vomiting	12	25	48%
Fever	23	25	92%
Chills	16	25	64%
Headache	23	25	92%
Myalgia	19	21	90%

TABLE 14.12. Attack Rates and Relative Risks: Foodborne Disease Outbreak Case Study Answer Key

Food Exposure	Attack Rate in Consumers	Attack Rate in Nonconsumers	Relative Risk
Shrimp salad	8/12 (67%)	15/35 (43%)	1.6
Olives	19/32 (59%)	5/18 (28%)	2.1
Fried chicken	19/42 (45%)	1/4 (25%)	1.8
Barbecued chicken	16/16 (100%)	6/30 (20%)	5.0
Beans	12/26 (46%)	12/22 (55%)	0.8
Potato salad	17/37 (46%)	8/14 (57%)	0.8
Green Jell-O	8/17 (47%)	11/20 (55%)	0.9
Red Jell-O	12/21 (57%)	9/16 (56%)	1.0
Macaroni salad	9/24 (38%)	14/24 (58%)	0.6
Root beer	23/46 (50%)	2/4 (50%)	1.0
Rolls	4/16 (25%)	18/32 (56%)	0.4
Butter	4/14 (29%)	19/32 (59%)	0.5
Deviled eggs	12/19 (57%)	11/28 (39%)	1.6
Potato chips	20/35 (57%)	5/15 (33%)	1.7
Pickles	12/21 (76%)	12/29 (41%)	1.4
Strawberry cream pie	10/13 (33%)	14/34 (41%)	1.9
Neapolitan cream pie	1/3 (20%)	21/42 (50%)	0.7
Cake	1/5 (24%)	19/38 (50%)	0.4
Tomato	5/21	18/28 (64%)	0.4

characteristically transmitted in poultry. The second most likely agent is *Shigella*, although *Shigella* is often characterized by the presence of blood diarrhea, which was absent from this outbreak.

Answer 6 Salmonella is often endemic in chicken populations. Contamination may spread during food handling, either at the butcher or at home.

Answer 7 Thorough cooking of all foodstuffs derived form animal sources, especially from fowl, can prevent such contamination. Also, cross-contamination with raw poultry must be avoided after cooking is completed. Food handlers should be educated as to the necessity of refrigeration, food preparation, and maintenance of a sanitary environment.

Answer 8 Proper cooking and heating of foodstuff will prevent illness.

15

Computing and Epidemiology

Andrew G. Dean

Division of Public Health Surveillance and Informatics,
Epidemiology Program Office,
Centers for Disease Control and Prevention (CDC)

B. Burt Gerstman

Department of Health Science,
San José State University

Computers play many important roles in modern epidemiology. Outbreak investigations and research studies require that the epidemiologist set up new databases and perform ad hoc analyses. Computerization of public health surveillance systems requires planning and knowledge of how computer and organizational systems are developed. Access to computerized medical records would be a quantum leap forward for epidemiologic research and public health surveillance and could have a profound effect on the future of epidemiology.

15.1 A BRIEF HISTORY OF EPIDEMIOLOGIC COMPUTING

The Mainframe and Minicomputer Era

John Shaw Billings, M.D., Director of the Army Surgeon General's Library, was partly responsible for the invention of the Hollerith punched card in 1882 for processing the U.S. Census. The Hollerith Company later became International Business Machines (IBM) Corporation (Collen, 1995).

ENIAC (Electronic Numerical Intregrator and Calculator), the first high-speed digital computer, was developed just after World War II for ballistic calculations. It contained 17,000 vacuum tubes that required a special staff just to change them as they burned out. Although ENIAC used enough electricity to supply 175 houses, the laptop computer on which this article was written is able to do addition 125 times faster and multiplication 600 times faster.

In 1963, the National Library of Medicine (NLM) developed the MEDLARS/MEDLINE bibliographic database, which was moved to an IBM 360 computer in 1965. The first minicomputer, the PDP8 of Digital Equipment Corporation, also appeared in 1965.

Computers and punch cards were used for epidemiologic studies in the 1960s and 1970s, but their use was generally restricted to academic and research centers. During this era, hospitals and health departments acquired access to mini or mainframe computers first for payroll and later for other administrative tasks. Larger databases, such as those used to keep mortality records, were gradually moved to computers. Most epidemiologists lacked the knowledge and resources necessary to interact with these early punch-card and FORTRAN-oriented systems. Setting up data entry for a data entry form could take weeks of planning, negotiation, and debugging.

In 1976, the first version of the Statistical Analysis System (now simply called SAS®) was released, providing software for managing and analyzing data on mainframe computers (*SAS Language Reference*, 1990). SAS® and SPSS® (Statistical Package for the Social Sciences) remain the most popular "big computer" languages for epidemiologists. Public-use datasets from the National Center for Health Statistics are still released in SAS format.

The Personal Computing Era

The Apple II computer in 1977 and the IBM-PC in 1982 were reliable, off-the-shelf computers that sold in large enough quantities to establish industry standards. Probably because of IBM's reputation in mainframe computing and because the presence of clones allowed for competitive bidding, most government agencies adopted the IBM standard. The Macintosh, released in 1984, was a favorite of graphic artists, students, and educators, but it never challenged the PC for more than a minority market share.

A few epidemiologists in the early 1980s wrote their own software in the BASIC or FORTRAN computer languages. Others used the dBASE database system, which could maintain records but lacked cross-tabulation and statistics. The 1975–76 "swine flu" emergency at the Centers for Disease Control (CDC) in Atlanta gave rise to software for cross-tabulation and simple statistics, written in BASIC on a minicomputer. Anthony (Tony) Burton adapted the programs to a smaller minicomputer for use by the Georgia Department of Health. EpiStat, the first general-purpose shareware program for epidemiologists on the IBM-PC, was written by Tracy Gustafson, M.D., then with the Texas Department of Health.

Epi Info™, written in Turbo Pascal at CDC, was first released in 1985 and is in the public domain (Dean et al., 1991, 1995). Subsequent versions evolved under CDC and World Health Organization (WHO) sponsorship. By 1997, more than 145,000 copies of Epi Info and the related Epi Map program had been documented in 117 countries. Translations of the program or manual are available in 13 languages, largely through the efforts of volunteer translators in other countries. Copies of the current version of Epi Info can be downloaded without charge from the CDC World Wide Web (WWW) pages on the Internet (www.cdc.gov, under "Publications, Software, and Products").

In the 1980s, SAS and SPSS became available on PCs. More recently, versions have appeared for Microsoft Windows®. Stata® (Stata Corporation, College Station, Texas) and

SYSTAT® (SPSS Inc., Chicago, Illinois) are other statistical packages that have since become popular.

By the mid-1990s, most students in schools of public health and most professionals in public health agencies used computers directly rather than through professional programmers. Typically, the computer was an Intel-based PC. Mainframes and minicomputers are still used but are often accessed from PCs through a Local Area Network that connects members of an organization.

The Age of Communication

The Internet developed gradually and then explosively in the early 1990s, as the Microsoft Windows environment finally brought the point-and-click ease of use that had been pioneered by the Macintosh® to the PC. Although the use of the Internet can be slow over standard telephone systems, large companies with fast leased lines find that doing business on the other side of the world can be almost as convenient as communication within a single building. Search facilities available on the Internet make it easy to locate Web pages on a particular subject from many parts of the world. Web pages are often indexed to related sites on the same subject.

The Internet is already playing a role in epidemiology, making it possible to search for information in National Library of Medicine databases (http://nlm.nig.gov) and to access epidemiologic resources from anywhere in the world. The University of California San Francisco, for example, has a Web page that provides point-and-click access to a host of epidemiologic resources (http://chanane.ucsf.edu/epidem/epidem.html).

The latest versions of Epi Info, Epi Map, and other public domain programs can be downloaded from the Internet, and information about commercial data management and statistical packages may be found by searching the World Wide Web with one of the many search engines accessible from popular browsers.

The WONDER site on the Internet (http://wonder.cdc.gov) offers epidemiologic databases from the CDC and other sources, while the CDC (http://www.cdc.gov), the WHO (http://www.who.ch), and more than 40 state health departments (http://www.astho.org/state.html) have WWW sites.

15.2 COMPUTING FOR INVESTIGATIONS AND STUDIES

Data Collection Forms and Database Structure

Ad hoc investigations and studies require the epidemiologist to set up new databases and perform statistical analyses. Most epidemiologic data are captured on a **questionnaire** or **data collection form** before being computerized. A separate data collection form is generated for each individual, household, or other sampling unit of interest. Each form is then entered into the computer as one or more related **records** consisting of multiple **fields.** For example, each subject in a study might be asked to fill out an individual questionnaire containing multiple questions. Each completed questionnaire becomes a computerized record, and each response to a question on the questionnaire is entered into a field. Records from a particular study are stored in **files** composed of individual records and fields stored in tabular form.

Common Types of Data Input

Questionnaires and data entry forms may contain items of various types. Common data types are:

- Text input (e.g., last name, diagnosis, comment)
- Multiple choice (e.g., years of education: 0–8, 9–12, 12–16, more than 16)
- Numeric responses (e.g., age, weight, years on job)
- Dates and times (e.g., date of birth)
- Yes/no responses (e.g., Do you smoke? Are you allergic to any medicines?)

Questions that allow for more than one answer (e.g., antimicrobial sensitivities: penicillin, streptomycin, tetracycline) should be divided into individual items, each with an entry, since each will be treated separately during analysis (e.g., penicillin sensitivity: y/n; streptomycin sensitivity: y/n; tetracycline sensitivity: y/n).

Relational Database Structure

Repeating groups of questions within a questionnaire also require special handling. A household questionnaire, for example, might contain a series of questions describing each person in the household with fields for subjects' names and ages. In the computer database, one might be tempted to create a series of fields called NAME1, AGE1, STATUS1, NAME2, AGE2, STATUS2, NAME3, and so on, for as many persons as might be found in the largest household. Analyzing such a database is difficult, however, because AGE1, AGE2, and AGE3 represent separate variables, providing no simple way to deal with the ages of all persons in the study. To remedy this problem, most database programs can create a separate **related file** for "questionnaires within a questionnaire" (e.g., PERSONs within a HOUSEHOLD). In this example, one file would contain HOUSEHOLD records, each with a unique household number identifier. A separate file would contain as many PERSON records as needed for each household, identified by HOUSEHOLD number. The software of a **relational database program** uses this common identifier to link records so that analysis can be performed on either PERSON or HOUSEHOLD characteristics. When PERSON records are analyzed, each is linked to the record for its own HOUSEHOLD, so that information on HOUSEHOLD (e.g., number of bedrooms) can be included in an analysis of PERSON records.

Full Screen Data Entry

Methods for setting up database files and entering data vary considerably among software packages. Epi Info, for example, uses the questionnaire designed by the user to create a computer **data entry screen.** Specifications can be added to the data entry screen for checking or modifying entries as they are made. Ranges and legal values can be checked, data can be automatically coded or mathematically transformed, and the cursor can automatically be moved from field to field depending on the response to a question.

Some programs use a **spreadsheet** or **grid format** for data entry. Spreadsheet format lists variable names at the top of columns in a grid and each record occupies one horizontal row. STATA, SYSTAT, and SPSS Windows use the spreadsheet input method. In SAS, a program must be written to specify the names, sizes, and data types of the spreadsheet grid using PROC FSEDIT.

Cleaning Data

During data entry, "**check programs**" can be used to limit entries to prescribed legal codes and values. For example, check programs can prevent the entry of male pregnancies and female prostatectomies. Because other items may offer more latitude for error, alternative data checking and validation procedures are also needed.

There are several methods for data verification, including:

- Reading the data from the screen or a printout and comparing with the original, preferably done by two operators
- Entering the data twice in different files and comparing the files using a special validation program
- Entering data a second time into the same file using a program that checks to see if the entries are the same, with errors presented for correction
- Analyzing the data to produce frequency counts and summary statistics so that values such as "*&!" and other "outliers" can be more closely inspected in the original record (This method has the same drawbacks as the male pregnancy checks mentioned earlier: it can only detect erroneous values that do not seem reasonable.)

Since the value of an epidemiologic analysis is only as good as the validity of its data, at least one of the above data verification methods should be used whenever a data set is created.

Converting Data from One Format to Another

In some cases, data for analysis may come from a colleague, from another center, or from a national dataset that has already been entered into another computer using a different software program. When this is the case, conversion programs are available to change data from one file format to another. dBASE files are often a good choice for an intermediary format when converting data from one system to another—dBASE files contain good descriptions of the data and are recognized by nearly all major programs. For example, Epi Info will analyze dBASE files directly and has IMPORT and EXPORT programs for this and other file formats.

Data Analysis

Interactive Versus Batch Processing   After data have been readied for processing, they can be analyzed one command at a time (**interactive processing**) or in batch mode by writing groups of commands into a file and running them as a **program.** Interactive processing has the advantage of providing immediate feedback so that syntax errors and analytic results become known before the next command is submitted. Batch programming is advantageous when complex logic is applied and tasks are required on a repeated basis.

Activating the Data Set The first step in preparing to analyze a file is to choose the file containing the data set. In Epi Info, this requires the READ command followed by the name and location of the file. In SAS, the SET, MERGE, or UPDATE statements are used for a similar purpose.

Variables As mentioned earlier, attributes or events that are recorded on a questionnaire or data entry form are called fields. In statistical jargon, the preferred term for a field is a **variable,** called such because the item takes on different values in different subjects. Variables are the fundamental unit of statistical analysis and are analyzed according to two broad types: categorical variables and continuous variables.

Categorical Variables Categorical variables are used to register characteristics that form predetermined, unordered categories. Examples of categorical variables include ethnic group (white, black, Asian, other), eye color (brown, blue, other), disease status (disease, nondiseased), and sex (male, female). Categorical variables are also called **discrete** or **coded** variables. Coded variables that can take on only two categories (e.g., diseased/nondiseased) are called **dichotomous** or **binary variables.** Coded variables that can take on more than two categories (e.g., racial/ethnic group) are called **polychotomous** variables. Common types of descriptive analyses for categorical data include line listings, frequencies, cross-tabulations, histograms, bar graphs, and pie charts.

   Line listings, or "lists," are simply columnar presentations of data with a variable name at the top of each column with each record occupying a line below. Output from a line listing might look something like this:

```
NAME          AGE  BIRTHDAY   ILL  ATE_HAM
----------    ---  --------   ---  -------
GERSTMAN J    07   03/02/90   N    N
ANKELE C      09   08/11/88   Y    Y
DAVIS N       14   09/20/82   N    Y
MARKEL D      23   11/03/73   Y    N
```

In most software systems, data can be sorted before listing. In Epi Info, for example, a SORT NAME command followed by a LIST command would list data with records sorted alphabetically by name:

```
NAME          AGE  BIRTHDAY   ILL  ATE_HAM
----------    ---  --------   ---  -------
ANKELE C      09   08/11/88   Y    Y
DAVIS N       14   09/20/82   N    Y
GERSTMAN J    07   03/02/90   N    N
MARKEL D      23   11/03/73   Y    N
```

Selected items from a data set can be listed by specifying variables in a LIST statement (Epi Info) or PUT statement (SAS). For example, a LIST NAME BIRTHDAY command in Epi Info would result in the following output:

```
NAME         BIRTHDAY
----------   --------
ANKELE C     08/11/88
DAVIS N      09/20/82
GERSTMAN J   03/02/90
MARKEL D     11/03/73
```

Frequencies take the place of sorting the questionnaires into piles based on a single item and then counting the questionnaires in each pile. In a survey of a single group, simple frequencies may be all the analysis that is needed, producing output similar to the following:

```
EVERSMOKED      Freq  Percent   Cum.
------------+---------------------------
Yes         |     32   31.1%    31.1%
No          |     67   65.0%    96.1%
Unknown     |      4    3.9%   100.0%
------------------------------------
Total       |    103  100.0%
```

Cross-tabulations are the computer equivalent of sorting the questionnaires into piles based on the value of one variable and then sorting each pile into additional piles (cells) based on the value of another variable. For example, we may want to calculate the attack rates of a foodborne illness in people who ate ham and those who did not eat ham. Output from a cross-tabulation for this purpose might look something like this:

```
                ILL
ATE_HAM |   +    -  |  Total
--------+----------+-------
      + |  29   17 |    46
      - |  17   12 |    29
--------+----------+-------
Total   |  46   29 |    75
```

Most statistical programs will add measures of association and appropriate inferential statistics to the cross-tabulation:

```
RISK RATIO(RR) (Outcome:ILL=+; Exposure:ATE_HAM=+)       1.08
95% confidence limits for RR                    0.74 < RR <  1.57

                        Chi-Squares   P-values
                        -----------   --------
          Uncorrected:       0.15     0.70170143
      Mantel-Haenszel:       0.14     0.70360201
       Yates corrected:      0.02     0.88899437
```

Continuous Variables Continuous variables represent measures or counts in which numerical values have a quantitative meaning. Examples of continuous variables include systolic blood pressure (mm Hg), age (years), weight (kilograms), and number of cases. For most descriptive purposes, continuous variables are adequately described by their mean, standard deviation, and sample size. The median, minimum, and maximum ("M & Ms") may also be reported. Less commonly, quartiles and the standard error of the mean (a measure of the mean's precision) are reported.

Output from a descriptive analysis of a single continuous variable may look something like this:

```
AGE
          Total       Sum     Mean   Variance   Std Dev   Std Err
            654      6495    9.931      8.726     2.954     0.116

        Minimum   25%ile   Median     75%ile   Maximum      Mode
          3.000    8.000   10.000     12.000    19.000     9.000
```

Data are summarized as follows: "The mean age in the 654 subjects is 9.9 years (standard deviation = 3.0 years)."

Inferential methods for continuous variables depend on the nature of the sample and study design. For example, pretest/posttest samples are analyzed with a paired t test, two or more independent groups can be compared with analysis of variance techniques, and relationships among continuous variables can be assessed with correlation and regression.

Graphical Analysis   High-resolution data visualization has become a routine part of exploratory data analysis. **Histograms, stem-and-leaf plots, dot plots,** and **box plots** are used to show the distribution of a variable. **Side-by-side plots** are used to compare groups. Two- and three-dimensional **scatter plots** are also used to visualize relationships. Producing publication-quality graphics may require saving the graph to a file of a suitable format and then using a page layout program to edit the final product.

Maps   The geographic distribution of cases is best displayed with a map. Maps can use dots or color/pattern combinations to show numbers of cases or rates for states, counties, or any geographical, regional, or floor-plan subdivision. In some cases, mapping software and suitable boundary files (the polygon descriptions that comprise a map) must be purchased as a separate program (MapInfo, ArcView). In other cases, statistical programs have mapping modules, usually at extra cost (SAS). Epi Info for DOS has a separate companion program called Epi Map that allows the user to draw maps of hospital floor plans or local outbreak settings. Epi Map can display more than one map on a screen to show both rates and counts simultaneously.

Missing Values   It is important to be aware of missing or unknown values in a dataset and how these missing values are handled by software. In Epi Info, missing values are created by leaving a field blank during data entry. Missing data may be included or ignored in an analysis by using the SET IGNOREMISSING = ON/OFF command. In some studies, it may be useful to have additional codes for missing values, such as 888 for "subject refused" or 999 for "not applicable." These additional "missing codes" can be included in the frequency analysis along with other information. For most purposes, however, it is adequate to treat missing values as "missing," regardless of cause—specification of a number of codes merely complicates the analysis without contributing useful information.

Data Management

Subsetting   Most analytic software offers methods for selecting or excluding records based on specified criteria. For example, particular records, perhaps only the cases, may be selected for analysis using the SELECT command in Epi Info or a subset IF statement in SAS.

Grouping and Mathematical Assignments   Values of a variable, such as AGE, can be grouped into categories, with values of coded data assigned descriptive text labels. This is done with the RECODE command in Epi Info and the RENAME or LABEL statements in SAS. New variables can be defined to hold the results of mathematical calculations and data can be transformed as necessary. IF statements can be used to make groupings and mathematical actions dependent on other conditions and results.

Immediate Processing Versus Pass Processing   In using data management commands, it is important to know whether the software being used executes commands immediately or during the next "pass" through the data. In Epi Info, for example, IF statements and assignments are not executed immediately unless preceded by the word IMMEDIATE. Without an IMMEDIATE statement, actions are performed once for each record during the next LIST, FREQ, or TABLES command.

Programming   Analytic software allows (and sometimes requires) commands to be saved in a program that is run in batch mode. Programs are started with a command like RUN <Name of Program>. Programs can ask for user input and do a variety of tasks that may be required on a repeated basis. Although it is possible to write programs to perform operations based on complex logic, like determining conformity of a series of symptoms with a complicated case definition, the time spent writing, debugging, and testing a program must be weighed against the value of the program for repeated use.

15.3 COMPUTING IN PUBLIC HEALTH SURVEILLANCE

Introduction

Epidemiologic surveillance is the "ongoing systematic collection, analysis, and interpretation of outcome-specific data for use in the planning, implementation, and evaluation of public health practice" (Thacker and Berkelman, 1988). Computer processing of data can contribute to the uniform methods necessary to detect trends and aberrations in disease rates over time and are well suited to the repetitive tasks required by surveillance.

Several computing concepts are particularly relevant to surveillance. These are updating of records, maintenance of "distributed" and "replicated" databases, and maintenance of links between original and replicated records.

One-Site Systems, Distributed Systems, and Replicated Systems

A simple **one-site surveillance system** can be maintained as a file on a single computer. Corrections can be made, as needed, and processing can be performed weekly or at other intervals to produce tables, maps, and graphs. A natural extension of this system is to have various peripheral agencies, such as states or provinces in a national system, maintain their own records and send these to a central national repository for processing. This leads to a **distributed database** or, in most cases, a **replicated database,** in which both national and state systems have copies of the same records.

Unique Identifiers

A **unique identifier** in each record—usually an ID number—is absolutely vital to a surveillance system that allows records to be updated after they are submitted. When corrections or comparisons become necessary, records are matched by this unique identifier. Changing or corrupting the unique identifier can cause data to be lost or incorrect data to be added as an update.

Individual Versus Summary Records

Another important concept for surveillance record keeping is that of summary and individual data records. Suppose that two reports are recorded in a state health department as:

```
ID      Disease     Onset
-----   ---------   ------
00011   Gonorrhea   3/3/97
00012   Gonorrhea   3/4/97
```

The reports may be sent to the central repository either individually, as shown above, or a summary record may be created as follows:

```
Count   Disease     Onset
-----   ---------   -----
2       Gonorrhea   3/97
```

Note that summary data carry an extra variable that represents a count. In processing summary records, the count variable is used as a multiplier ("weighting factor") so that final counts will be reported correctly. Most database programs have special commands for producing and handling summary records. For example, Epi Info uses OUTPUT FREQ for producing summary records and SUMFREQ for handling them.

Standards for Data Aggregation

When data are sent from one computer to another, there must be an agreed-upon data format to enable merging and updating of records. This agreed-upon format must include specifications for file names, file sizes, file types, and coding practices.

In most surveillance systems, some of the information needed at peripheral levels is not transmitted to the next level. For example, names, addresses, telephone numbers, and other information needed for local case follow-up may not be sent to the national level.

The question of how to establish and maintain records for data aggregation is an important one. The minimum information necessary for data aggregation includes a description of file names, variable formats, coding practices, and record structures. In some systems, local health departments are required to use standard software issued by the central agency. Although this enforces uniformity in transmitted data, the required software may not be consistent with local standards or skills, thus hindering the addition of data of local interest to be added to the database. Focusing on transmission standards for aggregation rather than on software allows more local control of data, at somewhat greater cost in testing and maintenance.

Data Backup

Record backup at each level of data management is very important. Since not all state data are sent to the national level, state records can only be partially restored from a national database in the event of a hard disk crash, computer virus, earthquake, fire, or other disaster. Tape or disk backups should be kept at each level, preserving several generations of backup to minimize the possibility that recovery will merely restore another corrupt copy of the database. At least one copy of the backup media should be stored off-site to cope with fire and other physical disasters.

Output and Reports

Surveillance system reports ideally include graphs, maps, tables, simple statistics, and rates. Surveillance results may be published in either traditional paper form, via the Internet, or by other electronic means (e.g., CD-ROM). In recent years, stacks of paper printouts have given way to hypertext reports in which many tables and figures are accessed from the computer screen by pointing and clicking at entries in an index. Similar methods are used in navigating through the pages of the Internet's World Wide Web with a browser.

15.4 MEDICAL RECORD SYSTEMS AND PUBLIC HEALTH

Electronic Medical Records

Lack of Acceptance   The electronic medical record has been anticipated as a possibility since the 1950s (Collen, 1995, p. 82), but it has been slow in coming. Despite substantial progress, the number of major medical care facilities with completely computerized medical records in the United States remains small. Reasons for this may include:

- The low cost, familiarity, and legal acceptability of paper records
- The lack of economic incentives for computerizing items not related to billing
- Difficulties in capturing data input from busy physicians, nurses, and others without an affinity for keyboards
- Lack of national or international standards for storing or transmitting clinical data from one institution to another, or even, in some cases, between parts of the same institution
- The tendency of computer systems to require certainty, while actual medical records are often highly sophisticated reflections of nuanced probabilities

Recording Uncertainty   As an example of the problem with recording uncertainty, the diagnosis on admission may be merely a symptom such as abdominal pain with a list of diagnoses to "rule out." Later on, a series of notes might contain an item such as, "feel this may represent an occult malignant process," signed by someone whose identity may mean little to the computer but whose word is either to be respected (chief gastroenterologist, 40 years experience, seldom wrong) or taken with a grain of salt (intern or first-year resident) depending on complex data not in the record. The ideal computerized medical record would, therefore, be created though a combination of text input, voice input (now approaching technical practicality), and other inputs from laboratory and other diagnostic sources (e.g., hematology, cytology, electrocardiography, radiology). Records would be immediately accessible from anywhere in a hospital or clinic and would be linked to other more traditional computerized databases for billing, laboratory results, pharmacy orders, and medical supplies.

Difference Between Medical Computer Systems and Epidemiologic Computer Systems   Even when complete electronic records exist, there are major differences between epidemiologic computer systems and clinical systems. An absolute requirement of clinical record systems is rapid retrieval of an individual record. In contrast, epidemiologic analysis (other than contact tracing or individual case follow-up) requires summarization of many records and aggregation of data over an entire population. From a computational point of view, clinical record retrieval requires a highly effective indexing system that links various parts of a single individual's record over a period of time (but not usually extending to encounters with another institution). Epidemiologic analysis requires rapid processing of selected items from many records, preferably without regard to how many different clinics are visited.

Clinical records must preserve uncertainty; epidemiologic analysis requires that everything, even uncertainty, be classified and distilled into as few categories as possible. An error in a clinical record can be life-threatening; errors in epidemiologic classification are expected, tolerated, and, if possible, eliminated. Billing systems in clinical facilities also require concrete categorization and may therefore provide records suitable for epidemiologic analysis, although with inevitable biases associated with financial incentives and requirements.

Risk Factors   Clinical records often provide only limited information about risk factors such as diet, smoking, and exercise that would interest an epidemiologist. Smoking is probably the best defined of such factors, even though there is no universal system for recording smoking history, particularly over a lifetime, and no coding system comparable to the ICD or other diagnostic codes.

Denominator Information   Finally, epidemiologists need denominator data to quantify the population at risk. Even health maintenance organizations with enrolled populations may have difficulty estimating the size of their population. Health maintenance organizations may have considerable turnover of clients, and, in some geographic areas, transference of clients from one clinic to the next prevents accurate counts of individual subjects. (Data are set up to count patient contacts, rather than people counts, as such.) This may seriously affect the availability of reliable denominator information.

Organizing Clinical Data for Aggregation

Computerizing clinical records for epidemiologic analysis will require many of the same kinds of coding and distillation practices that are required during an outbreak investigation or research study. The simplest level of analysis is to use visits or hospitalizations as the sampling unit of interest rather than persons. This removes many problems of linkage and follow-up but still requires coding of diagnoses and categorization of other variables that will be analyzed.

Detecting the occurrence of words or phrases in **free text** can be aided by the use of search engines. However, human intervention is still required to impart meaning. Meaning is dependent on the location in the text, and the relationship to words such as "rule out," "excludes," "not," "consider," and other modifiers. Hence, proper **abstraction** of records will require expert human assistance for some time to come.

Fortunately, partial abstraction of records is already being done by many facilities for purposes of billing and quality control, so that the burden of abstraction will fall only partially on the epidemiologist. The principles of record abstraction are similar to those used in capturing data during an outbreak investigation, and data collection forms for the two purposes have many parallel features.

Capturing **longitudinal data** on individuals, particularly those who visit more than one facility, is more complicated and often involves matching of names and addresses to make up for lack of other identifiers. Special software and analytic methods may be needed to perform longitudinal studies of this kind.

15.5 THE FUTURE

Networked Computers

The Internet, or whatever replaces it, will offer even more abundant epidemiologic resources and will become a medium for collaboration among epidemiologists worldwide. The searching capabilities of the "net" offer methods for the dissemination of ideas and for locating surveillance information from other parts of the world.

Targeted Communication

The dissemination of epidemiologic information via the Internet has already begun, generally in a form available to the entire Internet audience. During the next few years, secure private transmission, already used by banks and other corporations, will become more widely available, so that WWW pages can be restricted to selected audiences (e.g., neighboring health departments, colleagues in a study) rather than being open to the entire Internet. Eventually this capability will extend to individual homes so that video interviews or other targeted communications can be conducted with individuals at particular addresses, as is now done by telephone.

Access to Clinical Databases

The computer industry is moving rapidly to make access to another computer on the World Wide Web as convenient as access to one's own disk drive on the desktop. If this occurs, and if secure transmissions to selected groups become routine, there are possibilities for a "quantum leap" in accessing epidemiologic data. Instead of sending a hoard of record abstracters to hospital record rooms, future epidemiologists should be able to access already-digitized records or, better yet, summaries of records.

Surveillance of Common Illnesses

As described earlier, connecting the databases will be easy in comparison with establishing the standards, codes, conversion software, confidentiality and access agreements, funding, and other necessities for combing and interpreting diverse clinical databases. Development of standards and of software to convert between standards is important. When such advances have occurred, public health morbidity surveillance will no longer be confined to "reportable disease" or expensive record abstraction. It should be possible to construct a radar screen image, however fuzzy, of the great mass of common ailments that come to medical attention, and not merely those that are amenable to direct public health intervention or mentioned in regulations on disease reporting.

Essential Nature of Epidemiologic Computing

Today, an epidemiologist without computer skills is as handicapped as he or she would be without statistics or laboratory analysis. In the near future, however, the epidemiologist without computer skills and resources may be unable to function. It is unlikely that the computer will assume much of an intellectual role in epidemiology, but it will greatly enhance our ability to search for and process data.

REFERENCES

Collen, M. F. (1995). *A History of Medical Information in the United States, 1950 to 1990.* Indianapolis: American Medical Informatics Association.

Dean, A. G., Dean, J. A., Burton, A. H., & Dicker, R. C. (1991). Epi Info: a general purpose microcomputer program for health information systems. *American Journal of Preventive Medicine, 7,* 178–182.

Dean, A. G., Dean J. A., Coulombier, D., Brendel, K. A., Smith, D. C., Burton, A. H., Dicker, R. C., Sullivan, K., Fagan R. F., & Arner, T. G. (1995). *Epi Info, Version 6: A Word Processing, Database and Statistics Program for Public Health on IBM-Compatible Microcomputers.* Atlanta: Centers for Disease Control and Prevention.

SAS Language Reference, Version 6. (1990). Cary, NC: SAS Institute Inc.

Thacker, S. B., & Berkelman, R. L. (1988). Public health surveillance in the United States. *Epidemiologic Reviews,* 10, 164–190.

Index